HOWARD HAWKS, STORYTELLER

HOWARD HAWKS, STORYTELLER

Gerald Mast

OXFORD UNIVERSITY PRESS
Oxford   New York   Toronto   Melbourne

OXFORD UNIVERSITY PRESS

Oxford   London   Glasgow
New York   Toronto   Melbourne   Auckland
Delhi   Bombay   Calcutta   Madras   Karachi
Kuala Lumpur   Singapore   Hong Kong   Tokyo
Nairobi   Dar es Salaam   Cape Town

and associate companies in

Beirut   Berlin   Ibadan   Mexico City   Nicosia

First published by Oxford University Press, New York, 1982
First issued as an Oxford University Press paperback, 1984

Library of Congress Cataloging in Publication Data

Mast, Gerald, 1940–
Howard Hawks, storyteller.

Includes bibliographical references and index.
1. Hawks, Howard, 1896–   . I. Title.
PN1998.A3H3478   791.43′0233′0924   81-22474
ISBN 0-19-503091-5   AACR2
ISBN 0-19-503233-0 (pbk.)

Printing (last digit): 9 8 7 6 5 4 3 2 1

Printed in the United States of America

For Baby

Acknowledgments

Although the title page of this book names only one author, there is no proper sense in which this book is the product of just one person. The author of a book, like the *auteur* of a film, is dependent on the contributions of a large community of talented and interested people, who offer their knowledge, their suggestions, and even their anger to help shape the final product. Before leaping into the matters of the book itself, I want to take this opportunity to acknowledge and to thank those people who have contributed to what this book has become. Think of these few pages as the opening credits.

My heaviest debt of gratitude falls on those who accepted the heaviest burden of work—reading the entire manuscript, probably more than once, and offering their detailed suggestions. John Belton, Leo Braudy, Tag Gallagher, and Sheldon Meyer suggested ways to cut, or add, or revise, or restructure, or rethink sections of the manuscript, and the ways that the present book is tighter, more accurate, more interesting, or more convincing than the initial manuscript is largely attributable to their insight. The ways in which the book may still disappoint them is entirely attributable to my own errors or my own unwillingness to accept their suggestions. Todd McCarthy, who is currently working on a detailed biography of Hawks, checked the accuracy of my biographical sections, helping me separate the biographical from the apocryphal, whose mixing seems an inevitable and incurable disease of "film books." Let me hope that my biographical assertions will stand well enough when Todd's major work appears.

Next I must thank those who steered me to useful sources of information: Jean Furstenberg of the American Film Institute and David Shepard of the Screen Directors' Guild. Through them I was able to contact Christian Nyby, the best film editor to work for (and with) Hawks, whose detailed descriptions of Hawks's working methods and concerns made such an important contribution to this book. I hope that I did not try Chris's patience overmuch with my many questions and that I have presented his views fully and fairly. Jean Furstenberg also directed me to the archive of Hawks's private papers at the Harold B. Lee Library of Brigham Young University. As you will see, this study is terribly dependent on comparing the finished Hawks films with the evolving scripts from which they were made—as a means to illuminate Hawks's method and process of creation. James D'Arc, the archivist of the Hawks collection (and of Special Collections at Brigham Young), was extremely gracious in providing me access to the Hawks materials and in providing me with both photocopies and photographic stills. He also made it possible for the two of us to triumph over the vagaries of the United States Postal Service, which seemed intent on severing the lines of communication between us.

All those photographs in the book that do not come from the Brigham Young archive were made by me personally, directly from frames of the films themselves. Although frame blow-ups necessarily lack the crispness and sharpness of glossy production stills, there is no other way to illustrate the actual content and composition of specific shots without them. I am extremely grateful to Michael Shields who printed the photographs I shot, attempting to compensate as best he could for the inevitable fuzziness of such images and for my own mis-calculations. I don't know how these photographs will look in this book, but I have never seen a sharper set of frame blow-ups than the ones Mike carefully custom-printed for me.

Many of the ideas in this book grew out of a graduate seminar on Howard Hawks which I conducted at the University of Chicago in the Autumn of 1979. Although I cite those specific contributions from members of the seminar which I can recall, it may be that I have for-gotten the sources of certain ideas and that other ideas grew commu-nally from the common soil of our discussions. In any case, most of the ideas in this book were first presented to and tested within that group and were certainly sharpened, clarified, and developed as a result. The contributing members of the seminar were Nancy Diamond, Thomas Feucht-Haviar, Mark Kay, Stephanie Kreps, Bill Monroe, Andrea Stas-kowski, and Charles Wordell.

Finally, let me thank Burnell Y. Sitterly who, as usual, took charge of preparing the manuscript and checking its details.

G.M.

Contents

HOWARD HAWKS, STORYTELLER

1

Life and Work, Stories and Machines

Hell, the first thing you've got to do if you're going to make a picture is to get a story. The next thing is to get a good script, the next thing is to figure out who the hell is going to play in it, your characters, and then after that to make it.[1]

McBride: Do you feel that the character in *Red River* was somewhat like your grandfather?
Hawks: No.
McBride: But he was a lumber baron, wasn't he, in Wisconsin?
Hawks: Yes, he was a lumberman.
McBride: Was he in the mold of the John Wayne tough guy?
Hawks: He had a great deal more sense of humor than John.[2]

McBride: Do you think today's directors think about it too much, get too many analyses of their work?
Hawks: I don't credit them with thinking.[3]

THE LIFE STORY of Howard Winchester Hawks winds around and through the history of American film itself. He was born on May 30, 1896, five weeks after a motion picture was first projected in public to a paying audience in America. The son of a wealthy paper manufacturer and grandson of a wealthy lumberman—Hawks could never bring himself to use a term like lumber *baron*—he moved with his family from Goshen, Indiana to Neenah, Wisconsin in 1898, then on to Pasadena, California in 1906 because of his mother's health. The family's move came at almost the same time that the movies themselves went west; the independent film companies began production in California one year later, and D. W. Griffith would bring his Biograph family to the sunshine of Southern California for the first time in the winter of 1910. Although Hawks began his education in Pasadena, he was duly sent

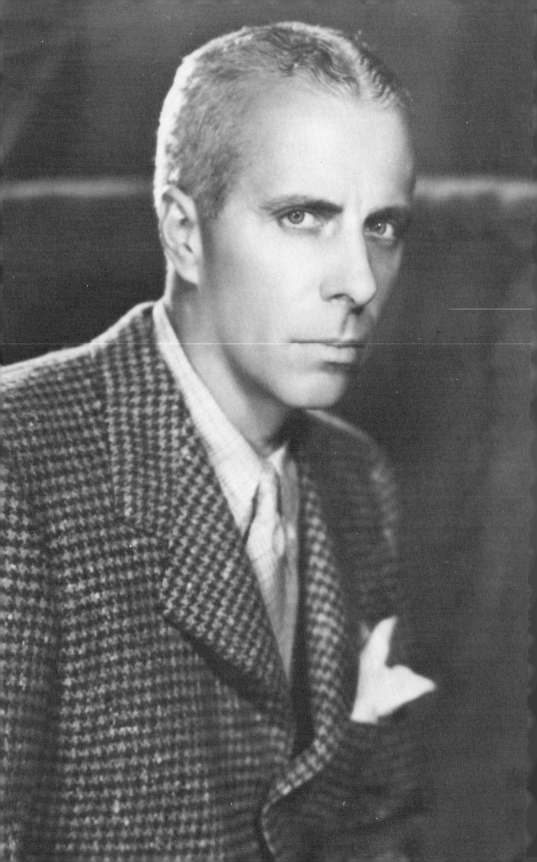

east to complete it at Phillips Exeter Academy and Cornell University, where he took a degree in mechanical engineering in 1917.

The young Hawks had two passions—reading stories and building machines—which he would combine in his adulthood by making stories with machines. Like Buster Keaton, that other film master with a passion for machines, born only six months before Hawks and in the same region of the country, Hawks would make the connection between the art of machines and a machine art. The differences in their machines would indicate the differences in their art. While Keaton's machines were bizarre and convoluted toys, Rube Goldberg contraptions that linked a myriad of intricate processes in order to accomplish absolutely nothing—machines whose ultimate function was simply to be admired in and for themselves—Hawks's taste was for sturdy, practical machines that efficiently got the job done—airplane motors, automobile engines.

Hawks's knowledge of flying machines would lead to many important experiences and acquaintances. He taught pilots to fly during World War I and would re-create his experiences with fliers in *The Dawn Patrol* (1930), *Ceiling Zero* (1935), *Only Angels Have Wings* (1939), and *Air Force* (1943). His love of flying would also lead to his turbulent sometime-friendship with Howard Hughes: "He [Hughes] flew my airplane and I flew his. . . . He could fly and he had a lot of guts. . . ."[4] Together Hawks and Hughes would make *Scarface* (in 1930, released 1932); then Hawks walked out on Hughes's production of *The Outlaw* (in 1940, released 1943) when their two egos bumped into each other and when Hawks refused to lavish unnecessary money on production values; Hughes then retaliated by threatening an injunction against the release of Hawks's *Red River* (1948), in which Hawks had devised a deliberate variation on a scene in *The Outlaw*; Hughes's RKO company, however, would release both *The Thing* (1950), which Hawks produced, and *The Big Sky* (1952). The relationship between the two men ended amicably enough when Hawks's son, David, won the Western Championship Motorcycle Competition in Las Vegas a decade later: ". . . there was a note from Howard saying, 'take him and a couple of the other boys to dinner and it's on me.' So that was the last time I saw Hughes."[5] Hawks's love of flying would also be one of the bonds be-

Howard Hawks in 1935

tween him and William Faulkner who, like Hawks, flew his own planes and who, like Hawks, had lost a brother in an airplane crash. Faulkner's brother Dean died flying the family airplane, while Hawks's brother Kenneth died flying stunts for a film Kenneth was directing, *Such Men Are Dangerous,* in the same year as his brother's flying film *The Dawn Patrol.* Faulkner's collaboration with Hawks would be the writer's most rewarding and most fruitful of his adventures in Hollywood.[6]

Hawks also loved machines that stayed on the ground. He built the racing car (for $3000) that won the Indianapolis 500 in 1936;[7] he rode motorcycles with Barbara Stanwyck and Gary Cooper—and taught both his sons to ride. Hawks continued to ride his motorcycle until he was 78. His knowledge of automotive machines would enable him to design and build the complicated camera car that would make it possible for him to shoot the extemporaneous hunting sequences of *Hatari!* (1962). And his knowledge of mechanics must surely have contributed to his design for Pharaoh's tomb in *Land of the Pharaohs* (1955), a complexly interdependent system of weights and counterweights for blocking the entrance to the ruler's crypt by sealing up the passageways of the labyrinth with stone blocks. Like the mechanical design for sealing that tomb, Hawks's stories themselves might be seen as complicated webs of causality in which each of the parts functions efficiently and effortlessly in producing the whole and in which the chain of narrative circumstances leads interdependently and inexorably to its fulfillment and culmination.

Hawks's career in films began in 1917 as a prop boy for Famous Players-Lasky, where he later served as an assistant director for Mary Pickford's pictures. He first had the opportunity to direct in 1917 when Miss Pickford's director, Marshall Neilan, fell ill, and Hawks shot several scenes of *The Little Princess.* During that Hollywood pioneer period, the young Hawks shared a house in the Hollywood Hills with several other young directors, writers, and producers of films-to-be; one of them was a young, "Jewish-looking"[8] man who turned out to be Irving Thalberg. Hawks remembers endless hours with Thalberg, discussing story ideas and story theory. In 1924 Thalberg recommended Hawks to Jesse Lasky when Famous Players needed a bright young man to run that studio's story department. Lasky hired Hawks to develop forty stories, and Hawks bought "two Rex Beaches, two Jack Londons, two Zane Greys, two Conrads" (one of which was *Lord Jim*).[9] Hawks "developed" these stories by first supervising the construction of their scenarios and then, in effect, producing the films made from them. Before he became a director Hawks was both writer and producer—two skills that served him well after he began directing his own films.

Hawks would never forget his debt to Thalberg; he tried to fulfill the three-picture contract he signed with MGM in the years just before Thalberg's death—*Today We Live* (1933), *The Prizefighter and the Lady* (1933), and *Viva Villa!* (1934). But Hawks walked out on the last two when Louis B. Mayer meddled with his directing. He explained to Thalberg that he simply couldn't work for Mayer. He also never forgot his debt to Jesse Lasky; he agreed to direct *Sergeant York*—and he convinced Gary Cooper to play the role—specifically as a favor to Lasky. He told Cooper that Lasky "has a story that I don't think it would hurt us to do, and he's broke and he's got the shakes and he needs a shave. So Cooper got an Academy Award, I doubled my salary, and Lasky made $2,500,000 from that thing and we had a good time making it." [10]

Hawks did not want to stay in Lasky's story department; he wanted to direct his own films rather than write and produce the films of others. He directed his first film, *The Road to Glory,* in 1926 for the Fox Company when Famous Players refused to let him out of the story department. For the next forty-five years the story of Hawks's life became inseparable from the stories he shot. Between 1926 and 1929 he directed seven more films for Fox, six silent, one part-talkie, none of striking artistic distinction or commercial success. With the coming of synchronized sound, Hawks wrote his own story of fliers in World War I, *The Dawn Patrol,* which he "paid John Monk Saunders to put his name on" [11] so that Hawks, who had never worked in the theater and who was therefore presumed to know nothing about dialogue, could direct it. The artistic and commercial success of this 1930 film—its underplayed, casual, offbeat, intimate dialogue, its willingness to toss lines off naturally rather than to orate them in the stiff, stentorian manner of many early, theatrical talkies—established Hawks as such a dependable, effective sound-film stylist and storyteller that he was able to make films for the next forty years without signing a single long-term contract with any particular studio.

In this forty-year career Hawks's best films were made for those companies which gave him the greatest freedom and allowed him to serve as the film's absolute and ultimate producer—in name, or at least in fact. Hawks's relationship with Jack Warner—one of the reputed ogres of the industry—was both cooperative and productive. As a matter of policy, Hawks refused to expose a frame of film while Jack Warner was on his set. After *The Dawn Patrol* for First National (by then a Warners subsidiary), Hawks made *The Crowd Roars* (1932), *Tiger Shark* (1932), *Ceiling Zero, Sergeant York* (1941), and *Air Force* for Warner Bros., culminating in the two Bogart-Bacall classics of the mid-1940s, *To Have and Have Not* (1944) and *The Big Sleep* (1946). Hawks also made his best late film, *Rio Bravo* (1959), for Warners as well as one of his worst, *Land of the Pharaohs*, although by the late 1950s Warners was only in name the same company that Jack Warner had run a decade earlier. Hawks did even better with an even bigger reputed monster of the industry, Harry Cohn. "A lot of people didn't like him but I thought he was good guy."[12] Hawks liked working for Cohn: "The guy thinks his salvation is a director because he can't get stars, but he can get directors who can get stars."[13] For Columbia, Hawks made his third sound film, *The Criminal Code* (1931), as well as three of the very best films of his most important period—*Twentieth Century* (1934), *Only Angels Have Wings,* and *His Girl Friday* (1940). That major period came to an end with a three-picture contract to Twentieth Century-Fox, which he satisfied with the two late screwball comedies *I Was a Male War Bride* (1949) and *Monkey Business* (1952), and the musical comedy *Gentlemen Prefer Blondes* (1953), as well as a single section, "The Ransom of Red Chief," of *O' Henry's Full House* (1952). Although Hawks's relationship with Darryl F. Zanuck at Twentieth was cordial and courteous, Zanuck would not approve the serious films Hawks wanted to make—in particular two Faulkner screenplays, *Dreadful Hollow* and *The Left Hand of God*—just after Faulkner had won the Nobel Prize.[14] During his major period Hawks had also made his classic screwball comedy for RKO—*Bringing Up Baby* (1938)—and released two independent films through the distributor United Artists—*Scarface* and *Red River.*

Hawks wrote, or supervised the writing of, every one of these films. He rarely received screen credit, however, because of the Screen Writers' Guild's prohibition against the director's or producer's receiving screen credit as writer. The credit cards for films frequently bear no relationship to the person or persons who really did the work. Most notorious, perhaps, is the writer's credit card for *Gone with the Wind,* its screenplay attributed to the noted playwright Sidney Howard (perhaps for publicity purposes) but actually written by David O. Selznick, Ben Hecht, and Howard Hawks (among others). Hawks contributed to the writing of any number of other major films for which he never received credit—most notably, three Josef von Sternberg classics (*Underworld, Morocco,* and *Shanghai Express*) and George Stevens's *Gunga Din.* In addition to writing his own films, Hawks also produced as well as directed most of them. And those he did not produce—among them, the three films for Mayer and the four Goldwyn films, *Barbary Coast* (1935), *Come and Get It* (1935), *Ball of Fire* (1941), and *A Song Is Born* (1948)—were among his least fulfilling and fulfilled ventures. Those were the films on which Hawks frequently "took a walk," or should have.

Hawks never considered his producing as important as his directing. Most indicative of his attitude are the title cards for *Red River, Rio Bravo,* and several other films, which read:

DIRECTED

and

produced

by Howard Hawks. Many of the other films he directed and produced credit no one as producer at all. But it was his producing that allowed him to write and direct his films as he wished. And to cast them. It was in his function as producer that Hawks became known as the discoverer of the stars who graced his films. Paul Muni, George Raft, Ann Dvorak, Carole Lombard, Frances Farmer, Jane Russell, Montgomery Clift, Joanne Dru, Angie Dickinson, James Caan, and, of course, Lauren Bacall all first attracted national attention as stars of Hawks films before they figured so prominently in anyone else's.

Among Hawks's closest personal acquaintances were the writers with whom he worked. Hawks claims to have "discovered" Faulkner—just as he discovered his stars—introducing the unknown Southern writer's first novel, *Soldier's Pay,* to the wits of the Algonquin Round Table before anyone else had heard of him.[15] In addition to working together and sharing an interest in flying, Hawks could keep pace with Faulkner, glass for glass, on drinking sprees, after which the two might awaken in some Culver City motel room where "Faulkner was fishing cigarette

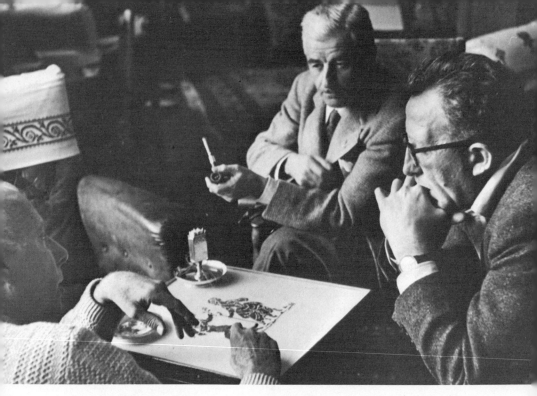

Hawks, William Faulkner, and Harry Kurnitz at work on the script of
Land of the Pharaohs

stubs out of a mint julep glass." [16] Faulkner not only liked the way
Hawks drank; he also liked the way he made films, so he asked Hawks
to teach him how to write them. [17] Faulkner wrote his first screenplay
for Hawks—an adaptation of his own *Saturday Evening Post* story,
"Turn About" (*Today We Live*)—and his last screenplay for Hawks
(*Land of the Pharaohs*). In between there were three other Faulkner-
Hawks scripts which became Hawks films.

Hawks was almost as close with another Nobel Prize-winning
American writer of his age, Ernest Hemingway, with whom Hawks skied
in Sun Valley and fished off Key West. Hawks and his second wife,
Nancy, even spent their honeymoon on Hemingway's *Finca* in Cuba.
Hemingway admired Hawks's films so much he wanted his friend to
direct the film version of *For Whom the Bell Tolls;* unfortunately he got
stuck with Sam Wood. Hawks admired everything about Hemingway's
life except his leaving of it; he refused to condone that final act of
"cowardice" or to sympathize with the obsession that drove him to it.

10

Nonetheless, Hawks's commitment to stoical endurance had melted enough for him to forgive his friend by 1972, when he began to plan a Hemingway project concerning the writer's friendship with the photographer Robert Capa. Like several other of his projects of the 1970s, Hawks was never able to film it.

In contrast to his associations with these two gentleman novelists were Hawks's close personal-professional relationships with two cynical, more popular and journalistic wits—Ben Hecht and Jules Furthman. Hawks always had a lot of "fun" (the word which appears most often in Hawks interviews) working with Hecht, thinking up crazy ideas to throw into a script while they alternated an hour of work and an hour of backgammon. Hecht admired Hawks's cool, quiet grace and elegance, describing him as a "mysteriously romantic fashion plate."[18] Hawks got on equally well with Furthman, who had been writing filmscripts since 1915 and whom few other than Hawks could stand: "Furthman wasn't hard for me to get along with . . . He's just such a mean guy that we thought he was great."[19] Furthman and Hawks made quite a pair—the director tall (six-one), thin, handsome, and silver-haired, the writer squat, dark, and oily. Furthman, who excelled in romantic stories of romantic figures in exotic locales—for both Hawks's and Sternberg's films (in collaboration with Hawks)—may even have had the handsome Hawks in mind as his image of romantic elegance and grace.

When Hawks was not busy developing scripts, finding stars, and shooting films, he enjoyed several hobbies, both indoors and out. He played golf and tennis—winning the United States Junior Tennis Championship in 1914. He sailed his yacht, the *Sea Hawk,* and raced his horses—as so many in Hollywood did. He was an expert carpenter and silversmith, making antique-type furniture out of wood. Christian Nyby, Hawks's editor from 1944 to 1952, recalls a baby's cradle carved out of a solid piece of oak and a "kibitzer's chair" with a high back on which the backward-seated kibitzer could rest his elbows.[20] One of Hawks's favorite art pieces was a silver belt buckle shaped into the design of the "Red River D" brand, which he made as a gift for John Wayne.[21]

Hawks's first marriage was to Athole Shearer, Norma's sister, in 1928. His old friend Irving Thalberg was now an in-law. There were two children: Barbara, and David, who has worked for years as an

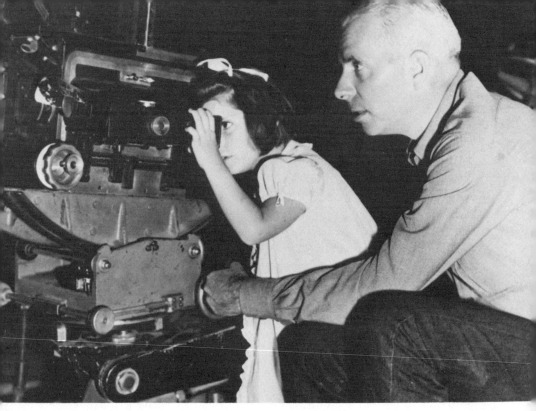

A Hawks family album: with daughter Barbara, son Gregg, wife Nancy and son David

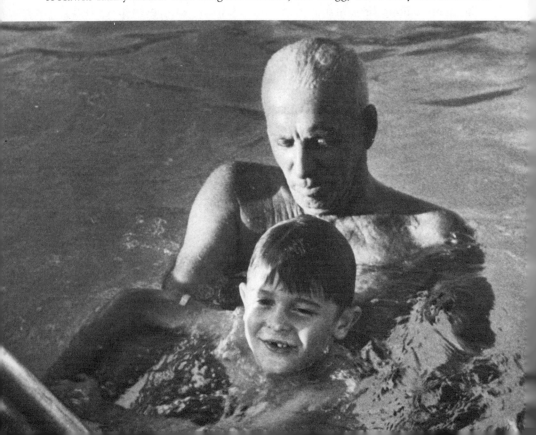

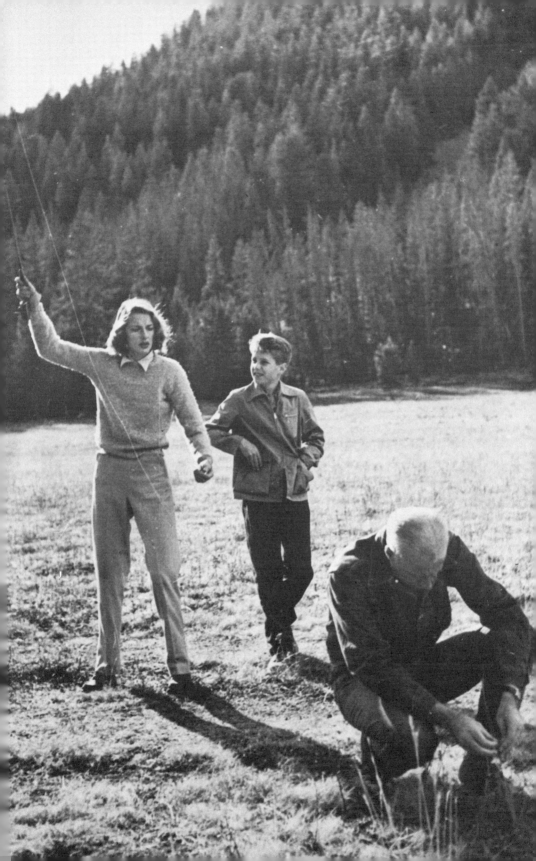

assistant director on the *M*A*S*H* television series. The couple divorced in 1940. His most celebrated marriage was in 1941 to the model and writer, Nancy Raye Gross, a beautiful twenty-four year old (nicknamed "Slim") who would be named the best-dressed American woman of 1947. They had a daughter, Kitty (her name a pun on the Wright Brothers' famous flight). After they divorced in 1948, Nancy married theater producer Leland Hayward; later she married the British financier Lord Keith. Hawks's third wife, Dee Hartford, was another twenty-four-year-old model; the marriage lasted from 1953 to 1959. They had one son, Gregg (named after the cinematographer, Gregg Toland). Hawks seemed to have liked his women tall and slender—like Bacall as "Slim." It is unclear whether the marriages ended because Hawks was a Don Juan whose sexual attentions perpetually wandered or because he was so committed to his vocation of making films that he had little time to play house. Perhaps it was a little of both. Carole Lombard is said to have warned a friend about Hawks's sexual prowess—that he was a very "sneaky" man who could get into a woman's pants before she knew it.[22] Unlike the men in so many of his films, Hawks was never able to find a woman who could be simultaneously his vocational and sexual partner.

The two primary qualities of Hawks's social manner seemed to have been a cool, paternalistic, gentlemanly—even lordly—detachment and a dry, droll sense of humor. Christian Nyby worked for Hawks for six years before he dared to call him anything but the formal "Mr. Hawks." He finally called him "Howard" after cautiously asking his permission to do so when directing *The Thing*.[23] Consistent with this report was the descriptive title of a *Look* magazine interview—"He Looks More Professor than Producer"—as well as Rosalind Russell's description of his eyes as "two blue cubes of ice," and Lauren Bacall's description of her feelings of intimidation and awe in his presence.[24] In any social or professional group, he was clearly the leader, director, father, boss, and king. According to Joseph McBride, he had the "highest self-opinion of any director I've met."[25] Despite the clearly conservative political implications of his social manner and his films—the dependence of the group on the paternalistic leader—Hawks never discussed political issues in public. Nor did he like to discuss religion.[26] For one thing, politics and religion were personal and private matters, not to be discussed openly—like all those thoughts and feelings characters refuse to discuss in his films. For another, political and religious discussions produce arguments, and Hawks did not like to argue. Unlike the argumentative energy of an immigrant director like John Ford, the patrician Hawks did not enjoy a good brawl.

Hawks's lordly sense of self was accompanied and qualified by a sly sense of humor that was as understated as the dialogue in his films. For example, there is Hawks's delivery of a story about the time Lee Marvin asked him to direct a western, *Monte Walsh*. Marvin's agent asked Hawks to go to Marvin's house to discuss the project with the star. Hawks replied that he never goes to stars' houses; they come to him. But Marvin's agent replied that Marvin himself had just told him that "he's reached a stage where people come to him." And Hawks replied simply, "Well, you tell him that he's not there yet."[27] Later in the negotiations (which took place at Hawks's office) Marvin pointedly informed Hawks that he wanted the film to be a Lee Marvin western, not a John Wayne western. Hawks drily responded that Marvin need have no worry about being as good as Wayne. Hawks did not direct *Monte Walsh*. A similar kind of Hawks wit can be seen in his assessment of the work of younger directors, like the slow-motion violence of Sam Peckinpah's *The Wild Bunch:* "I can shoot three people, put 'em on a cart, take 'em to the burial ground and bury 'em by the time he gets one person down to the ground."[28]

Hawks's wit and keenness of mind remained with him until his death. After *Rio Lobo* (1970), the last of five films he made after 1960, he continued to plan further projects—the Hemingway story and "Now, Mr. Gus," a globe-trotting comedy of two male friends in search of oil and money. In December 1977 Hawks was at his Palm Springs home alone; his housekeeper had the weekend off, and his son Gregg, with whom he lived, was off motorcycling.[29] He stumbled over one of his dogs, struck his head on the stone floor, and lay unconscious and unattended for over twenty-four hours until a friend discovered him and called an ambulance. Hawks spent two weeks in the hospital, attempting to recover from the concussion and the complications, but even a very vigorous eighty-one year old cannot easily shake off such a shock to the system. Hawks wanted to spend his last days at home, slyly making a date with his nurse as he was leaving the hospital. On one of his final days, which he spent sipping martinis and watching football games on television, Hawks played a farewell scene with his daughter Barbara that might well have come directly from one of his films. He told her he loved her, and she began to cry. It was the first time she'd heard him say it. Then Hawks tossed off one of those flippant, comically defensive comments that always undercut the sentimental force of such moments in his films: "Oh, get on with you." He died on December 26, 1977, one day after the death of another film master and pioneer whose life had also spanned the life of the cinema itself, Charles Spencer Chaplin.

Although his life and career coincided with what was to that point the entire history of cinema, there is considerable disagreement and controversy about the value of Hawks's life and career and its contribution to cinema. On the one hand, Hawks's reputation within the industry was enormous; no other Hollywood director—not Ford, not Capra, not Hitchcock, not Lubitsch (the directors with whom Hawks liked to be compared)—enjoyed greater freedom from the power of an individual Fox, Paramount, or MGM than Hawks, who worked for every major Hollywood studio. No director could win his independence from the industrialized studio system as Hawks did except by earning it. It is also impossible to discuss the power, value, richness, and importance of the American genre film and American film genres without reference to at least a half-dozen of Hawks's films, which seem the ultimate embodiments of those genre aspirations and that same tradition. Finally, given the fact that Hawks spent so much personal and professional time with two of the greatest American literary minds of his age, it seems quite probable that those minds accepted Hawks as "one of us."

On the other hand, although the industry honored Hawks with favorable contracts on his own terms, it never honored him with its artistic awards. Hawks was nominated only once by the Motion Picture Academy for best director (for *Sergeant York*—no doubt for its pious seriousness), although like Chaplin he received a special Oscar (in 1975)—one of those belated honors that the industry, in a mood of nostalgia and guilt, awarded its overlooked giants in the 1970s. Despite his importance within the film industry, Hawks received very little attention in the national press; his two biggest public-relations splashes came in 1944 when his most celebrated discovery, Lauren Bacall, made the cover of *Life* and in 1947 when his wife Nancy was named best-dressed American woman of the year. Lewis Jacobs does not even mention Hawks's name once in his classic history of the American film, *The*

Rise of the American Film, published in 1939, although hundreds of directors of lesser fame, ability, and reputation (then and now) received brief mention if not full discussion. Howard Hawks was not considered worthy of listing in *Who's Who* until 1971 (Ford was first listed in the edition of 1936, Capra of 1938) and not worthy of *Current Biography* until 1972. There is only one major critical book devoted exclusively to Howard Hawks in English, by Robin Wood; written over fifteen years ago, it has been out of print for a decade.[30] The Hawks career reveals an almost total lack of public recognition, not only of what he did but even of who he was. As the title of an article by Robin Wood put the problem in 1969, "Who the Hell is Howard Hawks?"[31] Only after he had finished making films did the general public come to discover who he had been—a belated discovery that perhaps led some critics to overvalue the importance of Hawks's last five films.

How could such a giant of such a public industry remain so invisible to the public? That question is certainly related to the value and interest of any book on Hawks, for to explore his neglect is to expose current artistic, cultural, and cinematic prejudices that prevent a recognition or even the discussion of the strength and value of work such as his. Even within the context of American studio directors, Hawks's work seems much less distinctive (*i.e.* much less idiosyncratic) than that of his more recognized and publicized colleagues—less allegorical than John Ford's, less political than Frank Capra's, less psychologically aberrant than Alfred Hitchcock's, less satirical than Preston Sturges's, less self-consciously clever than Ernst Lubitsch's, less grandiose than Cecil B. DeMille's, less cynical than Billy Wilder's, and so forth. The seeming "less"ness of his films, their seeming artlessness and ordinariness, not only tends to make their creator invisible but also makes it exceedingly difficult to evaluate them according to the existing standards, terms, and values for discussing films.

Hawks's films reject the dazzling visual displays of intellectual montage which propel the films of Sergei Eisenstein, nor are they committed to subverting normal perceptual reality with those unique visual properties of cinema articulated by Rudolf Arnheim. His films take little interest in recording and revealing the physical matter of the material world as urged by the realist theory of Siegfried Kracauer or in surveying and exploring the world in deep focus as urged by the realist theory of André Bazin. Even those Hawks films photographed by the deep-focus cameraman *extraordinaire,* Gregg Toland (*The Road to Glory, Ball of Fire, A Song Is Born*), who shot the Welles and Wyler films on which Bazin based his theory, do not demonstrate a remarkable commitment to deep-focus compositions. Hawks's films reject the modernist aims of Ingmar Bergman, Alain Resnais, Federico Fellini, and Jean-Luc Godard, filmmakers whose urge was not so much to tell a story but to inquire whether it was possible or desirable for stories to be told at all. The self-conscious, self-reflexive quest in films like *Persona, 8½,* and *Contempt,* whose subject is the making of that very film itself, seems totally absent from the films of Howard Hawks, which go about their cheerful business of telling lucid stories (although upon closer inspection and deeper reflection, it becomes clear that every human vocation in a Hawks film is a conscious parallel with or metaphor for the vocation of making films).[32] Finally, Hawks's films take little interest in the explicit examination of contemporary social problems as did the films of Eisenstein, Pudovkin, Renoir, or DeSica and such American films as *I Am a Fugitive from a Chain Gang, Our Daily Bread, Mr. Smith Goes to Washington, The Best Years of Our Lives, Gentleman's Agreement, Marty,* and *Twelve Angry Men.*

There is something uniquely American about the artistic aspirations of a Howard Hawks, whose urge was not to do something apparently difficult (both for the artist and his audience) but something apparently easy, something fun. It is perhaps because American critics themselves have a taste for the difficult that the artistic achievements of a Hawks and so many other similar American filmmakers were first fully appreciated by European critics, who possessed the objectivity and the temperament to perceive the value, energy, and density of the apparently easy and fun. Hawks did not make art for himself or itself—as opposed to the prevailing aesthetic standards of Romantic and modernist art—but to make a "connection" (to use Leo Braudy's term) with others.[33] Hawks was a typical American pragmatist of his age (the same spirit that produced the motion picture machines in the first place), applying that ethic to the purpose of art—a building and a sharing of community with others. He built stories the way he built machines—to accomplish the task that entertaining stories are supposed to accomplish in our democratic culture: not to exclude all except the specially equipped but to include as many as possible.

In this attitude toward art the aspirations of Howard Hawks parallel those of two other film masters, born almost in the same year and in the midwest, Buster Keaton and Fred Astaire. Like Hawks—and quite appropriately for this machine art—both revealed a passion for machines and a perception of the relationship of people and machines. Keaton's mechanical tinkering rivaled that of Hawks, while Fred Astaire's dance numbers (for example, "Slap that Bass" in *Shall We Dance?*) occasionally reveal an equally acute desire to wed human flexibility to mechanical precision. Like Hawks, both of these creators were midwestern, WASP pragmatists with both an urge and a knack "to get things done." Like Hawks, both of them felt that the thing that needs getting done in an art that entertains is entertainment. Like Hawks, both of them made films that seemed fun and easy. And like Hawks, both of them were "discovered" by a later generation of cultural critics to have created fun and easy works that, upon closer inspection, were also extremely careful and complex.

The urge to make and to respond to difficult art is understandable; it links the artistic impulse to its origins in the religious impulse: the agonizing struggle to purify the spirit. Experiencing this kind of art is like going to church: it may be trying but it is good for the soul. The urge to explicate difficult art is also understandable; its very difficulty demands explication—like the difficult biblical passage—so it can be apprehended and understood. To understand Spenser, Milton, Joyce, Beckett, or Eliot requires special learning so the reader can become worthy of the work. But the opposite kind of art that is easy and fun requires explication precisely because it is not apparently difficult, because—like some simpler biblical passages—its accessibility can mask its depth, precision, complexity, and implications. The apprehension and understanding of art that is fun and easy require not special learning but special sensitivity to complicated essences that have been translated into perfectly elegant, graceful, brilliant surfaces, and special care not to be fooled by those simple surfaces into believing the art is simple. They also require a certain immunity to the Puritanical suspicion that something fun cannot be very good for you.

Let me illustrate this claim with two very familiar examples from films by Keaton and Astaire. The montage sequence of Keaton's *Sherlock Jr.,* in which the dreaming projectionist first enters the looking-glass world of the film screen itself and suffers the persecution of the laws of that world, is one of the more celebrated passages in Keaton's (or anyone else's) films. In the most natural, casual, and unself-conscious of manners, the Keaton figure merely stands (or sits, or moves) in the apparently identical space of every frame while the scenery behind him (i.e. the physical universe surrounding him) changes at will—from doorstep, to park bench, to lion's lair, to city street, to desert, mountain, ocean, and so on. Now it is simple enough to stop a camera, substitute something in front of its lens, and then start it again—so that during projection something seems to have been removed from or added to the filmed world as if by magic. This kind of magic had been well known since 1896—the year of Hawks's birth and the year after Keaton's—with the films of Georges Méliès. But the essential technique for creating this kind of magic is that the filmed space must appear to remain absolutely stable; the camera cannot move—not one fraction of an inch—while it is stopped, or the illusion of appearance, disappearance, or conversion would be lost. The being or thing must change, appear, or disappear while the space surrounding it remains absolutely constant.

But for Keaton's montage sequence, there was simply no way to push different physical spaces in front of an absolutely still camera and behind an absolutely still man. In order to record a man in those shifting spaces, the camera and the man themselves had to move. So Keaton (and his special effects man, Fred Gabourie) had to calculate mathematically his precise position in each frame—relative to the camera and to the sides, top, and bottom of the frame—so he could recreate the impression of standing in that identical position in the next frame after the camera had been moved. Only then would the audience believe that the camera and Keaton had stood stock still while the spaces of the world obliged the artist by shifting themselves into the camera's gaze. To create the audience's absolute conviction in this absolute impossibility is precisely the goal of the entire sequence. Ironically, the sequence could only betray the difficulty of its conception and execution if it were imperfect in achieving this conviction: if Keaton's position in each succeeding frame were so imperfectly related to his position in the preceding frame that we could see that he and the camera had both moved and could thereby realize how difficult the stunt was which he had tried to accomplish. But by succeeding perfectly in making us believe the impossible, by our seeing him in precisely the same relative position in every changing frame, Keaton makes the sequence appear terribly ef-

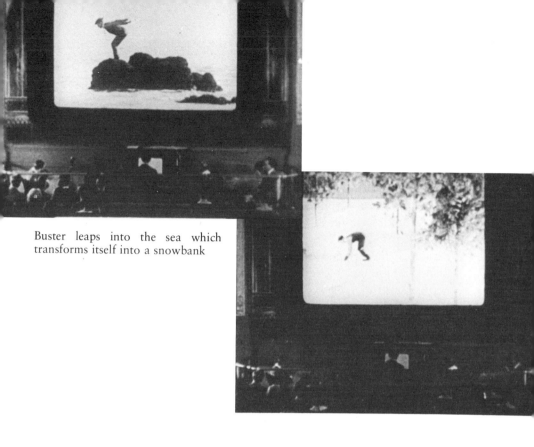

Buster leaps into the sea which transforms itself into a snowbank

fortless and easy. What could be easier than a man standing in the same place all the time?

Precisely this appearance of absolute easiness produces the conviction that permits the delightful comedy of the sequence—a helpless, ordinary, natural being at the mercy of a universe he cannot control and whose laws he cannot understand. But our conviction in a natural impossibility also produces the sequence's brilliant abstract disquisition on the differences between cinema space and natural space, as well as the cinema's reversing and refuting the normal, natural definitions of stillness and motion. That Keaton's magnificent accomplishment in the sequence was simply accepted as absolutely easy and unremarkable in its day seems proven by the fact that no one did remark on it until some forty years after Keaton made it.

The celebrated "Top Hat, White Tie, and Tails" number from Astaire's *Top Hat* reveals a similar masking of difficulty behind easiness. On its surface, the number is another of those typically graceful, per-

21

fectly elegant weddings of song and dance for which Astaire is famous. But a careful examination of the sequence reveals that Astaire carefully planned the number around a musical pattern inherent in the structure of the Irving Berlin song, that the visual principle of costume and decor in the number can be traced to the same contrapuntal pattern of the song's structure, and that all of the dance steps Astaire executes in the number are themselves the result of this musical and visual synthesis. Like most popular songs, Berlin builds "Top Hat" in a 32-bar pattern, with two A sections (the refrain) of eight bars each, a B section (the release) of eight bars, and a final A section which repeats (or slightly permutes) the original eight-bar refrain. The refrain of "Top Hat" is built on sustained, lengthily held notes, producing a flowing, liquid rhythm, and the release, in deliberate contrast, on brief, syncopated, staccato notes, producing a percussive rhythm. In the introductory first chorus of the song, Astaire's pattern of movement (and that of the men behind him) is built on the same rhythmic principles: languid, flowing, liquid movement during the refrains, percussive, tapping "breaks" during the release.

The visual patterns of the costumes and decor also establish the primary terms of the number's construction, which the later choruses will develop and permute. As in many Astaire numbers, both the set and the people are designed as sharp contrasts of black and white. The men all wear black suits with white shirt fronts, black top hats with white shirt cuffs, and even their canes are black shafts with white tips. The background behind them is deliberately gray—a middle tone that sets off the chiaroscuro extremes in front of it. But even the gray background contains reminders of the visual extremes with its circular globes of white light on white lamp posts. These lights on the lamp post indicate the second visual property of the number's conception, the deliberate contrast of the circle and the line. The men stand erect as linear figures, but their top hats are round; like those hats, even their canes synthesize the line (in their length) and the circle (in their tips). A circular white carnation dots the black lapel of every dancer's jacket.

Once Astaire has established the essential musical and visual contrasts in the number's opening chorus (which is what opening choruses of musical numbers are supposed to do)—liquid and percussive, black and white, circle and line—the remaining choruses of the dance can combine and permute these polar opposites. In his first solo dance cho-

22

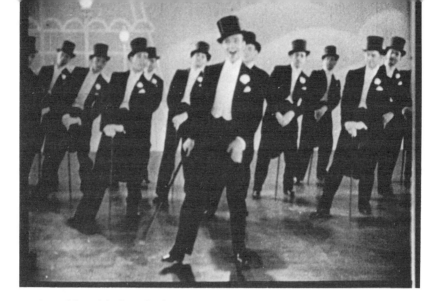

Circle and line, black and white.

rus, Astaire suppresses the legato qualities of the Berlin refrain by syncopating and percussing the entire song, converting this entire chorus into a complexly rhythmic conversation between his tapping feet and the syncopated taps of his cane on the floor. His taps and cane have literally become percussion instruments. The primary visual figure that Astaire's motion describes in this chorus is a synthesis of the circle and the line—his body traces a circular pattern while he raps his linear cane on the floor. The linear cane becomes the literal center of that circle of movement. The line has become equated with the song's staccato qualities (syncopated rapping on the floor), the circle with its legato qualities (flowing movement in an unbroken circle). But in his next solo dance chorus Astaire takes an opposite tack. The lights dim (a shift away from white and toward black), the sounds of the accompanying orchestra fade, and Astaire performs a whole chorus of the song without any tapping noises at all. The number has gone from pure percussion to pure legato, emphasized by the silently circular leaps of Astaire's choreography.

The line of male dancers returns for the number's final chorus—in which Astaire converts that line of tuxedoed dancers into sitting ducks in a shooting gallery. This trope elevates the purely geometric issues of the number (circle and line, liquid and percussive) into matters of the human spirit and imagination. Astaire's trope—that identically attired men are like identical, mechanical objects in a shooting gallery—arises from the very perfection of their identical attire and their ontological obligation to be mere members of a chorus (to be not people but a geometric figure—a line). But Astaire is also attired as they are. Unlike so many lead dancers in films and on the stage, he does not wear a slightly more elaborate, more attractive, or more noticeable variation of the chorus member's costume; Astaire wears exactly the same costume they do. The difference between Astaire and the mechanical ducks behind him is not one of outer dress but inner spirit. It is Astaire who has the imagination to see the visual connection between chorus men and mechanical ducks, to transform them into those ducks, and then to shoot them dead for their deadness. It is Astaire (and his collaborator, Hermes Pan) whose imagination has conceived and executed the entire musical number based on legato and staccato, circle and line, black and white. Astaire's weapon for killing these ducks is a combination of his linear cane and percussive taps, a synesthesia whose terms have been built into the number from its beginning. With this final trope, Astaire asserts that it is not dress, not outer attire, that distinguishes supple, spontaneous, imaginative human beings from mechanical, identical, inanimate dolls. Spontaneity and individuality are matters of the imagination alone. Dancing itself is not a physical activity but a material projection of the mind and spirit (like movies). An attentive examination of the plan and structure of this "elegantly easy and pleasant" musical number will convince the attender that there is no possibility that Astaire did not intend every one of these musical, visual, and spiritual connections.

Although these detailed discussions of two contemporaries may seem to have wandered very far from the stories of Howard Hawks, they serve as warnings and reminders that the perfectly easy (in direct proportion to its approaching perfection in its apparent easiness) is never easy. Without the ease, such a work or sequence could never be so widely and instantly enjoyable. But the ease, the *sprezzatura*, which captures our imaginations so forcefully and immediately is both a ruse and a mask for something terribly difficult in both conception and execution. The ease represents a kind of midwestern, James Whitcomb Rileyish, American humility—"Aw shucks, 'tweren't nothin' "—that wishes to deny anything very grand or grandiose about an accomplishment. It is the accomplishment, not its maker, which must speak its worth. It is the critic's business to listen carefully—particularly since these kinds of works deliberately do not proclaim but speak very softly and subtly. The energetic perfection and vitality of Hawks's greatest genre films imply that they represent the same accomplishment of ultimate easiness in storytelling as Keaton's in visual comedy and Astaire's in dance and song. The mask of easiness deliberately disguises the complex accomplishment of this American storyteller's American art.

2

Auteur or Storyteller

All I'm trying to do is tell a story and I just imagine the way it should be if you tell it and so I do it.[1]

In America . . . they're just beginning to appreciate the work of directors. They're beginning to find out that some directors put a stamp on their work and some don't. Some are good storytellers and some aren't.[2]

Above all in a motion picture is the story.[3]

He is one of those directors of whom it is said: I will go see everything he does because he is a good storyteller.[4]

ONE APPROACH to film criticism has specifically set itself the task of articulating the unique artistic qualities of this uniquely American art: the *auteur* theory, first advocated in France by the young François Truffaut in 1953 (as the *politique des auteurs*), then developed in America a decade later by Andrew Sarris and others of his persuasion. The name of Howard Hawks has been inextricably linked to the *auteur* undertaking, and if there is a single concrete accomplishment that can justify that entire undertaking it is the resuscitation of the reputation of Howard Hawks and the rediscovery of his films. The original *auteur*ist aim (an aim which has been both broadened and softened with the passage of time)[5] was to identify an individual artistic personality in a Hollywood film's director, a personality which could be distinguished from both the film's script and its stars. The undertaking works particularly well with a director like Douglas Sirk, who made domestic melodramas (also called "women's pictures," "weepers," "soapers," and several other derogatory synonyms) at Universal-International for producer Ross Hunter in the 1950s (among them, *All That Heaven Allows, Tarnished Angels, Written On the Wind, Imitation of Life*).

A careful look at Sirk's films reveals that the director built as many scenes as possible around hard, reflective visual materials (glass, mirrors, window panes, the shiny surfaces of furniture); that he used ordinary domestic objects (teapots, television sets, cups, saucers, clothing, sofas, pictures, tablecloths) as symbolic commentaries on the lives and values of the people who lived with those objects; and that he filled his motion picture frame with frames-within-the-frame (doorways, archways, window panes, mirrors) so that his films refer not only to life but also to imitations of life—in particular to the way life is imitated in movies themselves. Despite the tawdry, melodramatic scripts of these films, despite their saccharine musical soundtracks, and despite the leaden embodiments of the characters by those dim "stars" under contract to Universal who peopled Sirk's world (Jane Wyman, Rock Hudson, Sandra Dee, Lana Turner, John Gavin, John Saxon), the unique, personal devices of a creator named Douglas Sirk can be identified—devices which perform a devastatingly ironic critique of the very bourgeois world which is the film's milieu. For such films, the *auteur* theory's urging us to perceive the "tension" between the director's personality and the script's demands is the only way to come to know that such a creator named Douglas Sirk exists.

But Howard Hawks did not make such films. He spent his apprenticeship as a scriptwriter and producer. He developed (if not actually wrote) every script he shot (and he rewrote whole chunks of them himself on the set). He produced most of the films he directed (and he walked out on many he did not produce when some meddling Mayer or Goldwyn told him what and what not to do). As a producer Hawks controlled all those decisions about a film project that the director (in his job as director) does not: he hired the writers and approved their work; he hired the set designer, editor, musical director, cinematographer and approved their work; and, extremely important in film, he hired the actors who would embody the characters. While the director (in his job as director) is responsible only for what happens in front of the camera on the set, the producer (as the title implies) is responsible for the whole production and the production of the whole. In his work on a film, Howard Hawks was as much a creative producer, like David O. Selznick, as a creative director, like Douglas Sirk. This confusion between the director's and producer's responsibilities on a film leads to an *auteur*ist inconsistency with Hawks—the acceptance of *The Thing* as a Howard Hawks film when in fact Howard Hawks did not direct the film (not one scene) but produced it.[6] The contribution of Howard Hawks to a film cannot be illuminated (as can Sirk's) by his separation from or antagonism to his content or script or performers. His contribution *is* the whole film: "his acting style, his script, and his visual style are all one."[7]

A second problem the *auteur*ist encounters with Hawks can also be illustrated by the treatment of Sirk. Proving the existence of reflective surfaces, symbolic objects, and frames within frames in every Sirk film certainly establishes the existence of a presence named Sirk—but little more. It in no way proves that the films are of any value—or even that Sirk is of any value. To prove the distinguishability of a director's personality (the heart of the original *auteur* undertaking) cannot demonstrate in itself the talent of a director or the excellence of his work. *Auteur* discussions of Hawks, insistent on demonstrating that there *is* a Howard Hawks beneath the genre conventions of his films, seize on the bits of themes and business that link the films: the exchange of cigarettes, the professionalism of his characters, the sexual role reversals and the use of animals in his comedies, male friendship and the rites of passage that allow a female entrance to the male group in the adventure films, and so forth. Picking through the Hawks films to reveal these consistent bits both fails to demonstrate the value of individual films and tends to collapse Hawks's career into one giant work, making little distinction between the concerns and quality of any one of them. This tendency to equate the identification of Hawks motifs with the artistic quality of a Hawks film perhaps led *auteur*ist critics to value Hawks films from *Rio Bravo* onward so highly, though Hawks himself found many of these films to be among his greatest failures.

What did Howard Hawks think made his best films best? If one reads the interviews he gave over the final fifteen years of his life, one encounters the term "story" repeatedly—"I'm just trying to tell a story," "that's the kind of story that interests me," "that makes a good story," "that's how I wanted to tell that story," and so forth. Many of Hawks's *auteur*ist admirers steer clear of this embarrassing term: story means script, story means characters, story means "literature" and not "cinema," plot, not camera angles, editing, composition, lighting, and decor. Stories are not unique to cinema but common to novels, plays, operas, ballets, poems, even paintings. In this view (which underlies almost every major theory of film as a medium), the story is merely the premise, the given of any cinema work, and the real stuff—the cinema—is what gets added on. This view works best with those directors who add the most on—and are easiest to discuss because of all that addition. But such a view will simply not work for Hawks, who does not add cinema to his stories but pours his stories into cinema. To demonstrate that Hawks is of any value is to demonstrate that he told good stories.

What is a good story? First, there is the construction of an action—not just enumerating a string of events but organizing those events into a coherent and powerful shape. The construction of a narrative action relies on a very interesting paradox, of which Hawks was well aware. On the one hand, the events in a narrative must seem to flow spontaneously, naturally, surprisingly; nothing must be expected, nothing foreseen. On the other hand, the events in a narrative must be prepared for, motivated, foreshadowed; nothing is unexpected, everything foreseen. On the one hand, everything that happens to King Lear is a surprise; on the other, everything in the play proceeds from Kent's command in the beginning to "See better, Lear." It is surprising that Emma Woodhouse discovers that it is Mr. Knightley whom she really must marry; yet everything in *Emma* points the way to this inevitable and inescapable discovery. The paradox of narrative construction is that it synthesizes the accidents of nature—which seem random—and the patterns of logic—which are fixed; the outcome of events is simultaneously inevitable yet surprising to the reader or viewer when the inevitable occurs. The narrative that is insufficiently spontaneous and surprising is familiarly condemned as contrived, overplotted, unnatural, and stilted; the narrative that is insufficiently patterned is familiarly condemned as random, wandering, arbitrary, and formless.

How does Hawks's story construction relate to this paradox of surprising inevitability? In over forty years of filmmaking, collaborating with over a dozen major writers, Howard Hawks builds every story in an identical four-part structure. The first part is a prologue that either (1) establishes the conflict in a past or present close relationship of the major characters (this is the usual pattern of Ben Hecht's scripts for Hawks) or (2) initiates a conflict by the collision of two apparently opposite characters upon their initial meeting (this is the usual Furthman-Faulkner pattern). The second and third parts develop the central conflict established in the first, either by letting one of the conflicting characters or life styles dominate in the second part, then the other in the third, or by letting one of the characters work alone in the second part, then both of them together in the third. And the fourth section resolves the central conflict, often by a return to the original physical setting of the prologue but in which setting the warring characters now see themselves and one another in a new light. Occasionally Hawks adds a very brief epilogue or "tag" to return the narrative full circle to its beginning. Whatever else one can say about this narrative structure, it gives a Hawks story the firmness of shape, the elegance, economy, and symmetry that allow surprising events to transpire within the firm logic and structure of a controlled pattern.

Then, of course, this narrative structure must be peopled (indeed propelled) by characters, human portraits that are consistent, credible, and motivated, either interesting and complex in themselves or viewed in an interesting and complex way by the storyteller. But as important as the vitality and complexity of the individual human portraits themselves is the necessity of creating those particular characters for that particular narrative structure in which they exist. The very structure of a Howard Hawks narrative requires a central pair of characters who, at its beginning, seem to be warring opposites but who, by its end, realize that they are somehow alike. The clashing opposites discover they are spiritual partners, extensions of one another, complements not antagonists. This interrelation of narrative structure and character has several consequences.

The first is that, despite the apparent conflict of this pair on the surface, beneath that surface the two really *do* belong together. An inevitable gap develops between what the characters seem to be and feel and what they really are and feel. Any storyteller must communicate this kind of gap to the viewer-reader from the beginning (for it is only by perceiving this gap that the viewer-reader will find the ultimate resolution credible). This communication requires great psychological subtlety and perception on the part of the storyteller—to convey from the outset the feelings that lie beneath the surface to the viewer-reader without the characters giving away these feelings at the outset to each other. Such stories can succeed only by developing the complex and careful texture of internal human psychology—usually by a counterpoint between what the characters say and what the characters do (which casts suspicion on whether they really mean what they say).

Second, this kind of story can be resolved only by the characters' discovery of the way each really feels about the other—often accompanied and accomplished by the character's discovering how he or she feels about himself or herself. This discovery closes the gap between appearance and feeling established early in the narrative and, in effect, allows the characters' knowledge of one another and themselves to coincide with the viewer-reader's knowledge.

Third, this kind of narrative almost inevitably demands an outside observer (or observers) emotionally attached to one (or both) of the central antagonist-protagonists and who, like the audience, has already discovered the genuine feelings beneath the surfaces but must allow the central pair's discoveries to happen for themselves, since people can only discover things by discovering them for themselves. If the outsiders are closely attached to one of the central characters initially, their acceptance of the other precedes and foreshadows the final reconciliation of the warring pair. In their sharing of the audience's knowledge about what lies beneath the surface these outsiders serve as a classic chorus and, in their providing the author's attitude toward the merely apparent antagonism, they serve as the classic *raisonneur*. There is something logically and theoretically inevitable about the consequences of this particular interrelation of narrative action and character—and almost every Hawks film is woven from this identical pattern of events and human psychology.

The discovery which brings the narrative pattern to its completion is a moral discovery as well as an emotional one. The characters not only discover their feelings about themselves and one another but also the moral bases that make such feelings and responses meaningful. In making this personal, emotional discovery the character implicitly discovers the entire moral system on which the narrative has been constructed. What does this mean? In Jane Austen's *Emma,* when Emma discovers that she loves Mr. Knightley and he loves her (something that he has known all along but which she must discover for herself), she also discovers that she has been very foolish to believe that she can regulate every other character's personal and emotional experience while so neglecting her own. She in effect learns that no one can order anyone else's personal life and that everyone has the responsibility of setting his or her own life and feelings in order. Similarly, when Othello discovers that he has murdered an innocent wife, he not only feels personal anguish and pain at his terrible mistake but discovers his own inability to separate the apparent and the real—real innocence from seeming innocence, real honesty from seeming honesty. The innocent Othello learns that he has indeed been innocent of the world's potential duplicity.

Now everything in the narratives of both *Emma* and *Othello*—their events, their characters, their speeches—have been built around the moral issues that culminate in the discovery. The female characters in the Jane Austen novel—Emma, Harriet Smith, Jane Fairfax, Mrs. Elton—represent a spectrum of moral and emotional awareness, both of themselves and of the world in which they live. The male characters—Mr. Elton, Frank Churchill, Robert Martin, and Mr. Knightley—represent a spectrum of male partners, each of whom appropriately belongs with a particularly fitting, matching female. Part of Emma's moral blindness is her emotional blindness about which man belongs with which female partner—including, and especially, her own emotional partner. And in *Othello*, all of the characters represent different shades of real or seeming guilt or honesty—from the Moor, whose outside is black but his inside white, to Iago, whose outside is white but inside black, to Desdemona, whose outside and inside are white but appear black to Othello, to Cassio, who is similarly guiltless but made to seem tainted. Without understanding these moral issues it is impossible for us to follow the narrative at all. As Wayne Booth has shown in *The Rhetoric of Fiction,* the moral system that the author has built into the work is an essential element of a narrative's rhetoric, of our understanding the progress of both the events and the characters.[8]

It is essential in *Emma,* for example, that we understand that Emma is committing a moral error by falsely assuming she can manage the lives of others and that she will never come to know herself and her own feelings until she discovers the precise moral error she has committed. But it is also essential to our understanding of *Emma* that we sympathize with her moral error (it is an all too common, human one) and feel confident that when she finally does see her error she will be morally capable of recognizing it as an error. We must believe she is capable of making the discovery that the book's narrative action requires her to make. We must similarly have the same confidence in Othello's ability to recognize his error once he sees it, and the reason that Emma's kind of error is called comic and Othello's tragic is that her error is reparable (no lives have been destroyed by her error and she herself will be a wiser person as a result of her discovery) but his is not (Desdemona cannot be brought back to life).

But if the author's creation of a moral system of characters and actions is essential to a story's rhetoric—without which there can be no story—the paradox of this moral system is that it then can be turned back upon itself and examined to assess the depth, complexity, and richness of that author's moral vision in general. The reason that certain stories seem morally superficial, hackneyed, and shallow is not that they lack a moral system (for no story could be told without one) but because the moral system on which the story depends is itself superficial, hackneyed, and shallow—an accumulation of the most banal, conventional, and formulaic moral clichés that pass for moral wisdom in the culture. Jane Austen's *Emma* is admired as a rich, important human work, not solely for its carefully structured action, deeply and subtly observed characters, and gracefully perceptive writing but for the very depth, ironies, and complexities of the moral system that permeates it. It is important for human beings to know what Emma discovers, for what she discovers is one of the essential principles that makes life meaningful, human, and livable. *Emma* was certainly not written to teach the reader a didactic lesson about manipulating other people's lives; the reader already knows what Emma discovers in the course of the story (if the reader did not, there could be no story of Emma's coming to know what the reader and the author already know). But part of Jane Austen's reputation as a writer can be traced to her ability to construct such a complex and insightful moral universe as her means to elaborate her story of one woman's discovery. The moral and philosophical seriousness of Shakespeare's *Othello* stems from the same source—the elaboration of a rich moral universe through action and character, based on human issues which are enormously complicated and important.

Yet there is probably no more ludicrous response to Shakespeare's play than Thomas Rymer's dismissing it on the moral grounds that the only lesson it teaches is that "women should be careful how they bestow their linen."[9] Rymer's response is ludicrous because it ignores the *implicit* moral system that underlies the entire narrative; instead, it looks only for some explicit, morally edifying homily. This point brings us back again to Howard Hawks after what might seem a very long digression. If Hawks is to be considered a great storyteller it is essential that he convey a view of human life and aspiration that is serious and complex. Since his stories are obviously neither explicitly didactic nor polemical, and since they appear to be merely escapist genre stories, if they display any moral or philosophical seriousness at all it can only be in the implicit moral system that underlies the films' characters and their actions. Since the narrative structures of Hawks's actions bring his characters to a discovery, the potential seriousness and intellectual richness of his stories can only reside in what it is they discover and why and how—if the moral system that allows Hawks's stories to proceed is a complex and stimulating one. And because Hawks has created so many stories,* each of them with its own action leading the central characters to a discovery, and therefore each of them with an underlying system of moral value to be discovered, the power of Hawks's moral vision becomes even more compelling if these underlying moral systems are consistently, carefully, and complexly related to one another. To demonstrate this consistency is to demonstrate the importance and value of Howard Hawks.

* Hawks received screen credit for directing 39 whole films, co-directing 2 others. But he worked on scripts he did not direct (like Josef von Sternberg's *Underworld* and George Stevens's *Gunga Din*); he directed parts of films for which he received no credit, and he produced several films directed by others.

3

Stories and Movies

[*Paid to Love*] was made right after Murnau's *Sunrise* which introduced German camera trick-work to Hollywood. I was beginning
to direct and was feeling around. They liked it; I didn't. I don't like
tricks. I've always been mechanically minded so I tried a whole lot
of mechanical things, and then gave them up completely.[1]

I'd say that what I do is very subjective. . . . Today any plot you
have is bound to be an old plot, everything has been done. So your
freshness, your creativeness is in your method of treating it, how
the character reacts in the situation. Subjective style is the only way
you can do a film intelligently as I see.[2]

THE CINEMA is Hawks's means for telling his stories, just as the drama
was Shakespeare's means and the novel Jane Austen's. A Shakespeare
or an Austen, in using this means to a narrative end, not only had to
understand its characteristics to accomplish that end but also discovered
or developed any number of interesting, effective, charming, graceful,
and beautiful qualities of that means in the process. So too Hawks
understood the characteristics of cinema which allowed him to tell stories as well as develop or demonstrate some extremely subtle and interesting qualities of cinema itself. It is because these qualities are so subtle
and often so inseparable from his narrative ends that so many critics
who talk about cinema find little to say about Hawks.

The first problem for any builder of cinema stories is to decide which
parts of the tale need telling and which do not, which scenes to shoot
and which to omit, which to develop in detail and which to summarize
in dialogue or montage, which to telescope in time and which to render
in careful temporal wholeness.

The difficult work is the preparation: finding the story, deciding
how to tell it, what to show and what not to show.[3]

If you've got a good scene you can let an actor stall and play
with it. If it isn't a good scene the quicker you get it over with,
the better off you are.[4]

And what is a "good scene"? Obviously one of those essential scenes of
emotional and psychological reaction and interaction on which the narrative of psychological and emotional discovery crucially depends.
Hawks's ability to select or omit, emphasize or skim over scenes becomes especially obvious in those projects that are adapted from other
narrative sources: *Twentieth Century* and *His Girl Friday* from stage
plays; *To Have and Have Not, The Big Sleep, Red River,* and *The Big
Sky* from novels. Hawks remakes these narratives—usually by adding a
large body of introductory material to the plays and eliminating huge
chunks of the expository stage material; usually by emphasizing a small
or nonexistent concern in the novel and building the entire story around
this new emphasis, thereby eliminating huge chunks of the original material. In remaking them in this way Hawks produces narratives that
not only differ in emphasis and tone from their originals but also are
essentially new narratives altogether. A film's story (like any story) is
not merely a sequence of events but a sequence of events with a particular shape, balance, emphasis, and principle of coherence (the semioticians call this the difference between the diegesis—the recitation of facts
in chronological sequence—and the discourse—the way the facts have
been shaped and structured into a communicative whole). To change
the shape, balance, order, emphasis, or principle of coherence is to
change the story.

The second problem for the builder of cinema stories is the handling and control of narrative point of view. This problem parallels that
of the novelist rather than that of the dramatist—since narrated stories
necessarily have narrators (either intrusive or invisible) while dramatized stories do not (except for the occasional narrated description of
off-stage action). The problem in cinema is even more complex than
that in the novel, since the term "point-of-view" carries a single meaning in prose fiction but a double meaning in filmed fiction. In prose
fiction, the term "point-of-view" is merely a metaphor; no one literally
views anything—not the author, his characters, or the reader. A novel's
"point-of-view" is a metaphor for mental attitude—from which character's attitude is the action "viewed"? In *Emma,* for example, Emma's

point-of-view controls the novel's construction—an extremely ironic choice since Emma does not always "see" particularly well. Further, what is the storyteller's attitude toward the action, characters, and events?* In prose fiction, one of these attitudes is perceptual (Whose "view" of the action is it?) and one is moral (What judgments do we make of the action?)—but both of them are abstract attitudes rather than literal, concrete views.

In filmed fiction, however, one of these two points-of-view is literally viewed—because we have shots, which are literal views. From whose physical and psychological perspective do we see the action? Whose physical and psychological perspective does the shot convey? The other type of point-of-view, the moral and judgmental sort, remains an abstract attitude in a film, not a concretely physical view, inferable from the entire moral system of the work as a whole. The handling of point-of-view in this second sense is obviously not unique to cinema; in certain kinds of works (like those of Austen and Hawks) it is never explicit, always implicit, inferable from the entire action and the universe of characters in the work. But the handling of point-of-view in the first sense is unique to cinema and plays a very interesting role in the works of Howard Hawks. We are familiar with a kind of shot that can be recognized as subjective: after a man has been knocked to the floor, we get a shot from a very low angle of the figure who knocked him down, towering above him; after a man has been drugged, we get a very blurry shot that gradually clears into focus as he revives from his stupor. Hawks uses such subjective shots very infrequently—the blurred visions of wounded men in *Air Force* and *Land of the Pharaohs*. The opposite of this kind of shot would seem to be an objective one—a shot of a figure or figures from some outsider's perspective where no other major human perceiver has been established to be. Since no one has been defined

---

* My use of the term "storyteller" is synonymous with the term "implied author," coined by Wayne Booth in *The Rhetoric of Fiction*. It describes the narrative condition that someone telling the story—not precisely the author but not precisely the narrator of the story either—takes a moral attitude toward the events and characters of the story (such and such a person or deed is in error, such and such a person or deed is honorable, etc.) without which there can be no story. Cinema semioticians make a similar point in very different language, distinguishing between the living human being and the creative persona who can be identified by a series of consistent stylistic codes and thematic motifs.

to be perceiving the action from this position, then no one (inside the story) literally is. We accept this shot as a kind of authorial privilege (and it is the kind of shot that seems to dominate most narrative films).

But even this authorial, objective shot can be a subjective one—controlled by the very attitudes and perceptions that the privileged camera is observing. The shot can be simultaneously subjective and objective. In *The Big Sleep,* for example, as Marlowe interrogates Joe Brody, Brody sits in a chair while Marlowe (Bogart) paces around him, in a semicircle, accompanied by the panning movement of the camera which mirrors Marlowe's stealthy walking, Brody's nervous turning. Both characters are objects in the frame, and no one other than the camera is inside the room looking at them from this position; therefore the shot is, by definition, "objective." However, the very solid, powerful motion of Marlowe and the evasive, restless twisting of Brody also reveal how Marlowe feels (the solid, authoritative master of the emotional moment), how Brody feels (a hounded man turning on a spit), and how the "storyteller" behind the camera feels about both of them (Marlowe's prowling power, Brody's shaky weakness). The fact that the camera pans with Marlowe's movement—maintaining the moving investigator as the moving shot's fulcrum—saturates the "objective" camera position with Marlowe's "subjective" power. The unison of camera motion and character motion saturates the shot with Marlowe's moral power as well. In both senses of point-of-view—as emotional participant and moral sympathy—this shot belongs to Marlowe, al-

Marlowe's power. Marlowe (Bogart) pacing, Brody (Louis Jean Heydt) squirming, Agnes (Sonia Darrin) observing.

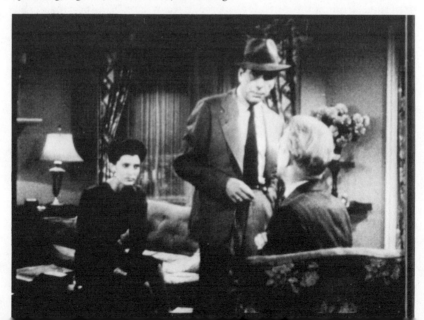

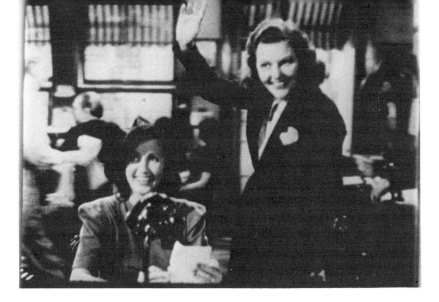

The workers in the pressroom address an implied Hildy, at least three feet to the camera's left.

though the camera itself occupies the perceptual point-of-view of an apparently objective, outside (*i.e.* nonexistent) viewer.

To take another example, when Hildy Johnson (Rosalind Russell) strides into the newspaper office where she formerly worked as a star reporter, at the beginning of *His Girl Friday,* the camera tracks along with her as she stalks through that space. Again the simultaneous motion of character and camera establishes how she feels about that space (it is her domain, her milieu—she "owns" it), how the others in that space feel about her (they agree that the space belongs to her), and how the storyteller feels about her in that space (he also agrees—which casts severe doubt on her stated intention to leave that world in which she so perfectly belongs). In handling his camera in this shot, Hawks takes very special care to establish that the camera's eye belongs to absolutely no one at all in that space; in addressing questions to Hildy when she is out of the frame, seemingly walking beside the camera, the interrogators never speak directly to the camera's lens (which would identify the camera's eye with Hildy's own) but slightly to the camera's left. The storyteller alone has given us our insight into the power and ease of Hildy's motion in that group of people. There is an alliance of storyteller and character (camera motion conveys her emotion) and another alliance of storyteller and viewer (we know more about the camera, her motion, and her emotion than she does). The gap between these two alliances will allow the story (in which that gap closes) to be followed. Of course, to equate motion with both emotional energy and moral force is itself a very interesting choice for a storyteller to make in a *motion* picture.

In a Hawks shot, not only the simultaneous movement of character and camera conveys this simultaneous objectivity and subjectivity. In *Twentieth Century* our first view of Oscar Jaffe (Barrymore) reveals him sprawling on the carpeted floor of his office, feathery quill in hand, as he floridly strokes a notation on a piece of paper. For the next shot, the camera has dropped down to the floor to observe him; it lies parallel with Jaffe's own body, which fills the frame's horizontal expanse. This low-angle shot conveys the way that Jaffe feels himself to occupy that space—its supine master. But in conveying Jaffe's perception of himself in that space, the storyteller disassociates himself from that impression (as he does not from Marlowe's and Hildy's filling of their spaces in those two previous shots) by commenting (satirically) on this man's grandiloquent view of himself (lying theatrically on the floor in a stereotypically romantic attitude, using a quill pen). The ridiculous extremity of the low angle both conveys Jaffe's impression of himself and mocks it (to work while stretched out on the floor is as deviant for a man as for a camera). Like the early traveling shot in *His Girl Friday,* this single shot in *Twentieth Century* establishes an essential piece of narrative, psychological information at the outset: this character *is* a character, a theatricalized person of poses rather than a sensitive, responsive human being; and he is unaware both that he is posing and that there is any difference between living and posing. To emphasize that both the camera's choice and the storyteller's attitude in this early shot are not accidental, the camera drops to the floor again, later in the film, when a black-caped Jaffe threatens suicide, revealing both the fine figure the man thinks he cuts and the ridiculous figure the storyteller thinks he cuts.

This kind of discussion has a number of implications. First, the whole issue of narrative point-of-view in the cinema is far more complex than the simple opposition—objective and subjective—implies. When an interviewer asked Hawks to discuss his subjective technique, Hawks replied rather skeptically: "What would your definitions be of subjective and objective?"[5] Whatever the interest of such questions theoretically, Hawks is their master practically, and the power and skill of his stories

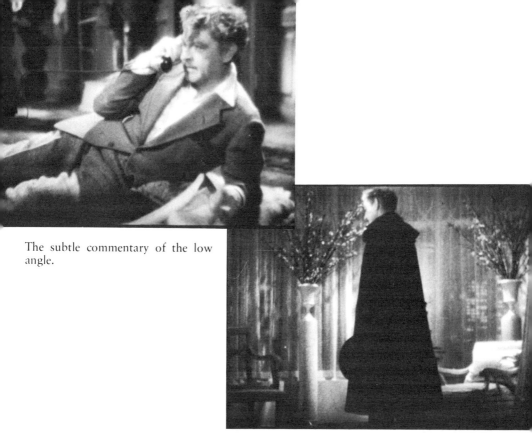

The subtle commentary of the low angle.

are partially attributable to this mastery. That Hawks can effortlessly and simultaneously establish both how his characters view the world and themselves and how the storyteller views their views goes a long way toward solving the central narrative problem of his films—a character making a discovery that the audience has discovered already.

Second, a very familiar description of Hawks's shooting style must forever be abandoned: that Hawks's camera works inevitably at eye level—an inevitability one can find hammered into the stone of the Hawks entry in *Current Biography* and his obituary in the *New York Times*. Hawks is himself responsible for this misconception, since he described his shooting as eye-level in his *Cahiers du Cinéma* interview: "I try to tell a story as simply as possible at eye level."[6] But what precisely is "eye level"? Andrew Sarris describes it as "at the eye level of a standing onlooker,"[7] but almost no shot in the entire Hawks canon seems to be from such a level. It is far closer to the chest or shoulder level of a standing onlooker, the camera tilted slightly upward at the object of its gaze. Or, to be more accurate, at the eye level of a *sitting* onlooker—which is precisely the audience's position as it looks on. This sitting position produces three general effects for those "eye-level" shots which might be defined as Hawks's "objective norm"—casual intimacy with the human figures (for sitting is a more casually intimate position than standing); the slight, subtle ennoblement of those figures, who loom ever so slightly above us mere audience mortals; and the alliance of the camera eye (the storyteller's view and values) with the audience eye, since we both are "equals," sitting together and observing these people in this world. But then the very notion of an "objective norm" is an inappropriate description of any Hawks shooting angle, since every shot carefully conveys the particular character's view of the moment and the storyteller's perspective on both that moment and that view.

The third implication is the way that such a handling of the camera must alter the common notions of cinema space. According to the traditional dogmas of film theory, the inherent paradox of cinema space is that it is simultaneously two- and three-dimensional.[8] Certain films (Michael Snow's experimental film *Wavelength* is probably the ultimate example) indeed set themselves the specific task of examining this paradox of cinema as physical space. But Howard Hawks films define space not physically but psychologically. Space is neither two- nor three-dimensional but saturated with the feelings, perceptions, attitudes, and values of the characters and the storyteller. Hawks's control of point-of-view makes his images represent not physical seeing but psychological feeling—and in doing so, he fuses the two senses of cinema point-of-view (as a character's seeing and a storyteller's judging) into one.

After the cinema storyteller decides which scenes to shoot and which not, and where to shoot them from, he must then decide what he will show within the frame and what he will imply from off-frame. In organizing his framed space, Hawks takes advantage of a fundamental difference between the theater's proscenium arch and the cinema's frame. Because the theater's frame is fixed of necessity, meaning on a stage can be generated only by the choices and arrangements of persons, objects, and light within that fixed space bounded by the arch. But because the cinema's frame is itself a completely flexible boundary to the space it encloses, simply to fix a particular boundary for a shot generates meaning. Multiple photographic objects, human or otherwise, within the same shot necessarily acquire a meaningful relationship to one another simply

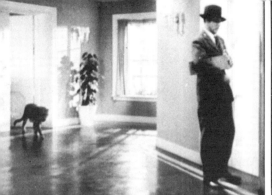
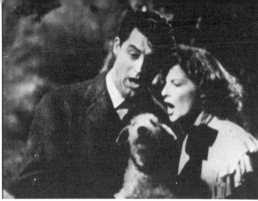
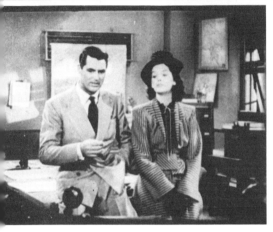

Making inferences from multiple pieces of contrapuntal or balanced data in the same frame.

by their common enclosure. Hawks's favorite framing device is to enclose multiple objects and actions within the same frame, allowing the viewer's eye to collect the individual pieces of visual data that generate inferences about the sense or meaning that arises from this particular juxtaposition. In shot after shot of *Bringing Up Baby,* Baby the leopard or George the terrier occupies the same frame with Susan (Katharine Hepburn) and/or David (Cary Grant), implying the attempted communication between humans and animals, and their attempt to get in touch with the animal impulses within themselves. In shot after shot of *His Girl Friday,* Hildy (Rosalind Russell) and Walter (Grant) occupy the same frame in perfectly balanced symmetrical compositions, implying the essential harmony and complementarity of the two regardless of their verbal warfare. But in a crucial shot of *Monkey Business,* in which Barnaby (Grant again) and Edwina (Ginger Rogers) occupy the same frame in perfectly balanced and symmetrical positions, each character remains completely oblivious to the actions of the other in the other half of the frame, implying a mental distance despite their physical proximity. Hawks's frames present multiple pieces of information in complex harmony or counterpoint, asking us to watch and infer, allowing the data, rather than the characters, to tell us what the people mean.

Another of the cinema's great narrative powers which differs from those of the theater is its ability to play with our awareness that the visual world enclosed in a single shot continues spatially beyond the framed limits of the shot, even if and when we cannot see that continuity.[9] The cinema allows two kinds of continuity between on- and off-frame space. The first is visual. That Hawks is aware of the visual interplay of framed and off-frame space can be demonstrated quite simply by discussing his pratfalls in and out of the frame in the two comedies *Bringing Up Baby* and *Monkey Business*. How can one frame a pratfall, other than show someone standing up, filling the frame, and then falling down, occupying only its bottom portion? Well, these two comedies develop a whole lexicon of framing pratfalls: the pratfall that begins off-frame and ends with the figure's sliding into the frame from the left; the pratfall that begins on-frame and ends with the figure's falling out of the frame—either at its bottom, or one of its sides; the pratfall that begins on-frame and then, after a cut, ends with a sound effect off-frame.

Or consider the way that framing alone produces a delightful moment in *Twentieth Century*. As a sheriff waits at the Chicago train station to arrest Oscar Jaffe, swearing he would recognize him anywhere,

The most important piece of data in the frame is the unidentified hand on the far right.

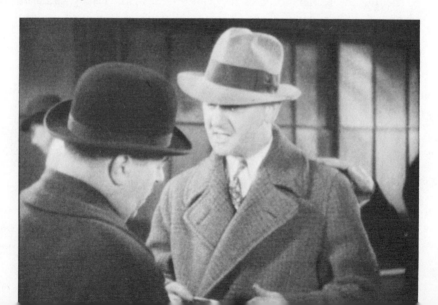

an unidentified hand slides into the frame from the right to tap the confident sheriff on the shoulder and ask for a light. Only a later cut reveals that the hand is attached to Jaffe himself in disguise. This slyly comic way of using the cinema frame is not merely a clever way to outwit a stupid but smugly confident character; it is a joke shared by Jaffe, the audience, and the storyteller, against the sheriff. The composition reveals that Hawks's use of the frame line parallels his use of the camera angle—to convey moral attitudes and narrative information. This Jaffe is a pretty clever strategist who should never be underestimated— much cleverer than the more respectable sheriff. Hawks's use of the frame itself becomes a vote for cleverness rather than respectability.

Even more complex is Hawks's use of off-frame sound—the second way of extending the frame beyond itself. In *Scarface,* for example, we see very few people who are horrified or injured by the gangsters' murderous battles; but we perpetually hear their shrieks, cries, and moans in response to the on-screen violence. Keeping these sounds off-frame allows Hawks to show that the gangster world indeed exists within the normal, social world and has an impact on that world; but, simultaneously, if we become too concerned about this normal world we could not savor (indeed strangely enjoy) the savagery of the gangster world. In *Scarface,* these off-frame sounds place the gangster world simultaneously within the normal world and outside it. The film's narrative could have no impact (since its goal is the paradoxically simultaneous condemnation and experiencing of this gangster world) without its counterpoint of on-frame visuals and off-frame shrieks. Similarly, the frame of *Only Angels Have Wings* is perpetually invaded by the sounds of airplane motors, usually revving up for the next flight that will take the flier away from the communal, social, relaxing world of conversation with others to his private world of dangerous solo flight. The counterpoint of on-frame society and off-frame motor is itself a metaphor for the film's contrast of communal and solitary human experience.

The usual way to talk about this contrapuntal contrast of sound and image is to claim that by using off-frame sound the filmmaker respects the fundamental visual integrity of the image and the cinema, using sound to supplement the visual image rather than to compete with it or repeat it. But Hawks's use of the frame as a visual or sonic barrier owes its obligation not to the integrity of cinema but to the needs of his narratives. Establishing multiple pieces of narrative information simultaneously is both economical and subtle (both of which qualities are virtues of any art).

The same approach to off-frame sound or space (or sound as space) determines Hawks's attitude toward his fourth tool of cinematic narrative: dialogue. Hawks did not become an important, or even very interesting, director until *The Dawn Patrol* and synchronized speech. The two silent Hawks films I have seen—*Fig Leaves* (1926) and *A Girl in Every Port* (1928)—are, with the exception of a few touches, thoroughly unremarkable films. Hawks himself admits that "I don't think that I learned what to do at that particular time,"[10] and he mentions several of his silent films in satirically deprecating terms (for example, about *Fazil* [1928]: "Charlie Farrell played a sheik, now you can imagine how lousy that was.").[11] In *The Dawn Patrol* Hawks used dialogue that, in contrast to the florid ranting of most early dialogue films (Hawks calls it acting in the "Riverboat" style), seemed restrained, natural, underplayed, understated. Perhaps more than any other single element, it is the spareness of Hawks's dialogue that gives his world its aroma, flavor, and texture. "Hemingway calls it oblique and I call it three-cushion."[12] To take Hawks's billiard analogy, the talk does not move directly at its target but bounces in several directions at several angles before reaching its mark.

The fact that Hawks's dialogue is so spare, so indirect, that it implies much more than it says, may again seem related to an abstract notion of cinematic virtue that can be expressed quantitatively—the less dialogue (and the more picture) the better. Hawks's use of dialogue owes its allegiance not to cinematic virtue but to the view of humans and human psychology that underlies his narratives. Hawks's characters don't tell everything they know. First, because it is dangerous or foolish to tell everything you know. "The men I like are not very talkative."[13] For Hawks, talk is cheap and actions speak louder than words—whether in personal or professional life. Second, because they aren't always sure what it is they know. That is why they must undergo the process of the narrative—to make their discovery of what it is they know. And once they make this discovery, they attempt to communicate that knowledge to another, not by speaking about it but by performing some concrete, often oblique, action.

If Hawks lacks faith in the ability of talk to reveal thoughts and feelings, he has great faith in it as sound itself, as a kind of music. One reason that Hawks's central couples—Barrymore and Lombard, Grant and Russell, Bogart and Bacall—belong together, regardless of what they say, is because their voices—as musical instruments—sing so well together. The rhythms of Hawks's dialogue scenes—the dizzying speed of the comedies, the laconic saunter of the westerns, the brittle crackle of the gangster and detective films—reveal the power of his ear for dialogue. Hawks admits that sections of *Twentieth Century* were so fast he couldn't understand them, so he depended on his sound man to inform him if all the words were intelligible. For *His Girl Friday* he deliberately attached brief verbal tags, before and after each articulate speech, so the actors could step on each other's lines, overlap one another, thereby increasing the dialogue's pace without destroying its intelligibility. But in *Only Angels Have Wings,* a climactic emotional scene between Bonnie Lee (Jean Arthur) and Sparks (Victor Killian), in which she wonders if Geoff (Cary Grant) really wants her to stay, is played entirely in a whisper, although there is no one else in the room to overhear them. The whispering makes musical sense and psychological sense—a delicate muting of sound in sympathy with Geoff's emotional sorrow for Kid (Thomas Mitchell), the best friend who has just been killed. But an opposite musical mood and psychology underlie the principle of dialogue for Tess Millay (Joanne Dru) in *Red River,* from whom words tumble in a torrent, a character who starts babbling every time she gets excited or frightened. The fact that she is babbling—as a means to release her energy—is far more important in conveying her meaning than any of the specific words she babbles.

The fifth and final cinematic tool Hawks uses to tell stories derives from the fact that filmed images are photographs of physical objects, and those concrete objects can accomplish many of the tasks of narration which verbal speeches or descriptions must accomplish in plays and prose fiction. Cleverly used, these external surfaces can reveal internal sensations, which tend to be the essential stuff of narratives of discovery, like those of Howard Hawks. These photographic objects become especially important in narratives in which the communicative power of speech is either suppressed (as in silent comedy) or undermined (as in Hawks films). And Hawks was a great student and admirer of the silent comedies. Those photographic objects can be of two kinds—inanimate and animate.

In thinking of a prototypically "cinematic" use of a material object,

I am reminded of the clock that the doctor, Chebutykin, holds while he speaks in the last act of Chekhov's *Three Sisters*. As Chebutykin attempts to talk about the waste of his life and talent, he plays with this antique clock, the gift of his dead mistress, which then falls out of his hand (or does he drop it deliberately?) and smashes to bits. Or in the same play, during the confessional "fire scene" when various characters attempt to confess their hopes, longings, and frustrations, their listeners all retreat behind a screen so they cannot be seen, hoping that this ruse of invisibility will also make the confessions, which pain them to hear, inaudible. Chekhov used such physical objects because he believed that they could express more feeling more subtly and with greater fidelity to the ways human beings with these psychological and emotional problems actually express these problems, than could explicit speeches. There may be other ways to use objects on the stage and in the cinema, but there is no question that Hawks's use of objects is very much in this Chekhovian tradition. The deliberate reduction of an explicitly communicative verbal text (in Chekhov and in Hawks) places an inevitable burden on the artist's use and the characters' handling of physical objects as the means to reveal the emotional subtext.

Hawks's films are full of objects—bracelets, hatpins, necklaces, coins, hats, coats, umbrellas, eyeglasses, boutonnieres—that mutely "say" what a character does not say simply by the character's way of holding, using, addressing, or passing such objects. The exchange and lighting of cigarettes is one of the most consistent Hawks gestures for communicating states of human closeness or distance, and the entire narrative of *Only Angels Have Wings* can be comprehended in the subtextual terms of who's lighting a cigarette for whom and when and why. Although the scripts by Jules Furthman tend to put the heaviest communicative burden on these exchanges of light and cigarettes, most Hawks films contain at least one crucial piece of cigarette business (including the disguised Oscar Jaffe's comic asking for a light from the sheriff). Cigarettes are important in Hawks not because they are a part of his "signature," a means merely of distinguishing his work, but because they perform the essential kinds of narrative functions that objects must perform in stories like those he tells—"saying" the important things that the characters he wants to tell about, the characters he likes, will not and would not say.

But it is in his finding animate photographic objects—movie stars—

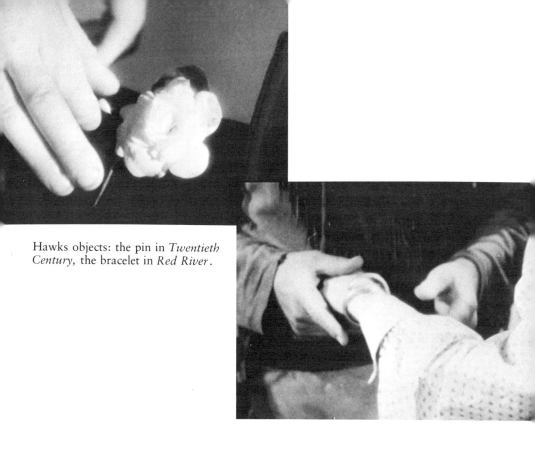

Hawks objects: the pin in *Twentieth Century*, the bracelet in *Red River*.

to embody those characters that Hawks makes his most important and perceptive narrative choice for the cinema. The list of Hawks's discoveries is a long one: Lombard, Muni, Clift, Bacall, and so forth. But it is significant that even many established stars who worked for Hawks played roles for him quite unlike any they had played before; but once they had played that role, it became an essential and assumed characteristic of that star from then on. Cary Grant had never played a character quite as doltish and flustered, unsuave and unmasculine as he did in *Bringing Up Baby*. Katharine Hepburn had never played a character as spontaneously babbling and dizzy as she played in that same film. Rosalind Russell had never played a character as aggressively brainy as she did in *His Girl Friday* (her previous comedy role, in *The Women*, was funny, dizzy, and gossipy but not solid, strong, and smart). And John Wayne had never played the character—rock-solid, firm, slightly over the hill, unbending in his stated commitments and intentions, using that inflexibility to mask his vulnerability and insecurity—that he played

51

in *Red River*. Once he had played it, he not only played it again in dozens of films, but that persona also came to represent such a powerful cultural archetype that it served for many as a symbol, if not the cause, of the American attitude that produced the Viet Nam War. True, Hawks used many stars—Barrymore and Bogart, for example—who brought their familiar personas with them. And when Hawks used Wayne, or Grant, or Bacall a second (or third, or fourth) time he capitalized on traits that they had already sketched together.

This kind of discussion may seem to have more to do with Hollywood glamor, press agentry, and fan magazines than the Art of Cinema, but this wedding of star persona and fictional character is one of the unique potential characteristics of the cinema as a narrative medium. As the art historian, Erwin Panofsky, pointed out in his famous essay on cinema theory, "[film] characters have no aesthetic existence outside the actors."

> Othello or Nora are definite, substantial figures created by the playwright. They can be played well or badly, and they can be "interpreted" in one way or another; but they most definitely exist, no matter who plays them or even whether they are played at all. The character in a film, however, lives and dies with the actor.[14]

Panofsky means that on the stage we would be able to make a meaningful distinction between say, Laurence Olivier and Hamlet, but in a film Humphrey Bogart *is* Philip Marlowe (or is it Marlowe who is Bogart?). Although one can make another film in which Elliot Gould or Robert Mitchum or James Garner is Philip Marlowe, that character is no more the same Marlowe than Cocteau's Oedipus in *The Infernal Machine* is the same as Sophocles'. The star's personality—either well-known from previous exposure or suddenly revealed to and discovered by an audience as a result of the camera's gaze—fuses with the scripted traits of the role which that personality embodies in that particular film. This complex fusion is one of the essential ways that the cinema creates deep, rich, consistent, credible human portraits—the ultimately desired goal for characters in any narrative medium. For this reason, Cavell believes that such human photographic objects should quite properly be called "stars," beings whose only functions are to be and to be gazed upon, rather than "actors," people who actively work to impersonate others.[15]

Howard Hawks was quite aware that great movie stars do not pretend to be others; they succeed at being completely themselves as an other. He is quite candid in his preferring personalities to actors.

> I usually like to work with a personality rather than an actor.[16]

> It's much better to be a personality and do it well. For instance, if I go home to work out a scene for Cary Grant, I know what he's gonna do.[17]

> One suggestion that I have in regard to Bacall is that I really believe the way to get the best out of her is not to ask her to do anything past her limitations. I'd much rather have her do less and do it well than to try and give her something she's not capable of doing.[18]

What does it mean to "work out a scene for Cary Grant"? Certainly to find something that Cary Grant can do well, and interestingly, and believably. But also, certainly, something that Cary Grant can do in the guise of a particular character in a particular scene of a particular story that will serve to illuminate that character and that story. It is Grant-Huxley or Grant-Geoff or Grant-Rochard or Grant-Fulton for whom Hawks is "working out a scene." Hawks is dependent on the personalities of his actors not only to enliven and reveal the characters they impersonate but also to propel the narratives in which those characters function. The conclusions of at least three of Hawks's greatest films— *His Girl Friday, To Have and Have Not,* and *The Big Sleep*—were worked out on the set. As Lauren Bacall observed in Hawks's obituary, "He gave actors their head and then used the reality of those situations."[19] The evocations, vibrations, and interrelations of the stars produced a higher narrative logic and wisdom, allowing Hawks to throw out some fifty pages of each original script as a result.[20]

In a filmed narrative, the actors are often not so much performers or interpreters of a character (as they are on the stage) but the characters themselves. The characteristics of the human figure do not (or do not necessarily) preexist and therefore predetermine any specific embodiment of that figure. The existence of the physical being precedes and determines the traits that the human figures will demonstrate in the story. The movie star does not merely embody a character in a text; the great movie star *is* a text. If Hawks had used Dick Powell or Robert Montgomery or Robert Mitchum as Marlowe in *The Big Sleep,* if he had used Randolph Scott or Joel McCrea or Gary Cooper as Dunson in *Red River,* we would not simply have a new interpretation of Marlowe or Dunson. We would have a different Marlowe and Dunson, and, therefore, we would have a different *Big Sleep* and *Red River.* No director-producer realized better than Hawks that the familiarity and the absolute believability of a star's personality (it is very easy to believe that Cary Grant is Cary Grant and John Wayne is John Wayne—and for good reason) contributed to the depth and credibility of the fictional character in a filmed story.

> When he'd hear the actors playing those roles, reading those lines, if they didn't sound correct to him, he would say, "Come on, let's straighten this out." He would try to word the same meanings in the lines as the actor's own vernacular. . . . To get the words to fit the actor rather than the actor to fit the words.[21]

Once Hawks had effected the perfect synthesis of star personality and fictional character he could (and would) eliminate or revise whole passages and events in the written script, so that the story that resulted remained true to the character-personality as well as to its original structural logic. Character inevitably produces credibility in stories, and for Hawks these credible star personalities were the characters.

Hawks's method of making cinema stories had two distinct processes—preparing the script for shooting and making changes on it during shooting as it grew organically into a film. In preparing the script he took special care to build the beginning sections of the story very solidly. The early sections of a Hawks film make the fewest alterations in its written script. When reading any script for a Hawks film—even the one marked "final shooting script"—one repeatedly observes the film's scripted story evaporate as the narrative progresses, dissolving into that other fuller and richer story which the film became. Hawks constantly reworked his ideas, both on the set and at home, as his filmed narration took shape, until he reached a narrative conclusion that frequently bore no relationship at all to the one in the script with which he began shooting. Hawks's procedure is a reminder that there is no single filmscript against which the finished film story can be measured; the filmscript itself undergoes several drafts, and even the "final" one is amended daily on the set—particularly by the kind of director who wants to tell his own story rather than decorate someone else's.

After approving the script that he will take with him to the set, Hawks got a strong feeling for the narrative's major sections by writing the titles and essential action of each of the script's sequences on index cards, tacking those cards to his office wall, and moving them around to examine how they might best fit and flow.[22] (It is interesting that a director like Hitchcock, who began as a designer, storyboards his films—sketches the look of shots on cards—while a director like Hawks, who began in a story department, writes the narrative sequences down.) Hawks then shot the entire film, usually in narrative sequence—each scene as it furthered the progress, flow, and logic of the narrative.[23] This shooting strategy was decidedly at variance with the Hollywood norm of shooting scenes according to their locations, rather than their narrative logic, for purposes of financial economy. By the time Hawks reached the end of a story, he had developed the narrative means— particularly his sense of the sequences, the actors, the characters, and the interrelation of all three—to have improved (and tightened) the shooting script, which he rewrote daily, allowing the narrative consequences to grow organically out of the process that produced them. Hawks working out a film narrative in practice was a bit like a logician working out a theorem or a composer working out the variations on a theme: he solidly established his givens, the premises, at the beginning, followed their consequences as they elaborated themselves, and then brought them to a conclusion when they had indicated where they could and must go. The one variable that Hawks could not know about before he began filming was exactly how each of the human participants would shape the evolving pattern and, even more important, what impact those participants would have on one another and, therefore, on the pattern.

> You sit in a room and you write the best scene you can, and it has an ending, and it has a place in the story, and you go out to film it, and everything changes.[24]

Hawks used his human participants—these personalities as characters and these characters as personalities—to slap the final breath of life into his stories.

Elegant and symmetrical narrative construction, depth of character, perceptive psychology, moral discovery, the psychologizing of cinema space, camera angles and framing that both reveal and suppress information, dialogue that frequently communicates more by its sound than its sense, inanimate objects that "speak" more clearly than people, and characters who are embodied by and inseparable from the personalities who embody them are the inextricable strands of Hawks's cinematic aims and cinematic attainments—stories in cinema and cinema in stories.

4

Stories and Values

I think that if they would do more of that type of relationship [Bogart-Bacall] they would do better with it, because it didn't come out and show what they were doing all the time.[1]

That's just a form of speech, Women's Lib. The woman that you admire is the one who, for years, has taken the liberties and done the things without doing a lot of talking. I hate these people who go around spouting—they're no good unless they can talk about the things they do. For instance, I can't stand Jane Fonda—I wouldn't want to get anywhere near her. . . . She talks too much, and about stuff she doesn't know about.[2]

To FOLLOW any story the reader-viewer-listener must know where to place his or her emotional and moral sympathies. We must be led to desire the achievement of certain results and the frustration of others. The storyteller can borrow the most familiar and prevalent moral notions of the culture in which and to which he tells his story to control our understanding of it through our placing of moral sympathies (for example, "thou shalt not kill"). But the storyteller whose moral system completely derives from the most common prevailing cultural values will never seem a complex or original thinker. His story's moral system will be so completely conventional, familiar, and unremarkable—indeed so obvious—that, ironically, the system will seem invisible. The story will appear to lack any moral system, the storyteller to lack any moral sense whatever. The other kind of storyteller, who provides his own personal terms of moral definition within the story, terms which extend, examine, or subvert the most commonly accepted values within the culture, is the storyteller who will also seem a "thinker," searching for personal and complicated definitions of meaning and value rather than accepting the most general and simple ones that the culture as a whole supports in order to remain a culture. The complexity of a story is at least partially dependent on the complexities of its moral system and definitions.

When Nadine Groot (Walter Brennan) tells Thomas Dunson (John Wayne) at a crucial turning point of *Red River,* "You was wrong, Mr. Dunson," the viewer must have received enough information from the storyteller to know whether Dunson was wrong or not—and exactly how or why that wrongness matters. The balanced disinterest of Groot in the story (he is one of those choric Hawks outsiders, the friend who deliberately indicates the direction of our sympathies), is one of the storyteller's means of supporting the moral validity of the character's assertion. Hawks's careful shaping of the incidents that precede Groot's conclusion also supports that conclusion; Hawks structures the action as three events which increasingly depict Dunson's growing harshness, irrationality, and imbalance. And our sympathies for Matthew (Montgomery Clift), the man who will correct the wrongness of Dunson, who will succeed Dunson as the group's leader, also support Groot's generalization. In a Platonic sense, the beauty of Matthew-Clift's eyes and face, the ease and grace of his casually comfortable body, become moral traits in the film. Matthew becomes the moral, physical, and emotional opposite of Dunson's wrongness, supporting Groot's judgment by Clift's very physical being. Because motion pictures are pictures—a recording of physical surfaces—the physical characteristics of the people who embody the characters become moral characteristics as well. The storyteller (if he has the power to select those physical presences—as Hawks did) deliberately uses those physical presences to control our moral awareness and sympathies.

But the fact that John Wayne is the physical presence who embodies the Mr. Dunson who "was wrong" complicates our moral sense of that wrongness in a way that the storyteller absolutely depends on to make his story come out the way he wants. In knowing that Dunson is wrong at this specific moment, we also know that Dunson is not essentially and irremediably wrong at the core. There is something essentially right about John Wayne (again the storyteller's dependence on the *moral* evocations of a star's presence), and what is right about Wayne is right about Dunson when Dunson is right. In film narrative, simply being a movie star is in itself a moral quality which plays a role in the storyteller's directing our moral sympathies. As the two morally right stars (both of whom have been morally wrong as characters at specific moments in the film) move steadily toward facing each other in mortal combat at the narrative's climax, the storyteller deliberately manipulates an extremely complex conflict within our moral sympathies: "We were walking a tightrope in telling a story like that. Are you still going to like Wayne or not?"[3] We fear that one of these morally right stars must be sacrificed because of the one erring moment of his character (this is a very painful fear). We earnestly hope that this sacrifice can be avoided (although we cannot see how) because we have felt the moral and emotional rightness which the storyteller has carefully defined in the union, the "marriage" of Dunson-Matthew and Wayne-Clift. The narrative's conclusion is able to preserve this "marriage," to avoid the painful killing, precisely because of the moral strengths embedded in the two stars and (as the specific discussion of *Red River* will demonstrate) the moral issues embedded in the film's narrative structure from its very beginning.

Our ability to respond to any single story depends on our being able to follow the moral path which the storyteller has charted. The task of attempting to understand an author's (or *auteur*'s) moral vision in general, however, can only be accomplished by comparing the moral system which the storyteller develops in one narrative with the moral system which the storyteller develops in others by that same author. Is the storyteller of *Red River*, for example, related to the storyteller of *The Big Sleep* or *Bringing Up Baby*? Is there some clear relationship between the moral systems required to tell stories that are so wildly different on their surfaces? Does each of these stories expand our knowledge of the storyteller for each individual tale, so that the result of "reading" all the tales is our knowledge of the composite storyteller that emerges from all of them together? Can we, in the end, understand how "Hawks" (not Hawks the man in the world but "Hawks" the composite storyteller who makes the moral distinctions within the stories themselves) sees the world and its values? The composite storyteller of any great author's many tales is larger, richer, and more complex than the single storyteller of any single tale.

Let me begin this probing of the dimensions of "Hawks," the storyteller of all Howard Hawks films, with that spiritual union of Thomas Dunson and Matthew Garth in *Red River*. This union is built on the apparent, superficial oppositeness of the couple and their underlying spiritual unity and complementarity. On the surface, Dunson is hard, strong, tough, and "male" while Matthew is soft, sweet, loose, and "female." Underneath the surface, both men are equally good at what they do. It is impossible to determine which is quicker on the draw or steadier of aim. Without either of them the task that they accomplish in partnership could not and would not have been achieved. Without Dunson there would have been no immense herd of cattle and no Red River D Ranch; without Matthew there may as well have been no herd and no ranch, for his driving that herd to Abilene guarantees the fertility and perpetuation of that ranch. The two apparently opposite men extend one another's capabilities beyond the limitations of either one of them alone.

The first general moral position which the Dunson-Matthew (and Wayne-Clift) union implies is that mere physical surfaces and appearances in no way indicate a man's spiritual worth and capabilities (an interesting value for movies, which are so dependent on physical surfaces to convey internal states). The contrast and complementarity of the hard Dunson-Wayne and soft Matthew-Clift can be traced to Hawks's first sound film, *The Dawn Patrol,* and the spiritual unity of the harder, tougher Courtney (Richard Barthelmess) with the sweeter, prettier Scott (Douglas Fairbanks, Jr.); despite their differences of physical appearance they are both close friends, equally good fliers, and equally resolute in the face of death. They work together better than they do apart. The sweeter, prettier, younger Eddie Greer (Eric Linden) contrasts physically with his harder, tougher, older brother Joe (James Cagney) in *The Crowd Roars,* but they both drive races equally well—and at the end of the narrative they drive a race together as extensions of one another. The sweeter, more apparently effete British sailors (Robert Young and Franchot Tone) contrast physically with the tougher, apparently stronger American flier (Gary Cooper) in *Today We Live,* but the narrative demonstrates that they are all equally competent and courageous, and to perform the film's climactic bombing, all three work together. The sweet and pretty Colorado (Ricky Nelson) in *Rio Bravo,* is, like Matthew Garth, as good with a gun as the tougher-looking John T. Chance, played by John Wayne. The tough Chance is even tougher to defeat with the pretty Colorado by his side.*

---

* I realize that "pretty" is a very strange adjective to apply to male attractiveness, but in searching for an alternative I discovered that there was no other word in our culture to apply to such males. "Handsome" implies a more mature

With this superficial contrast of hard and soft males, Hawks plays deliberately with cultural stereotypes of beauty (particularly male beauty). Beautiful males are somehow not supposed to be masculine males, while Hawks reveals that their masculine competence is irrelevant to their physical beauty. The manipulation of this cultural stereotype of masculinity leads directly to a parallel manipulation in Hawks's comedies and the Bogart-Bacall films. Having demonstrated the worthlessness of superficial definitions of maleness in the adventure films, the storyteller can demonstrate the worthlessness of superficial definitions of femaleness in the comic and Bogart-Bacall films. Lily Garland (*Twentieth Century*), Susan Vance (*Bringing Up Baby*), "Slim" (*To Have and Have Not*), and Vivian Rutledge (*The Big Sleep*) all comment (implicitly, of course) on the cultural stereotyping that women are somehow less female if they are smart, shrewd, talented, and tough. They talk as well as the men in their stories, walk as well, work together with them, compete as equals, complete as pals. This reversal of sexual stereotyping becomes explicit in *His Girl Friday* and *I Was a Male War Bride*, in which a woman wears the literal or figurative pants, the male might wear a dress, and the spiritual oneness of the male-female couple (like the "male-female" couples of *Red River* or *The Dawn Patrol*) is far more important and essential than their physical, sexual differences. That oneness allows them to get a difficult job done—done well and done together.

The ironic culmination of these stories built on the reversals of sex-

---

and more rugged kind of male beauty, like the other, older male in each of these Hawks pairings. The younger male's good looks are attributable both to very smooth, regular features and extreme youthfulness—in effect, a pretty boy (as in "Pretty Boy" Floyd). Hawks was unable to complete his "Billy the Kid" movie, *The Outlaw*, a most explicit study of a tough male who became a legend because he was pretty. Although Hawks used this kind of man for the entirety of his career, pretty boys became especially popular in American films of the 1950s with such icons as Troy Donahue, Tab Hunter, Edd "Kookie" Byrnes, Ricky Nelson, Dwayne Hickman, and Frankie Avalon. While Hawks gives this kind of man a dignity by allowing him to be good at something other than looking pretty, most of the pretty boys of the 1950s were good for nothing (including acting) except to be observed as beautiful objects. The linguistic difficulty of describing such men reveals that Hawks's use of them was as culturally surprising as was his use of the strong, shrewd woman. See note 17 on page 380.

ual stereotyping is *Gentlemen Prefer Blondes,* in which the two women, journeying aboard ship across the seas, play precisely the same sexual games with men that the two male sailor-buddies play with women in Hawks's silent *A Girl in Every Port:* "We pulled a switch by taking two girls who went out looking for men to amuse them: a perfectly modern story."[4] The two "girls" themselves (Jane Russell and Marilyn Monroe) demonstrate a likeness in difference and a difference in likeness which reveals the storyteller's subtle psychological shading. The major alteration which Hawks's film made in this stage musical was building its story around these two female poles, while the stage version revolves around the single center of Lorelei Lee. And one of Hawks's two poles is not even blonde—although Jane Russell impersonates a blonde in general and Marilyn Monroe in particular near the end of the film. The two poles, Russell and Monroe are superficially different physically (one dark, the other blonde) but essentially one spiritually (like Wayne and Clift in *Red River*). Hawks emphasizes both their superficial differences with color (Russell's costumes tend toward black or yellow, while Monroe's toward lavender or red) and their similarities with color (deserted in Paris, both women wear sailorish navy-blue dresses with white collars, although Monroe wears white gloves while Russell is barehanded with bright red nail polish). Such subtle similarities/differences of costume and color are Hawks's deliberate (and typically subtle) physical symbols of spiritual qualities.

Hawks also conveys the essential spiritual similarity of the two women with his camera, which balances them perfectly in every frame they share; they occupy symmetrical halves of the frame, sitting still or stealthily moving (underscored by the familiar movement of Hawks's tracking camera) in perfectly framed unison. The perfect compositional symmetry implies an absolute spiritual symmetry. True enough, the perfect balancing of the two stars in Hawks's frames may well have originated in their contracts, which demanded that Hawks balance their screen time. Hawks's symmetrical frames certainly make sure that each gets no more exposure than the other. But Hawks was able to turn this legal necessity into a narrative virtue. He succeeds not just in balancing their contracts, but in equating the two women's spirits with his balanced frames.

The storyteller's collapsing of superficial stereotypic sexual differentiations between characters to reveal their underlying spiritual unity and complementarity is parallelled in other stories by the collapsing of other merely apparent physical differences. First, the storyteller frequently demonstrates that a man who might not be physically whole remains spiritually whole. Hawks builds several stories around men who have been crippled, characters who have lost a physical part of themselves to an injury which has not impaired or damaged their spiritual wholeness. Mike Mascarenhas (Edward G. Robinson) has lost a hand in *Tiger Shark;* Jim Deakins (Kirk Douglas) loses a finger in *The Big Sky,* Ned Arp (John Robert Crawford) loses a hand in *Red Line 7000.* None of these physical losses keeps these men from asserting their physical power or demonstrating their physical competence in their vocations. The bullet that has lodged near the spine of Cole Thornton (John Wayne again) in *El Dorado* and which paralyzes his gun-arm is the culmination of Hawks's depictions of physical handicaps and the victory of the human spirit over those handicaps. Thornton deliberately manipulates his enemy's stereotypic presumption—that the man with one arm is a helpless cripple—as a strategy in defeating him.

Growing out of the physical loss which is overcome by spiritual exertion are those stories in which the storyteller depicts a spiritual debilitation which takes physical form, but is then overcome by a greater determination and revival. The most obvious sign of apparent spiritual decay in Hawks films is drunkenness. Joe Greer's spiritual nadir in *The Crowd Roars* and Pancho Villa's in *Viva Villa!* both show them withdrawing from the world of men to inhabit the world of the bottle. Judy in *Only Angels Have Wings* has beaten a similar retreat. In both *Villa* and *Only Angels* a friend awakens the sodden drunk with an identical act—pouring a jug of baptismal water over the drunkard's head (a "slap" of water that parallels other friendly slaps in Hawks's films). Eddie, the rummy in *To Have and Have Not,* is also introduced with an awakening bucket of water; he was a good man once and is still a good man, if only because he uses others' presumptions of his drunken incompetence (as Cole Thornton uses those stereotypic presumptions in *El Dorado*) to outwit them. Dude (Dean Martin) of *Rio Bravo* has also become a rummy, a "borachon," and he, like Eddie, first uses his enemies' presumptions to catch them off guard, then conquers the need and the desire to drink altogether. J. P. Harrah (Robert Mitchum) in *El Dorado* fights a similar and eventually victorious battle of spiritual and physical redemption.

The storyteller of a Hawks film is dependent on a contrast between "is" and "seems," between the surface appearance and the underlying reality. This ironic and paradoxical contrast of outside (often dependent on the deliberate manipulation of some cultural stereotype) and inside leads directly to the storyteller's problem (and method of solving the problem) of revealing the differences between surface and essence. Films, by definition, depict physical visual surfaces; explicit verbal utterances (one of the advantages of the synchronized-sound film) are also surfaces which may or may not refer sincerely to the essence beneath. How can the storyteller convincingly reveal to other characters and to the viewer when a character's thoughts and feelings are really real? The storyteller's answer to this question is an ironic and paradoxical interplay of words and physical actions which also plays with cultural expectations and stereotypes.

Despite the cultural assumption that people should mean what they say, Hawks's stories are built on the existential premise that people mean what they *do*. Dunson (*Red River*) might say that he is going to kill Matthew, but he cannot kill anyone—much less his "son-wife"—in cold blood. Harry Morgan (*To Have and Have Not*) may say that his sympathies are minding his own business, but his sympathies will not allow him to sit by and watch Renard torture Eddie, his friend. Hildy Johnson (*His Girl Friday*) may say that she wants to be "a woman" but cannot tear herself away from the Press Room when Earl Williams tears himself out of jail. Lieutenant Gates and Henri Rochard (*Male War Bride*) may say that they cannot stand one another—but they work well and inseparably as a team. The two British sailors may speak effetely, in *Today We Live*, but they behave bravely every night in their tiny torpedo boat. "The language is confusing, but the actions are unmistakable," as one of Hawks's own characters, Hank Entwhistle, observes in *Monkey Business*.

One possible exception to this Hawks rule of doing rather than saying is *Barbary Coast*, in which the two most sympathetic moral citizens are talkers—the newspaperman Cobb (Frank Craven) and the poet James Carmichael (Joel McCrea). But the irony of this film is that the storyteller builds his tale on another cultural reversal—that talking is a kind of doing, speaking is an action (especially for a journalist or a poet). Louie Chimalis (Edward G. Robinson), the mobster who runs Old San Francisco, makes the presumptuous mistake of underestimating the power of speaking as a form of social and moral action. He appreciates the sounds of words ("I like the way he talks") without realizing the power of words to stir emotions and provoke actions.

The relationship of Hawks's characters to objects is an extension of their doing rather than saying. Many of his characters either are not consciously aware of their internal feelings—they simply feel without a self-conscious awareness of that emotion, as so many people do—or refuse to expose those feelings openly to every eye. These Hawks characters play very dead-pan poker, refusing to wear the heart on the sleeve. The storyteller, however, can reveal the heart to the viewer by the way the character handles the sleeve—as Hildy Johnson does in *His Girl Friday*. Either Hildy is able to put her coat on properly or she is not. Either Harry Morgan lights "Slim's" cigarette or he does not. Johnny Lovo in *Scarface* plays with a saltshaker and reveals something (to himself and to us) about his feelings; almost thirty years later, John T. Chance in *Rio Bravo* plays with a deck of cards unconsciously until it informs him (or he informs himself of what he did not consciously realize before) that someone at a poker table has been cheating. Guino (*Scarface*), Kid (*Only Angels*), and Canino (*Big Sleep*) flip coins, Lily Garland worships a hatpin, Dunson gives away a snake bracelet, and both Lorelei Lee and Princess Nellifer (Joan Collins in *Land of the Pharaohs*) covet a dazzlingly large and expensive piece of jewelry. The tossing of a coin in a spittoon is a sign of human contempt in both the silent *Underworld* (directed by Sternberg, but co-written by Hawks)[5] and in *Rio Bravo;* Tony Camonte announces the arrival of the new "president," Johnny Lovo, by tossing a spittoon through a glass door, while the poet of *Barbary Coast* is degraded by his job of polishing spittoons. And perhaps one of the most memorable Hawks objects for revealing and "saying" the unsayable can be seen in his very first sound film, *The Dawn Patrol*—a blackboard with a list of the fliers' names chalked upon it. The annihilation of one of those fliers is announced silently (to us and to the group) by merely erasing the line of chalked letters from the board.

The storyteller requires both the story's characters and his audience to make complex inferences about internal feelings from clear yet subtle pieces of physical data. Sounds are one kind of physical data, and Hawks characters and audiences must make inferences from such off-frame sounds as the buzz of airplane propellers (*The Dawn Patrol, Only An-*

gels), the hoot of train whistles (*Twentieth Century, Red River*), the crack of gunshots (*Scarface, Tiger Shark, Twentieth Century, Only Angels, The Big Sleep*), and the scraping of a metal coin in a metal spittoon (*Rio Bravo*). The inferential process from visual signs might be quite simple. From a row of bullet holes in a door we infer the presence of O'Hara's gang in *Scarface* and Eddie Mars's men in *The Big Sleep*. From drops of blood in both *Rio Bravo* and *Land of the Pharaohs,* Dude and Princess Nellifer infer the presence of a wounded man.

Or the inference can be quite complicated—for example, understanding the significance of a slap across the face. "Slim" and Harry have no difficulty "reading" the meaning of the Gestapo's contemptuous slaps in *To Have and Have Not,* but Eddie "reads" the meaning of Harry's slap only after stowing away on Harry's boat and finding himself entangled in a very dangerous job. In *Red River,* Matthew the boy cannot "read" the meaning of Dunson's slap, but he can as a man at the film's climax. Princess Nellifer "reads" the contemptuous and possessive assumptions of the Pharaoh's slap upon their first meeting. Although she returns the same verbal response to that slap as the boy Matthew, "Don't ever do that again," she never changes her "reading" of it, eventually taking revenge on the Pharaoh (as Harry takes revenge on the Gestapo) by causing his death. These bits of physical data are the most solid pieces of evidence that the storyteller provides his characters for "reading" one another and the most solid evidence for his viewers to "read" beneath the surface data along with them. By implication, the storyteller believes that such physical data are the only solid evidence that real human beings can use to "read" one another as well. For people, like characters, mean what they *do*. A Protestant director like Hawks puts his faith in action, while a Catholic director like Frank Capra puts his faith in public confession.

The storyteller supplements this physical action as data with another kind of action as data from which the viewer makes inferences. The overall pattern of the narrative's action, what the characters do—not from moment to moment but within the evolving pattern of the narrative structure as a whole—provokes another kind of "reading" from physical data. The symmetrical patterns of Hawks's stories, the actions that carefully and deliberately mirror one another, not only provide the narrative with its solid shape but also serve as a moral and psychological road map—concrete, external signs of both the characters' and storyteller's more abstract intentions. The recurrent slaps in *To Have and Have Not* and *Red River,* the recurrent calling out of numbers in *Only Angels Have Wings,* the recurrent use of the word "right" in *The Dawn Patrol* (signifying a character's acceptance of an unpleasant but unavoidable task or situation), the recurrent welcoming speech to each group of new recruits in *The Road to Glory,* the recurrent loss of a night's sleep in *I Was a Male War Bride*—each of these cyclical actions provides a systematic context for "reading" the significance and meaning of any single action.

Hawks's narrative constructions resemble the labyrinthine corridors of the tomb conceived by Vashtar, the enslaved architect, in *Land of the Pharaohs.* Once Vashtar sets the first stone of the mechanism in motion, it necessarily activates each of the other stones in turn, linked in an irreversible and unbreakable chain of logical succession. The machinelike perfection of the narrative structures is underscored by their circularity, in which the beginning leads not only irreversibly to the end (as with Vashtar's tomb) but the end leads back again to the beginning. *The Dawn Patrol, Barbary Coast, Today We Live, The Road to Glory, Twentieth Century, Bringing Up Baby, Red River, Hatari!* and many other Hawks films end in the same physical setting, or with the same physical action, or with the same thematic motif with which they began. These narrative machines, like Vashtar's tomb, suggest the existence both of an architect and of an architectural plan, which allows the meaning and function of any part of the structure to be "read" by its place and function in the whole. To make such a narrative machine is another way to mean by doing rather than by saying.

The storyteller's principles of psychology (that people reveal themselves in action, not words), of morality (that people must be judged by their actions, not their words), of character interaction (that characters "read" each other's actions, not their words), of audience participation (the viewer also "reads" the characters' actions, not their words), and of narrative construction (to imbed the story's values and significance in its system of actions, not its words) are all identical. The words of these dialogue films are significant only in that they are actions: physical sounds (Hawks's care to depict talking musically, as a kind of singing), elliptical and incomplete phrases (the ability of Hawks's characters to communicate not only through their words but around, over, and under the words as well). Talking becomes a deliberate strategy either to avoid, to provoke, or to expose (the exchange of words becomes a deliberate game for Oscar Jaffe and Lily Garland, Geoff and Bonnie, Walter and Hildy, "Slim" and Harry Morgan, Vivian and Marlowe). In *Barbary Coast,* Cobb the newspaperman and James the poet manufacture words; Potts, the professor in *Ball of Fire* (Gary Cooper), collects words; and Lorelei Lee (Marilyn Monroe) in *Gentlemen Prefer Blondes* fractures words. For the storyteller, words themselves are things, concrete objects, like all the other things in the world of his stories.

The general moral attitude which pervades this storyteller's world is a respect for the concrete, the tangible, and the specific, a distrust of the abstract, the vague, and the general. The stories expose several of our culture's familiar moral and psychological oppositions as either false or facile abstractions. It is perhaps in the nature of both our language and our culture to organize meaning paradigmatically; a word or a value can be known only in contrast with its opposite: male and female, adult and child, human and animal, and so forth. Although such polarities may be both linguistically and culturally necessary, Hawks exposes their artificiality by collapsing these abstract dichotomies into specific human actions which reveal that the tidy verbal oppositions are neither so tidy nor so valid as the existence of the words suggests.

The first of these is the clear opposition of the terms *male* and *female,* which Hawks's stories collapse by depicting male-ish females and female-ish males who still, despite their superficial characteristics, respond, feel, and act like males and females.

The second of these is the opposition of the terms *external* and *internal,* or body and spirit, which in Hawks's stories are complexly and subtly linked rather than simply and diametrically opposed. Hawks's dependence on the faces and bodies of movie stars to convey essential psychological and moral information is itself a sign of the link between the outsides and insides of human beings.

Third, there is the opposition of the terms *work* and *play,* which Hawks collapses by revealing that, for those who love their work (from gangsters to actors to newspapermen to detectives to cowhands to sheriffs to fliers to big-game hunters to race-car drivers), work is as much "fun" as play.

Fourth, there is the collapse of the terms *childhood* and *adulthood,* for those adults who play at work (as in the adventure films) or who work at play (as in the comedies) experience the naive and innocent joy of children.

Fifth, there is the opposition of the terms *human* and *animal,* for humans can act like animals and animals (from Baby the leopard in *Bringing Up Baby* to Baby the elephant in *Hatari!*) like humans.

Sixth, there is the opposition of the terms *words* and *deeds,* which Hawks collapses by showing that words are deeds and that deeds speak more clearly than words.

Seventh, there is the opposition of the terms *love* and *friendship,* which Hawks collapses by revealing that those who love can, should, and must be friends if their love is to mean anything at all, and those who are friends are also a kind of lovers.

The ultimate synthesis of love-friendship, work-play, speaking-doing, outside-inside is that those characters who find their spiritual complements are capable of being and doing more than they could alone. They are completed by their opposite who is not really opposite but one. Like the circular snake bracelet in *Red River,* these ultimate Hawks "marriages" produce a two in one that is one in two.

In the entire work of Howard Hawks there are no characters, no scenes, no lines of dialogue that explicitly articulate or advocate the synthesis of any of these seven abstract oppositions, no characters, no scenes, no lines of dialogue that explicitly attack these cultural and linguistic polarities as somehow abstractly invalid and inapplicable to the genuine, concrete, and specific interrelationships of human beings. But Hawks's stories, in their characters, their scenes, their shots, their structured actions, and their implicit use of dialogue surely attack our cultural confidence in these pure and simple polarities, suggesting a more complex and more vital series of shades of human sameness and difference that lie between these two clear poles. This moral attitude may or may not reflect the real beliefs of Howard Hawks, human being, but it surely reflects the beliefs of Howard Hawks, storyteller.

These large and general claims can only be substantiated by examining some of his specific stories.

5

Dangerous Professions:
Scarface and *Only Angels Have Wings*

Professionals are the only people I'm interested in. Amateurs I'm not interested in. Flying, driving races, anything like that—I'm interested in the guys who are good. I hate losers, and the ones who are not good are bound to be losers. So I just don't pay any attention to them.[1]

I make movies on subjects that interest me: That could be automobile racing, airplanes, a drama, or a comedy, but the best drama for me is the one which shows a man in danger. There is no action where there is no danger.[2]

ON THEIR SURFACES, Howard Hawks's *Scarface*, his second film of 1930, and *Only Angels Have Wings*, his last film to be released in the decade, have little to do with one another. The one is set in the reality of urban America—with its newspapers, police, and crime—the other in a campy, self-contained banana republic, sealed off from the rest of the real world by ocean liners, palm trees, and never-lifting fog. The one is peopled by brutal criminals whose business is extortion, theft, and murder, while the other is peopled by young fliers who are at least legitimately (if also rather romantically) employed. The one seems a world in which human relationships are merely matters of convenience, expediency, and power, while the other seems a richly emotional world of human feeling in which people work as hard as possible to hide their feelings. While the earlier film seems to contradict the very narrative pattern of psychological, emotional discovery that lies beneath every Hawks narrative, the other fulfills it perfectly. But that avoiding of a moral and emotional discovery in *Scarface* is merely apparent, for Tony Camonte makes an emotional discovery (that destroys rather than com-

71

pletes him), although he is incapable of discovering the full moral system which has generated these two films.

Both *Scarface* and *Only Angels* are built around the work of professionals, men who are committed to their jobs and good at them. Hawks suggests the subtle parallels between the two vocations of gangstering and flying with the geographic fact that the private office of the boss —whether the gangster boss or the fliers' boss—is to the far right of the room where the other "boys" or men hang out. In Hawks's films, the boss's office (in *The Dawn Patrol*, in *His Girl Friday*) is usually on the far right of the public room which contains the other members of the films' vocational societies. Although both bosses, Geoff and Tony, are devoted to their work, the very work to which Tony Camonte is devoted makes it impossible for him to fulfill another kind of human need. This difference leads Robin Wood to classify *Scarface* with Hawks's comedies of "social irresponsibility" rather than with the dramas.[3] But like Geoff Carter in *Only Angels Have Wings* (and like Howard Hawks himself), Tony Camonte is a man who believes in his work, who defines his life as his work, and whose life becomes meaningful only in and through his work. Unlike flying the mails, the work of a gangster contradicts another value in Hawks's films—the need for a man to complete himself in love and friendship with another, a completion that then refuels and enlivens his appetite for work and his ability to work. Tony Camonte becomes a kind of Hawksian freak (like Thomas Dunson later in *Red River*), embodying only one side of the commitment to a human vocation (the side that stresses the vocation and ignores the human).

Scarface was Hawks's favorite film;[4] it is not difficult to see why. It was the film in which he first hit his full creative stride. Despite the success of the previous *The Dawn Patrol,* that film is much flatter, more stilted, less exuberant than the film that immediately followed it. *Scarface* seems packed with those qualities that best exemplify the work of Howard Hawks—surprising psychology, elegant structure, superb performances, the counterpoint of violent action and savage comedy, of perceptively revealing visual imagery and crackling talk—and seethes with the energy and "fun" of its making. Long withdrawn from circulation by its copyright owner, Howard Hughes, for years the film could only be seen abroad or in private screenings of pirated prints. *Scarface* has returned to public circulation with the death of Hughes, and the existence of an authorized copy is a testament to Hawks's love for it: he personally preserved its original negative (the only film of his he so carefully guarded).

Despite Hawks's understandable affection for the film, *Scarface* is a shadow of what it might have been. It is one of the few—perhaps the only—Hawks film whose script offers more interesting possibilities than the finished film was able to develop. Almost every other Hawks film goes far beyond and digs far beneath the blueprint sketched by its script. But the script of *Scarface* contains scenes and suggestions that the film simply could not make; and the film—particularly its added didactic scene that banally lays the social responsibility for eradicating the gangster evil on the American voter, and its butchered ending—contains elements that the script did not suggest (and that Hawks did not shoot).[5]

The cover page of the *Scarface* script attributes its authorship to one Seton I. Miller; this name (like the name for the author of *The Dawn Patrol*) was a cover: for Hawks and Ben Hecht, who wrote the script in eleven days (based on a preliminary draft by Miller, W. R. Burnett, and John Lee Mahin).[6] The title card of the film uses a similar ruse—the claim that the film was based on a novel by Armitage Trail. But *Scarface* bears few traces or scars of that source. This attribution, like the official title of the film—*Scarface: The Shame of a Nation*—was merely a public-relations tactic to make a highly controversial film seem more respectably literary. Hawks and Hecht, created this script in the same spirit of "fun" that shines through the film.

> When Hecht . . . and I used to work on a script, we'd sit in a room and we'd work for two hours and then we'd play back-gammon for an hour. Then we'd start again and one of us would be one character and one would be another character. We'd read our lines of dialogue and the whole idea was to try and stump the other people, to see if they could think of something crazier than you could. And that is the kind of dialogue we used, and the kind that was fun.[7]

Scarface is truly "crazier" than the more conventional and familiar films in the gangster cycle that followed it—Mervyn LeRoy's *Little Caesar* and William Wellman's *Public Enemy*. For Hawks, Hecht, and company the gangster life could be both "fun" and funny. Tony Camonte is no "Caesar," no tyrant like Rico; he doesn't command by threat and threaten by command. A major source of Rico's power is his snarling voice (that voice which is a major source of Edward G. Robinson's power as well). But Tony, like most Hawks men, talks very little. When he does talk, it is likely to be an "oblique," "three-cushion" joke rather than a direct verbal and vocal attack. He doesn't snarl, he quips. As opposed to the sociological emphasis of *Public Enemy,* which examines the poverty and unemployment that produce public enemies rather than public defenders, Hawks-Hecht's gangster comes from no clearly defined sociological background at all; we first meet him fully sprung. He does not come to be a gangster; he already is. And while Wellman's film defines gangsterism as an aberration, in opposition to the mainstream of American social and moral life, *Scarface* defines gangsterism as one current in that very mainstream.

The original script of *Scarface* sets the aberrant gangster world of Tony Camonte even more firmly within the American mainstream than the film the Hollywood censors finally allowed Howard Hawks to make. A character in the script named Benson, the State Attorney (state unnamed, but Illinois implied), is on the take. He engages in private and friendly conversations with both gangsters—Johnny Lovo and Tony Camonte—but he proclaims in his public campaign speeches: "The gangs must go. Prohibition must be enforced." No such hypocritical character, speeches, or scenes exist in the film. The character of Tony's and Cesca's mother differs radically in the script from her film embodiment, a prototypically immigrant mother who spends her time wrapped in a "colorful" peasant's shawl, stirring the spaghetti on the stove, making pious remarks about the brutality of her son and the evil of his money. In the original script she is quite content to receive and enjoy the money Tony makes. She becomes his silent accomplice by taking no moral stand against his activities at all, merely enjoying the fruits of his brutal labors. She even sends her son vacationing in Florida the telegram that summons him to commit the final crime that leads to the death of both her children. There is a major (and ironically comic) scene in Florida with Tony and his moll, Poppy. As Tony fishes aboard his yacht, he serves as host for a large group of society swells and the intellectual elite—particularly a lady novelist who writes dirty books. These proper members of respectable society find the murderous gangster a perfectly pleasant host and an intriguingly interesting personality. These scripted motifs make it quite clear that gangsters and their brutal world exist because they are in fact thoroughly accepted by the very moral, political, and cultural life of modern America, which deplores them only in theory.

Finally, there is the defiant existential assertion of the script's ending which the film's compromised conclusion completely subverts. While Tony Camonte displays an obligatorily whining cowardice and impotence in the film—obviously developed to undermine the myth of the gangster's courage and power—his death in the film's script is a mammoth act of existential assertion in the face of impossible odds and inevitable defeat. The battle he fights single-handedly from his metal-shuttered lair rages for several paragraphs, ending not just with tear gas (as it does in the film) but with the entire building ablaze and ablasted. As Tony stalks out of his lair, down his secret stairway, his body receives what seem to be hundreds of rounds of bullets from police machine guns—and yet he continues to walk (like the impregnable vegetable monster in *The Thing,* the film Hawks produced twenty years later), refusing to fall. Tony stalks toward his private nemesis, the police officer Guarino—on whose badge Tony struck the match to light his cigarette early in the film. Tony raises his pistol to Guarino's face and fires at it point blank. But the gun has no bullets. It merely makes an empty click. Then Guarino raises his own gun, fires point blank at Tony, and the gangster falls at the policeman's feet. But even as he falls, Tony continues to pull repeatedly at the trigger of his empty gun, making it click perpetually with his last ounce of ebbing strength.

No wonder the industry would not let Hawks make this film—with its general indictment of social and political corruption and its heroically defiant gangster who asserts his satanic will and energy until the last breath of life leaves him altogether. Although made in 1930, the film's release was delayed two years because a battling Howard Hughes refused to surrender to the censor's scissors. Hawks and Hughes had fun flying airplanes together; they thought they might have fun making films together. Hawks was looking for the means to produce films independently; Hughes was looking for the means to learn more about making movies. Their collaboration turned out to be more learning experience than fun as Hughes fought for two years to get the film released. "Hughes was fighting them. He'd fight anybody." [8] Perhaps they received additional pressure from the studio industry for their temerity in making the film independently.[9] To get the film released, Hughes was forced to compromise the ending (Tony becomes a coward without a gun in his hands) and to add a scene in which a conscientious newspaper editor (Ben Hecht would have a good laugh at this one) sententiously lectures a representative civic group of "responsible social citizens" (precisely the kinds of people Hawks and Hecht burlesque in *Twentieth Century* and *His Girl Friday*) about the voter's duty to eradicate the gangster menace. The more general indications of social corruption (the corrupted politician, mother, and society swells) would have to go altogether. Hughes would resume his defiant battle against industry regulation in 1940 with the depth and the evocations of Jane Russell's plunging neckline in *The Outlaw*, but Howard Hawks had probably learned from *Scarface* that there was no point trying to tell a story that the censors (and the public) would not allow to be told. Even in its expurgated version, *Scarface* enraged the moral pillars of the Hollywood Temple. In *Decency in Motion Pictures*, the devout Catholic publisher of the *Motion Picture Herald*, Martin Quigley, described the film as a perfect example of Hollywood's moral sins *before* the enforcement of the official Hollywood Production Code:

> A gangster picture which presents heroically the exploits of a criminal, showing him as rich, courageous, and cunning against contrasting characteristics on the part of the guaradians of the law. It glorifies crime, presents methods of crime and familiarizes the audience with them. Even though the criminal is brought to justice in the final scenes it is an influence against law and order . . .[10]

As opposed to the more general moral and social issues of the *Scarface* script, Hawks's film concentrates exclusively on the energy and vitality (not the courage or cunning) of the single gangster. His story in the *Scarface* that survives is built in the usual four-part Hawks structure. The film's first section, a prologue in seven scenes, establishes the gangster world in which the characters live and "work"—and the narrative issues that follow from it: (1) The murder of "Big Louie" Costillo in a restaurant by a whistling shadow whom we later learn belongs to Tony Camonte, Big Louie's own bodyguard; (2) The newspaper office where the city editor stimulates public interest in buying his papers by devising loudly lurid headlines about the developing "Gang War" (this is the genuine Ben Hecht view of publishers, as opposed to the sententious public servant in the added scene); (3) The barber shop where we first see the Scarfaced Tony, as that face unwraps itself from a swatch of towels, like a mummy come to life; (4) The police station, where Tony avoids the law with the legal machinery of a writ of *habeas corpus* (which Tony jauntily christens a writ of "hocus pocus"); (5) The apartment of Johnny Lovo, Tony's new boss, distinguished for its garishness, expensiveness, and the pretty female possession, Poppy, who occupies it ("Pretty hot," says Tony; "Expensive, huh?"); (6) A brief scene in an automobile between Tony and his friend, Guino, for whom Tony articulates the "one law you gotta follow to keep out of trouble: Do it first, do it yourself, and keep on doing it"; (7) Tony's home where we meet the immigrant mother and the attractive sister, Cesca, whom Tony "protects" by chasing away one of her suitors.

Everything the film's narrative will require has been effortlessly and effectively introduced in this opening prologue: Tony has switched bosses from the one that he has killed to the one that he will eventually kill; their battle will center upon the possession of Poppy, the sex object whose possession signifies the wealth and power of her keeper; Tony's two closest relationships, with Guino and Cesca, already contain the seeds of their destruction—the gangster ethic that denies the existence of friendship, the sexual jealousy that denies his sister's right to experience life as he does. All these personal motifs are surrounded by the social system that nurtures them: the legal system that lacks the machinery to control the gangster world; the newspaper business that feeds off the public's interest in that world.

The most remarkable of these seven sequences is the first one, a single traveling shot that sets the style and tone of the whole film. This lengthy moving-camera shot, the longest single tracking shot (in both time and space) in the entire work of Howard Hawks, can partially be attributed to the style of Lee Garmes, Hawks's cameraman for *Scarface*. The most "Germanic" of Hollywood studio cinematographers, Garmes is noted for his use of the moving camera and expressionistic shadows. *Scarface* is the most shadowed of Hawks's films, looking very much like Sternberg's *Underworld* (1927), the silent film that Garmes shot and Hecht wrote with Hawks's help. This opening traveling shot combines humor and violence, irony and information, subtlety and clarity. It also initiates the strategic handling of point-of-view that will allow Hawks to tell this story.

The shot and the film begin with a streetlamp (the off-frame clop-clop-clop of a milkwagon's horse), the yawn of a waiter (dawn is clearly implied), and a printed sign: "First Ward Athletic Club, Stag Party." The camera tracks with the waiter, who walks into the restaurant, from our left to our right, picking bits of litter and strewn confetti from the floor and potted palms (another parallel with the after-party litter of *Underworld*). The waiter pauses (and the camera stops with him) as he picks a brassiere off the floor with his left hand (some stag party!), while in his right he picks up another, smaller object, scrutinizes it quickly, and tucks it inside his shirt for safekeeping. Although this object is very difficult to see, particularly since our eye has been attracted by the larger dangling brassiere in the man's other hand, close observation reveals it to be a falsie, an even more subtly salacious (and comic) sexual object than the surprising brassiere.

The sound of conversational male voices drifts into our hearing from off-frame, and the camera takes its leave of the waiter and continues the move to its right toward the source of the sound. The point-of-view of this particular traveling shot might be described as detachedly analytic and probingly curious; rather than moving with any single character—a type of traveling shot in Hawks that almost always emphasizes and sympathizes with the power of a character who fills a particular space with his or her motion—it moves horizontally, parallel with the world it is observing, establishing both the physical geography and the

The waiter with his comic objects.

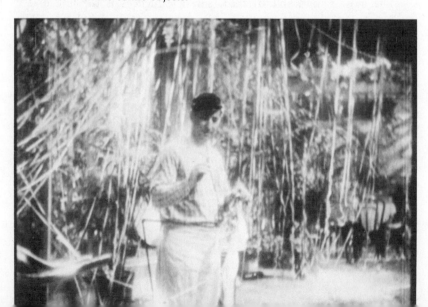

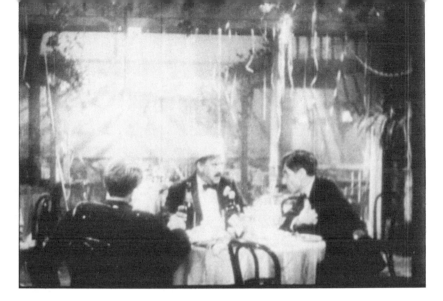

Big Louie and party.

spiritual topography of that world for the disinterested observer. The camera (like the audience at this point of the film) is not quite sure what should interest it—noting what it can in the process of seeking out what is important, hovering on the outside of a world, seeking a way into it.

Perhaps these conversing voices will be the key. The detachedly curious camera moves closer to the table of these conversing men, so we can both see and hear Big Louie, the physically "biggest" man in the center of the group (Harry J. Vejar), and the man who does all the talking while the others only listen and laugh. "Look at me. I gotta plenty. I gotta house. I gotta nice girl. (Then he belches.) I gotta stomach trouble too." Louie sits contentedly at the "top of the world," as he calls it—that top of plenty, house, and girl to which all gangsters aspire. Unfortunately, Louie is going to fall from that top because his "stomach trouble" is going to get a lot worse, filled by the bullets from Tony's gun.

As Louie walks to our right to make a telephone call, the camera continues its tracking movement from left to right with him. But when he stops the camera does not, taking its leave of him, as it did of the waiter earlier. The very fact that Hawks's camera is willing to detach itself from this man informs us that he is indeed detachable. Neither our interest nor our sympathies need linger with him any longer than the camera does. Instead, the camera is attracted by the shadow of an

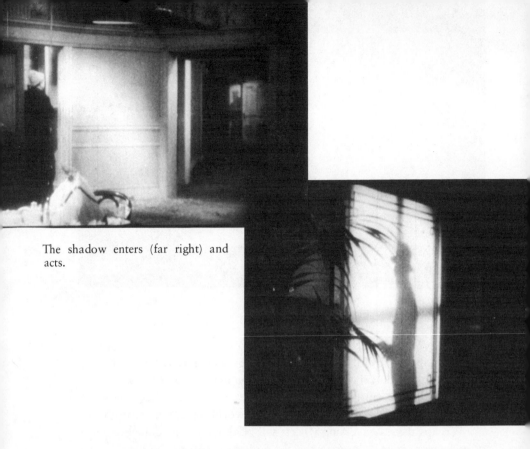

The shadow enters (far right) and acts.

opening door and the figure who occupies that light-filled doorway. It continues its deliberate movement from left to right until it finally comes to rest on this arresting shadow, in full-figure; the shadow whistles (or we hear the whistling while we watch a shadow) an aria from *Lucia di Lammermoor* and holds a gun, flanked by the leafy shadows of respectably potted palms. The camera (and the viewer through it) have found the final and focal subject of its search—signified not only by the awesome sight and sound of this shadow but by the fact that the camera itself, by stopping, implies it has reached the culmination of its left-right journey. It has reached its limit of both distance and interest; it will now retrace its journey in the opposite direction with that walking shadow as its (and our) traveling companion.

Although the film's devotion to shadows may seem a clear function of its Germanic style and mood (recalling especially Fritz Lang's *M*), Hawks would always find shadows useful and effective—for effects as diverse as the vigilante hanging of a brutal henchman in *Barbary Coast*, the comic suspense to hide Cary Grant's changing into a negligee in the bathroom of *Bringing Up Baby,* or the isolation of Bunk Kennelly, the man who causes the stampede in *Red River,* standing alone as the shadows of his comrades troop past him without pausing to speak to him. This shadow does pause, however, to speak to Big Louie: "Hello, Louie." It follows this verbal sally with the physical volley of shots that eliminates the man Tony has been hired to protect. By staging and shooting this first murder in shadow, Hawks manages to begin the delicate balancing of point-of-view that allows this story to be told—we see the murder clearly and are capable of recognizing its brutality; but we do not experience that brutality fully, distanced by the murder's shadowy indirectness, so that we do not come to loath or detest the man who performs it. It is a shadow, a two-dimensional shape, not a man, who is the brutal murderer. Nor do we feel deeply for the shadow's victim, since the victim's moral and emotional life is as vague and blurry as the shadowy killer. The victim is physically repulsive, selfishly materialistic, and comically vulgar (the belch). The story of *Scarface* requires our simultaneous judging of Tony's acts and our strange attraction to his charm, energy, directness, and humor. Hawks's murder in shadow-show permits this balance since the three-dimensional man (when we meet him) will be so much more engaging than this flat shadow and since the shadow's victim is far less appealing and attractive than that man.

After the shots and the sound of Big Louie's fall, Hawks's camera again asserts its cool detachment and discretion. It continues moving back in the opposite direction, retracing its path from right to left, discovering the body on the floor—just as the waiter, the man who opened the shot, comes into the frame to discover it. The waiter puts on his jacket and moves toward the door through which he entered at the shot's beginning, this time moving from right to left, as the camera tracks with him, completing the perfect circle that encloses this shot. Significantly, in the next shot, inside the newspaper office, the camera continues this counter-movement (right to left), traveling with the newspapermen who are also moving like the waiter, in that right-left direction. Throughout Hawks's career, tracking camera movements from left to right are consistently the active, assertive strophe, while the reverse movement from right to left serves as the reaction, the echoing antistrophe.

This opening traveling shot is not only a complexly graceful perfect circle of human action and camera motion. It is a metaphor for the whole film in its demonstration that, as in every Hawks narrative, the end is the beginning. The shadow who shoots Louie will aspire to the same "top of the world" that Louie occupied; he will betray any personal and professional associates, just as he betrayed Louie, to get there; and he will end exactly as Louie did—fallen and motionless. This opening shot's contrast of movement and stasis is another significant metaphor, both for the film and for Hawks's work as a whole. Johnny Lovo, Tony's new boss, later observes that "Costillo slowed down too much," in response to which Tony playfully quips, "Yeah, and now he's come to a dead stop." Tony, like the traveling camera in this opening shot, equates movement with life itself—for no particular reason, in no particular direction. To move is itself to be alive. This view in one way or another underlies all of Howard Hawks's *motion* pictures, which contrast the vitality of movement with the lifelessness of coming to a dead stop.

In addition to establishing this energy, the vital Hawksian equation of motion and life, the film's prologue also establishes the two emotional triangles on which the remainder of the narrative will be built. The first triangle—the conflict of Tony (Paul Muni) and Johnny (Osgood Perkins) for possession of Poppy (Karen Morley)—is established simply and early with both visual triangulation and editing in the first scene in Johnny Lovo's apartment. As Tony and Johnny sit, discussing their plans, at opposite sides of the frame, Poppy sits behind and between them, a perfectly symmetrical triangle of the two men and the

Triangular tension: Tony, Johnny, and Poppy between them.

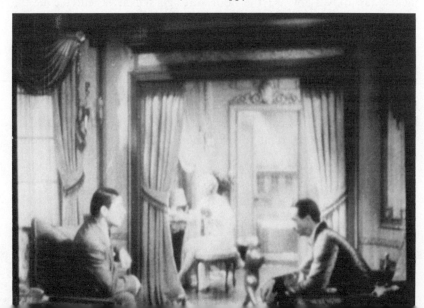

woman. The symmetrical stability in the relationship of this triangular composition reveals the apparent but false stability in the relationship of Tony and Lovo. Hawks punctuates the apparent placidity of these triangular three-shots with tensely conflicting close-ups—of Johnny, of Tony—when an argument about strategy erupts between them. Johnny wants Tony to confine his gang's power to the South Side, to keep away from the rival O'Hara gang's territory on the North Side. Tony will follow Johnny's orders in the film's second major section—when he sews up the South Side for his new boss. But Tony will take the North Side in the film's third major section and, in the process, eliminate Johnny and take Poppy for himself.

But the film's second triangle, Tony and Guino's (George Raft) covert battle for possession of Tony's own sister, Cesca (Ann Dvorak), is far more complex psychologically and far more disturbing for both the audience and for Tony. Hawks establishes this triangle, whose resolution will occupy the film's fourth and final major section, by more complex means. When Tony chases away the man he sees kissing Cesca he is doing far more than protecting his sister's "honor"—as "Old World" ethnic types were wont to do in Hollywood films. Hawks meant to imply Tony's incestuous longings for his own sister. Hawks's original idea for the film was to depict the Chicago Capones as if they were the Florentine Borgias.[11] In the original script's Florida scene one of Tony's guests aboard his yacht specifically parallels him with Caesar Borgia, asking if he has a sister. Hawks would consistently remove such overt and obvious scripted symbols when he went to shoot his films. Instead, in the film, Tony erupts irrationally, immediately, instinctively (protesting too much, one thinks) to his sister's rather casual embrace. Then, feeling guilty about this eruption which he himself does not (and cannot) clearly understand, Tony offers Cesca a handful of money. The exchange of money in a Hawks film always serves as a material sign of a desire to exchange less tangible thoughts and feelings. In some films (*To Have and Have Not, Red River*) the acceptance or refusal of money is a concrete sign of personal honor and integrity. But in *Scarface*, Tony gives Cesca money because he cannot give her anything else, and she accepts his money because it is really his way of life—Tony himself— that she wants to accept.

Hawks, however, does not let the emotional currency exchange stop here but gives it the one additional twist that will embrace the final member of the triangle. As Cesca sits in her bedroom, on her bed, holding that money, she hears the music of an organ-grinder on the street below. Looking down from her window, she catches her first glimpse of Guino, who returns her gaze as he casually, pointedly, tosses his coin in rhythm with the music. This coin tossing was to be the first of many pieces of coin business in a Hawks film as well as becoming an archetypal gesture for George Raft that he himself would live to parody twenty-seven years later (in *Some Like It Hot*). Cesca completes the sexual circle when she tosses a coin out her window to the organ grinder below. Originally the script called for her to toss one of Tony's bills, but the simple word Hawks wrote in the margin of his script—"Coin?"—shows him improvising a much subtler (not one of the bills Tony just gave her, but a piece of money nonetheless) and surer (coins fall, bills float) link to Guino below, who has been defined by his coin tossing. Guino catches Cesca's coin, flips the musician his own, and holds onto hers, which he then begins to toss exactly as he did his own, staring and smiling up at the coin's sender. The juxtaposition of the circularly turning handle of the street musician's organ (Hawks may well have known the lurid 1920s' jazz tune, "Organ Grinder," made popular by Ethel Waters), the repetitive, hypnotic tossing of that metal object, and the lingering close-up of Cesca's face firmly lock Guino and Cesca in a circle of mutual desire. Hawks has used a piece of inanimate physical matter to make the internal, emotional point—Cesca and Guino share a sexual energy that is more than the mere exchange of metal. His grasping her coin in his hand is the closest he can come to grasping her hand.

The second and third major sections of this narrative grow from the simpler of these triangles—the tension between Tony and Johnny Lovo, his boss and rival. In the film's second section, Tony rises to power and wealth *with* Johnny (selling his orders for bootleg beer to the South Side taverns, as Johnny instructed) and in its third he rises to power *against* Johnny (taking the North Side from O'Hara against Johnny's instructions). Hawks-Hecht demarcate these middle, mirror-like sections with careful symmetrical patterning. The second section begins with Tony's breaking a glass door, hurling a cuspidor through the outside door of the First Ward Athletic Club that bears the departed Louis Costillo's name as "President." The third section ends with the breaking of a second and similar glass door that now bears Johnny

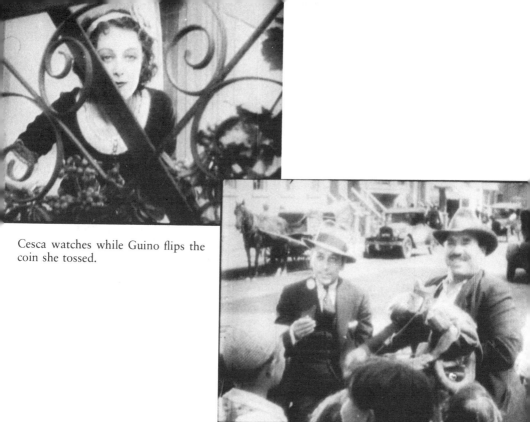

Cesca watches while Guino flips the coin she tossed.

Lovo's name; its shattering will signal Lovo's death (just as the shattered door previously signaled Big Louie's) and the termination of the Tony-Lovo relationship. These middle sections contain wildly energetic montage sequences which mirror one another. The first telescopes the taking of the South Side (selling beer by such intimidating methods as arm-twisting, pistol-whipping, shooting, beating, and bombing); the second telescopes the taking of the North Side (a gang war of machine-gunning, racing, careening, and crashing automobiles). This symmetrical punctuation of the two montage sequences is so percussive and so energetic that their spirit can best be understood by the final image of the first one: a firing machine gun superimposed over the flying pages of a wall calendar. The metaphor is that of machine-gunning time itself, making time pass by blasting it away. But the second montage sequence ends with a much subtler and ironic image of death. The death of O'Hara (who owns a flower shop) is simply announced—without a word—when Guino shows Tony a flower; Tony jauntily fingers the rosebud in the

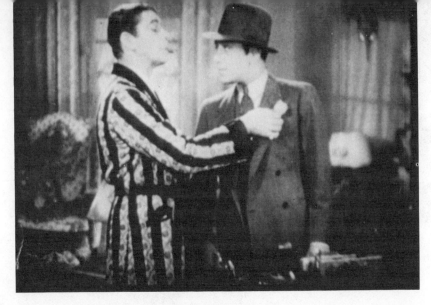

Approving of murder by arranging a flower.

button hole of Guino's lapel. By translating a human death into a boutonniere Hawks maintains our sympathy for the murderer (what else do
you do with a flower?), removes our sympathy from the victim (a human being has been translated into a comic object).

Like the two montage sequences, the dominant tone of these two
symmetrically patterned middle sections is a counterpoint of gleeful,
childlike comedy with the brutally violent acts of murder, extortion,
bombing, and beating. Hawks was struck by the childishness of the
gangsters he met.

> I get awfully tired of a lot of the gangster stuff that I see where
> everybody is growling at somebody and the toughest guy in the
> world. These fellows were not that way. They were just like
> kids. We had fun doing it.[12]

Just this gleeful "fun" and lack of growling distinguishes *Scarface* from
those other, more familiar films of the gangster cycle—more familiar
perhaps because they were more socially palatable; more palatable precisely because they took the gangster world seriously, not as sport. Tony's
most deliriously gleeful, childish reaction is his discovery of a new toy—
the light, portable machine guns that the rival O'Hara gang has im-
ported (in crates of apparently innocent pineapple boxes) for use in its

war against Lovo and Camonte. "Lookit, Johnny, you can carry it around like a baby. . . . Out of my way, Johnny, I'm gonna spit." Whereupon Tony playfully empties the machine gun into a rack of pool cues (a brilliantly visual piece of physical business which Hawks devised during shooting), making the wooden sticks dance to his percussively deadly tune. The physicality of bullets in this film (and in many others of Hawks)—biting into wood, knicking stone, ripping newspaper, pitting plaster—is another of the film's consistent visual motifs. For Tony, biting bullets are kiddie's spitballs. Tony takes a similarly childish delight in the metal shutters he has installed on the windows of his apartment, with sliding peep holes so he can "play peek-a-boo" with any uninvited callers. But if Tony delights in these merry games of death, Hawks has great fun playing them too—and asking the viewer to play with him.

Perhaps the most childishly playful and bizarrely funny scene in the film is one of its bloodiest, when the O'Hara gang, with their new machine guns, seeking revenge for their murdered leader, sprays the restaurant where Tony hangs out. Juxtaposed with the sights and sounds of rattling bullets and crashing glass is a comic telephone conversation between Angelo, the incompetent "Dope" of a secretary (Vince Barnett), and some anonymous caller who has obviously tried to lure Tony to the telephone where he would make an easier target. Angelo is the perfect example of Hawks's and Hecht's thinking of "something crazier than you could." Nicknamed "Dope," Angelo is a "seckatary" who cannot write (just as twenty years later Hawks and Hecht will give us another secretary, Miss Laurel—played by Marilyn Monroe—who cannot type). "Dope" perpetually asks, "who is this?"—one of his running gags in the film since he is as comically incapable of getting an answer to this simple question as he is of writing that answer down. Because the rattle of machine guns makes it impossible for "Dope" to hear, he keeps asking the caller to repeat the inaudible name. Then Hawks tops this comic business when one of the bullets pierces the huge coffee urn standing behind Angelo, sending a steady stream of coffee onto the seat of Angelo's pants (the coffee urn ironically—and probably deliberately—seems to be pissing on Angelo's backside). Who but Hawks would juxtapose deadly bullets with a pants-wetting burlesque gag? And who but Hawks would top the sequence as playfully as he does? While the injured, moaning people who have suffered this devastation are led off frame,

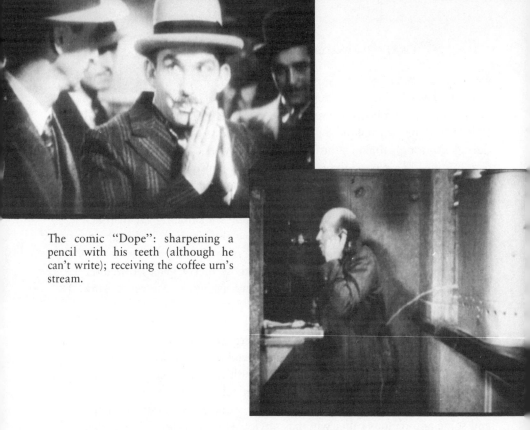

The comic "Dope": sharpening a pencil with his teeth (although he can't write); receiving the coffee urn's stream.

Angelo matter of factly apologizes to Tony for not getting the caller's name because there was too much noise, totally oblivious to the destruction around him.

Not only is the scene a dazzling combination of the brutal and the comic, not only does it re-create the exuberant, energetic fun of the gangster's world of danger as the gangster existentially experiences it, and not only does it transmit that expression of fun to an audience who would never want to experience it in social reality; it also shows Hawks's masterful control of point-of-view in continuing the simultaneous condemnation and enjoyment of this world. Hawks transfers our visual attention from human death and destruction to a comic object—a "pissing" coffee urn. He keeps the painful reactions of the innocent humans off-frame (until the final shot of the sequence), using the counterpoint of violent sound and comic picture to remind us that this comic conversation is deadly destructive at the same time. A note Hawks writes to himself in the margin of his script, "There shouldn't be anyone in restaurant but Tony and his henchmen," also indicates his awareness that the normal adults must be heard but not seen if we are to enjoy his gangster children at play.

A similarly playful juxtaposition of death and laughter generates the film's comic visual symbolism, a plague of "Xs" that litter the scene of every murder. Hawks explains that newspaper reports of gang murders always marked the location of every murdered mobster with a tidy X. Newspaper readers were as avid to experience the gangster world vicariously as moviegoers; Hawks-Hecht's editor, with his "Gang War" headlines, would seem nearer the truth than the schoolmarmish editor Hughes was forced to add. Hawks decided to mark each of his movie murders with an X, offering a $100 reward to any member of the crew who invented a clever way to pin a new X on a murder.[13] To convert murdered humans to mere Xs (two-dimensional shapes; a letter of the alphabet) is yet another (and consistent) way to convert our potential sympathy for humans into our enjoyment of comic objects.

The playfully comic symbol of death reaches its ironic apex in two scenes that signify the total obliteration of the O'Hara gang. For the famous "St. Valentine's Day Massacre," a neat row of seven silhouetted Xs signifies the tidy deaths of seven thugs all in a shadowy row. We hear the machine gun on the sound track but we watch mere two-dimensional shadows and letters. The death of Gaffney (Boris Karloff), the last surviving member of the O'Hara gang, takes place in a bowling alley. Just before his death, Gaffney bowls a strike, whereupon the scorer marks an appropriate X in Gaffney's column. As we watch Gaffney's next bowl, he is machine-gunned (off-frame sound again) immediately after the ball leaves his hand. Hawks's camera deserts the victim, for whom we might feel some sympathy, to follow his bowling ball, merrily continuing its journey toward the pins, as if its prime mover were still alive to view its success. The ball knocks all of them down, except for the single pin that keeps willfully spinning, obstinately refusing to fall. A second burst of off-frame machine-gun fire seems to settle the pin's hash (rather than Gaffney's), for it finally collapses and drops, coming (like the man we cannot see) to a dead stop. Not only does the pin become a comic symbol of the dying Gaffney, who apparently required a second dose of bullets, but also the transferring of our attention to objects and away from humans has been Hawks's consistent method for making these murderous antics seem antic rather than murderous.

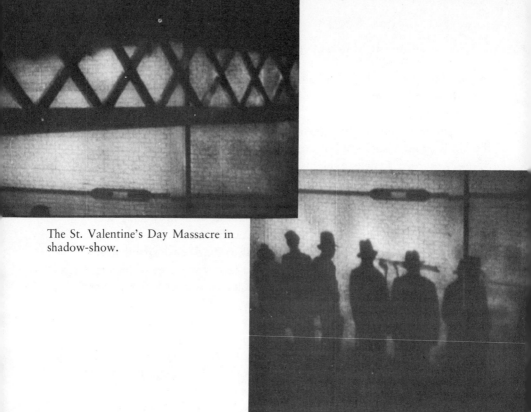

The St. Valentine's Day Massacre in shadow-show.

Bowling balls do not feel pain. Xs are not alive and cannot feel anything at all. Dehumanizing the victims maintains our respect (if not our sympathy) for those who have been clever enough to convert their victims into markers in a game. Perhaps the only way that gangsters can play the gangster game at all (just as the only way Hawks can make his gangster film) is to think of their victims as objects, not as people. Such playful reductions may still seem as socially unacceptable to some viewers today as they did to the censors of fifty years ago. This film (and Hawks as a whole) will probably not appeal to them.

The second and third sections of *Scarface* adopt a playful attitude toward language that also reduces words—the medium of human thought and emotion—to objects. Tony's malapropisms reveal his ignorance of the subtle shadings of words. Tony uses words succinctly and directly—the same way he uses bullets. Big, fancy, subtly shaded words mean as little to him as fancy, subtle moral shadings. When Poppy tells him that his new ring seems kind of effeminate, Tony's response is,

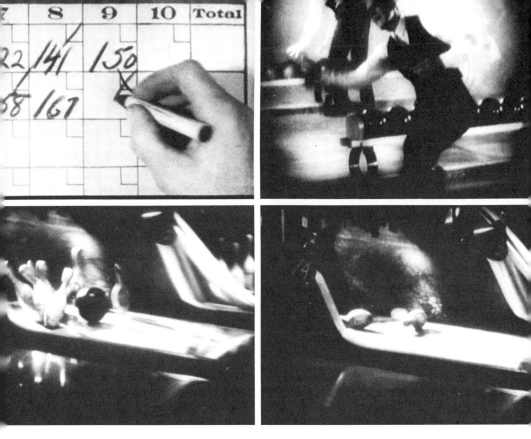

The death of Gaffney.

"Yeah, I got it in an auction. A real bargain." When she remarks that his new apartment is "Kinda gaudy, isn't it?" Tony replies, "Ain't it though. Glad you like it." *Tiger Shark* (which was not written by Hecht) uses the identical play with "effeminate," while *His Girl Friday* (which was written by Hecht) uses a similar one when an Italian thug, whose blonde girlfriend is described as an albino, replies, "No, she isn't, boss. She was born right here in this country." Fancy words and fancy talk become a subtle leitmotif in many of the scripts Hecht wrote for Hawks (most pointedly in *Barbary Coast*), not surprising for a newspaperman for whom words are the tools of the trade. Hawks's fondness for fractured speech would culminate in his two Marilyn Monroe films, whether written by Hecht (*Monkey Business*) or not (*Gentlemen Prefer Blondes*). The fractured words in *Scarface* function like the film's comic visual devices—broken objects are funny, broken people are not.

The verbal humor in *Scarface* parallels the intellectual humor that arises from a night at the theater when the gang of slickly tuxedoed hoods takes in a performance of *Rain*. Despite their deadly vocation, the thugs look at least as proper as everyone else in the theater. And they respond to the play's issues as any other theatergoer might. Tony finds Sadie Thompson's experience uplifting and edifying; he excuses her behavior because she's a girl who's been "disillusioned." Hawks and Hecht provide no such bromide to excuse Tony's behavior. The untalkative Guino, however, asks a more pragmatic question: "Why's a girl wanna hustle in a place like that for?" (This line could never have sneaked past the Production Code Administration four years later.) "Dope" agrees: "Yeah. It's always raining all the time." "Dope" prefers a show with a lot of jokes. This playfully abstract aesthetic discussion immediately precedes the murder of Gaffney in the bowling alley. Indeed, Tony faces a difficult decision: does he catch the last edifying act of *Rain* or does he remove the last troublesome member of the O'Hara gang. Is art more interesting than his own adventurous life? He resolves the dilemma by going to the bowling alley but leaving Angelo behind to inform him of the play's outcome. Just before killing Gaffney, Tony receives "Dope's" review: "She crawls back in the hay with the army." (Another line that could never have survived four years later.)

The playful second and third sections of Tony's rise culminate with Tony's elimination of Johnny Lovo and his seizing Lovo's kingdom for himself. First, Lovo moves to eliminate Tony—but Tony escapes the sedan of pursuers who want to take him for a ride. After Tony discovers Johnny's responsibility for the move, he makes his counter-move in response to it. Hawks conveys Lovo's initial decision to remove Tony with the effortlessly communicative use of a tiny, ordinary physical object in a gesture and a scene that do not exist in the film's script. Johnny, Poppy, and Tony sit together at a table in the Paradise Night Club, another symmetrical triangle that recalls their first scene together. Again the gangsters are all carefully groomed and dressed in evening clothes, just as at *Rain*, the elegant and polite surfaces which cover the violence beneath. When Poppy picks up a cigarette, both Johnny and Tony reach toward her with a light. Poppy considers Johnny's lighter carefully, then turns deliberately to Tony to take her light from his match. The inevitable Hawks cigarette serves the very particular purpose of revealing who feels what about whom. Soon after Poppy tips her hand toward

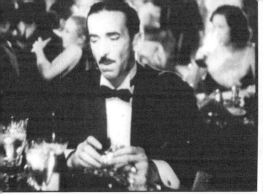
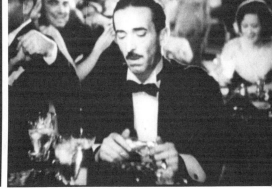

The conversation with the salt-shaker.

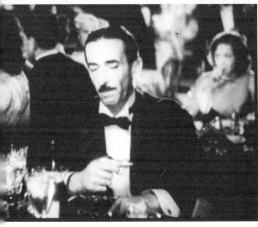

Tony, he asks her to dance and she consents—although she previously told Johnny she didn't feel like dancing. By accepting both Tony's match and his dance, Poppy has informed Johnny Lovo both who is her "boss" and who is *the* boss.

Now Johnny sits at the table alone, deserted by the woman he considered his possession. As Johnny sits there, he fiddles nervously and unconsciously with the silver saltshaker he holds in his right hand. As his fingers play restlessly with the object, they come to grasp the shaker by its metal handle, pointing it as if it were a pistol. Then Johnny looks down to take notice of this shaker in his hand and, while looking at it, he pulls his index finger against the handle, exactly as he would pull the trigger of a pistol. He then carefully sets the shaker down, knowing what he must do. This handling of the saltshaker and the transforming it into another kind of object to reveal Lovo's intention (both to himself and to us) takes three definite steps: (1) unconscious, nervous fingering of the object, realizing he is upset but unsure what to do about it; (2)

unconscious transforming of the saltshaker into a pistol, as his fingers evolve a strategy of what they unconsciously want to do; (3) the conscious realization (by looking down to notice what his fingers have been doing by themselves) that he must take some concrete action to do what he wants to do. This brief, simple, subtle, psychologically revealing manipulation of a very simple, ordinary object is as indicative of Hawks's fundamental views about human psychology, complex characterization, and credible storytelling as any moment in Hawks's entire work.

Tony's counter to Johnny's move, in which he eliminates the boss and rival who betrayed him, is another of the film's most powerful sequences—like the opening shot of the murder of Big Louie, which this later murder deliberately recalls. Tony stands facing Johnny in Lovo's office, the very seat of power that Tony's killing of Big Louie allowed Johnny to occupy. Hawks's camera stares at Tony's face in a tight close-up. Hawks has repeatedly stated that he prefers to use close-ups sparingly, saving them for moments that really count.[14] Here the close-up really counts as both the camera and Tony's facial expression remain absolutely, firmly still; nothing moves in the frame except the smoke that drifts across it from Tony's cigarette, the sign of those feelings which stir beneath the still surface. Then Hawks cuts to Johnny, who nervously pours himself a drink; Hawks reveals that Tony now is the scene's and the office's emotional "boss," contrasting Tony's solid stillness with Johnny's weak, evasive movement. The camera—like Tony—is solid and still, his emotional ally. As Johnny jitteringly pours his drink, the sound of Tony's whistling—the same aria from *Lucia* he whistled in the film's opening murder—floats in from off-frame. Hawks's editing pattern here, deliberately keeping Johnny and Tony in separate frames (as opposed to the earlier compositions of their tensely and somewhat uncomfortably sharing the same framed space) reveals that Tony and Johnny now occupy absolutely separate emotional spaces. Tony's calm control is reinforced by the occasional cut to Guino, who sits coolly and quietly, tossing his coin in a deliberate, measured, metronomic rhythm which also contrasts with the stuttering, unrhythmic pattern of Johnny's scattered movements. The issue is settled when Tony viciously and pointedly jabs out his cigarette in an ashtray, transferring his emotion to a Hawks object, then turns and silently walks toward the glass office door which now bears Johnny's name. The camera again stands still, merely watching Tony's receding back, until he stops and suddenly

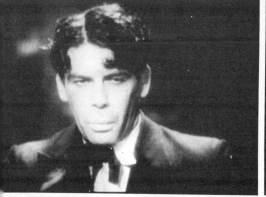

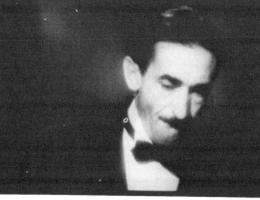

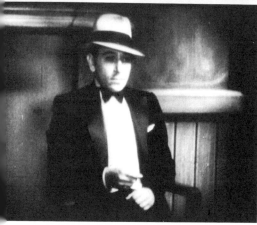

Tony whistles, Johnny squirms,
Guino flips his coin.

smashes his fist through the glass barrier. As Tony turns around violently to face his betrayer, Hawks makes an equally violent cut—precisely on that whirling movement—back to Tony's face in tight close-up, brilliantly capturing the eruption of both feeling and intention in the act of smashing an inanimate object.

Johnny Lovo knows, without a word's being said, that Tony knows who tried to kill him; the camera, the cutting, and the objects all condemn Lovo for his betrayal, just as Tony does. Johnny begins babbling, pleading, begging, offering Poppy to Tony in exchange for his life, one of those torrents of sound in Hawks that betrays the excitement and desperation of the speaker. Without saying a word (Tony's silence contrasts with Johnny's sound, just as his earlier stillness contrasted with Johnny's nervous movement), Tony simply walks toward the door as Guino moves in the counter direction toward Johnny, drawing his gun. Hawks continues to watch Tony's departure, not Guino's execution of Lovo. Tony moves toward the outer door of the office while a still

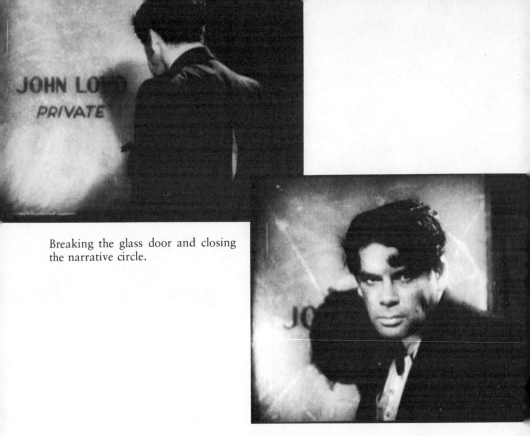

Breaking the glass door and closing
the narrative circle.

camera watches his back recede. Its choice of stillness, as opposed to
the alternative choice of traveling with him, emphasizes the fact of his
departure and his lack of interest in the event to follow. It also emphasizes that the event is settled and the settlement is just.

As we continue to watch Tony's walk, we hear a single off-frame
shot (another delicately and indirectly managed murder that conveys its
information without forcing us to watch it in detail). Tony, without
missing a step, continues to walk out the door (the very door through
which he threw the cuspidor that signaled Johnny's arrival as "President") and the shot fades out. Like the opening shot of Big Louie's
murder, the film's two middle sections (which begin with Tony and
Johnny walking in together through a door and end with Tony's walking out alone through that door) describe another completion of a perfect circle. The very coolness of this departure and the camera's detachment emphasize Tony's strength and control, but ironically the moment
signals another kind of departure in the narrative. The removal of Lovo
is to be Tony's final act of strength and control, for when Tony returns

to the story in the final section of the film, this particular cool Tony has departed from it.

The film's fourth section—Tony's fall—returns to the other triangle established in the prologue—the relationship of Tony, Cesca, and Guino. Hawks has kept this narrative issue alive in the film's middle sections with a scene in the Paradise Night Club, just preceding Johnny's conversation with the saltshaker. Cesca seductively dances for Guino during the playing of "Some of These Days" (this song will return in *Only Angels Have Wings*), as Hawks's camera simply and detachedly observes her lithe body in full frame, watching her without moving, just as Guino watches without moving. Ann Dvorak, the first of Hawks's woman discoveries, is a prototype of the kind that would repeatedly return: smart; determined; her sex appeal transmits itself through humor and her humor transmits itself as sex appeal; tall, thin, not much bust but a lot of leg. In film after film, Hawks finds a woman's legs the most interesting part of her anatomy (even of Marilyn Monroe's). Guino, like Hawks's camera, remains detached from Cesca's dance; he knows and respects the fact that she is Tony's sister. But he likes to look at her, just as he looked at her from below as he tossed her coin in that previous "dance" to the organ grinder's tune.

The argument between Tony and Cesca that follows this dance in the nightclub also prepares us for the film's final section. Hawks shoots their violent confrontation in back-lit silhouette, specially devised by Lee Garmes when Hawks felt that the clash didn't play well full-face and fully lit.[15] It plays much more mysteriously in back-lit silhouette

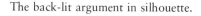

The back-lit argument in silhouette.

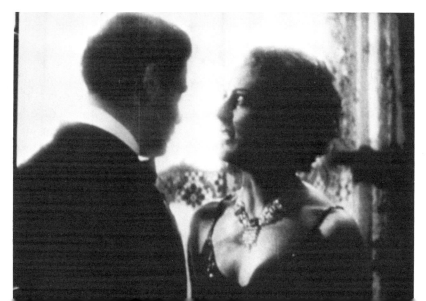

because it paradoxically plays one kind of verbal scene (a loud argument between a brother and sister) off against an opposite kind of visual scene (the intimacy of two close, silhouetted heads bathed in moody "moonlight"). The result is a very curious love scene that furthers the exploration of their very curious love. Hawks himself refers to this moment as their love scene:

> We had a scene in which Muni told his sister that he loved her, and we couldn't play it in full light. We wound up playing it in silhouette against a curtain with the light coming from outside.[16]

Muni does not in fact tell her that he loves her in this scene. The tight composition of the two shadowy heads and the streaming light from behind "say" what Tony cannot say; his words are quite the opposite of a declaration of love. Hawks remembers what is meant, not what is said.

Finally, Hawks prepares for the film's concluding section by defining Tony's view of Guino as a sexual "tomcat." When Tony tries to locate Guino for their visit to Lovo's office, a series of phone calls ironically and effectively reveals the number of shady women's apartments in which Guino might be found. Guino's presence in one of these ladies' lodgings is announced, even before we see him in the frame, by the smoke that drifts into the frame from two tell-tale cigarettes in an ash tray. This same kind of smoke will later drift into the frame inside the apartment which Guino and Cesca share. The appearance of this identical smoke will lead the viewer to assume (just as Tony assumes) that Guino's relationship with Cesca is identical to that of all the other women he smokes with.

Cesca, like her brother Tony, is persistent, determined in getting what she wants. And she wants Guino. She strides into what has now become Tony's office at the "Athletic Club" while her brother is out of town (this is the point where the Florida scene occurs in the script) and where Guino now sits alone. As is common in Hawks, the office, the seat of power, remains; only its occupant changes—from Louie to Johnny to Tony. The fact that Guino now sits in the boss's seat may imply its potential future inhabitant—if Cesca's own plans of sexual conquest hadn't intervened. Hawks has built this ironic love scene between Guino and Cesca around yet another physical object—Guino sits in Tony's chair cutting a string of paper dolls. The identical, symmetrical dolls (neither the object nor the business appears in the script) is perhaps a metaphor for Guino's love life—a series of faceless, identical, flat physical objects, each of them different but all of them alike. Cesca manages to lure Guino's attention away from these dolls with her provocative humor: "The one on the end is cute." Because Hawks was dissatisfied with the scene between Guino and Cesca in the original script—his notes in the margin are "not the right key" and "rotten"— he again uses the concrete physical object to allow the expression of more subtle, interesting, and sincere feelings. Guino will decide to add Cesca to his string of paper dolls. Perhaps she will be the cute one on the end. Or perhaps she will replace that string of dolls altogether. This uncertainty—of whether Cesca will be the one in Guino's life or merely the one of many, an uncertainty produced by the ironic suggestion of those paper dolls—will play an important narrative role in the action to follow.

Hawks establishes the mood, the happy harmony, of Cesca's and Guino's life together with a third use of song. Like the earlier organ grinder's tune and "Some of These Days," and like the songs in later Hawks films, this bouncy, cheery tune which Cesca sings while accompanying herself on the piano conveys essential psychological and emotional information about the community of feeling which the characters share. (I have never seen a script that indicates the use of song.)* Hawks's framing and composition work with the cheery music to emphasize the stability of this happy home with a carefully symmetrical

---

* I am not by any means claiming that Hawks was the only major Hollywood director of the period to use music metaphorically. One of the generic expectations of films in the period is that they would use music and song in this way. Music, for example, is equally important and effective in the films of Capra ("The Man on the Flying Trapeze" in *It Happened One Night*, "For He's a Jolly Good Fellow" in *Mr. Deeds*, "Polly Wolly Doodle" in *You Can't Take It With You*), McCarey ("Home on the Range" and "My Love Is Gone with the Wind" in *The Awful Truth*), and Ford ("Red River Valley" in *The Grapes of Wrath*, "My Darling Clementine" in that film, "She Wore a Yellow Ribbon" in *Fort Apache*). Such shared conventions are what make genres generic. My argument relates to the specific uses to which Hawks puts music and song, as opposed to the specific uses to which other directors put them.

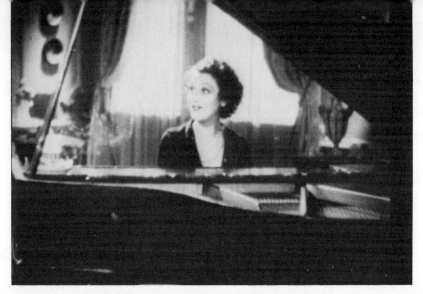

Cesca at the piano as Guino's smoke drifts in from the left.

image that places Cesca perfectly within the triangle (yet another visual triangulation) formed by the piano's lid. But the cheery stability of this happy ménage is invaded by the suggestion of danger and disruption. Into this stable image drifts that smoke of Guino's cigarette from off-frame, suggesting not only Cesca's nearby listener but the ominous approach of that other character in the triangle whose own cigarette smoke last drifted into the frame when he condemned Lovo to death.

Tony indeed returns to invade the happy home, directed there (as in the original script) by their mother. She also assumed the moral worst about sharing an apartment with Guino. Tony's appearance at the apartment's door (to continue the film's symbolic Xs, its number is the Roman numeral X) puts an abrupt end to the home's harmony: a look of confusion spreads across Tony's face when he discovers that his friend Guino is the man with whom his sister has been living. He follows that brief confusion almost immediately by shooting him, without either asking for or permitting a word of explanation. Again Hawks depicts this shooting with the same imaginative indirectness that marked Tony's other three major killings (Louie, Gaffney, and Johnny). This time, however, the visual concentration on a physical object, accompanied by an off-frame shot, condemns the act of murder and attaches our sympathy to the victims rather than to the murderer. Hawks keeps his camera on Cesca's face (not a shadow, not a bowling ball, not a receding back, but a human face). She screams, "Tony don't," followed by the crack of an off-frame shot. Then Hawks cuts to an extreme close-up of the coin that Guino has just tossed in the air, while Guino slowly sinks out of the frame, shaking his head "no." Like Gaffney's final toss of the bowling ball, the person who tossed the object is no longer alive to view the completion of that action and the end of its motion. As opposed to the stranger Gaffney, we know much more about this victim, this object, and this woman (who first met the man by the exchange of such an object). Indeed, this coin is, by implication, that very token of love. With Cesca and Guino, the people have a history, a life, through the history of the object, unlike Gaffney's bowling ball which has a life of its own. As Cesca kneels over the body of her fallen lover and Tony tries to pull her from it, Hawks's camera emphasizes the narrow enclosure of the apartment corridor; its low angle mirrors its continuing sympathy for the fallen man and sobbing woman and its detachment from the standing man who murdered his best friend.

Cesca's moral defense of her life with Guino, "We were married yesterday, Tony," casts her brother adrift on the sea of emotional confusion that has surrounded his relationship with his sister. Not only has he killed his best friend, but he also lacks the moral platitude of outraged honor as an excuse for his act of human betrayal. This confusion infects Tony both physically and mentally from this point in the film; his body stoops, his walk slows. And Hawks's camera conveys Tony's physical and emotional breakdown by returning to its detached strategy of the opening shot, observing Tony's final retreat into his apartment lair as a horizontal movement across the frame, perpendicular to the camera's position, just as it watched the unimportant waiter and Big Louie in the film's opening shot. Tony's walk has lost its purpose and direction—stumbling and halting. His talk has also lost its staccato punch—stuttering and mumbling. Tony mutters irrelevantly and illogically over the telephone to Poppy, "I didn't know, I didn't know." In his bent body, his purposeless walk, and his muttered, incoherent words Tony Camonte comes as close as this character can to an emotional and moral discovery—the crime of destroying the lives of the two people who were closest to him in the world, simply because, as he lectured Guino earlier, he "did it first," and he did it too fast.

This final section of Tony's fall displays the overall strategy of a stripping away, of loss, of the central character's being denuded of his immaterial assets (essentially human relationships), so that in the end he stands alone with his things. Although this is a typical pattern of gangster films (as recent as *The Godfather II*), it has a special relevance to the films of Howard Hawks, who finds things important only in so far as they suggest, reveal, and imply the immaterial. First Tony loses Guino—by Tony's own hand; then the comic but loyal "seckatary," Angelo, struck in the stomach by a bullet meant for Tony. Angelo, a thorough professional despite his comic incompetence, continues to do his loyal job in his quirky comic manner (carefully locks the door of Tony's hideout, takes the final phone call from Poppy, and this time even manages to transmit the name of the caller), even to the moment of death. Finally, it is Cesca's turn. She has come to the hideout with a gun specifically to revenge Guino's death (women who unsuccessfully attempt to use guns recur in *Viva Villa!*, *Only Angels Have Wings*, *The Outlaw*, *The Big Sleep*, and *Red River*). In what might seem a stunning reversal, she decides to fight with him rather than against him in his final hour, serving as his moll, loading the guns for his use (just as Tess Millay would do for Matthew Garth in *Red River*). The motivation for Cesca's act arises from the whole complex of unstated feelings between the brother and sister throughout the film (particularly that shadowy, back-lit argument).[17]

Cesca's appearance in his besieged lair seems to revive the sagging gangster (just as the reunion with Lee, again played by Ann Dvorak, revives the broken Joe Greer in *The Crowd Roars*). But a bullet from the machine guns of the police surrounding Tony's fortress specifically to arrest him for the murder of his friend, Guino, ricochets off one of Tony's protective metal shutters as he pulls it closed, careening into Cesca's vulnerable body. The physicality of Hawks's bullets is again so concrete (the bullet leaves its scuffmark on the metal shutter) that one can almost trace the path of the projectile. The armor of Tony's defense produces the opposite of its intended result, killing rather than protecting the inhabitants of the fortress. There is a difference between flesh and metal, living beings and dead things, that Tony does not understand.

From the moment of Cesca's death, Tony will not fire another shot. In the script he was to have kissed her full on the mouth, a communion that refuels his defiant energy and provokes his final act of mammoth assertion. With Cesca's death in the film, his defiance collapses, the tear gas drives him sobbingly out of hiding, and the tough mobster is killed in cowardly flight by the coolly professional, impersonal detachment of an anonymous policeman's machine gun—not, as in the script, by his cop nemesis Guarino in brutal and personal revenge. As Tony lies in the gutter, the camera tilts up for a final look at the flashing electric sign that serves as the film's obvious moral symbol.[18] Although the shot of this sign closes another Hawks circle (from the electric streetlamp that opened the film to this arrangement of electric lamps), it is the kind of obvious symbol Hawks would eliminate from his later films. The sign flashes, "The World is Yours"; then below it, "Cook's Tours." Tony, who had beamingly showed the sign to Poppy earlier in the film, indicated the direction of his intentions for the world.

The camera's return to the sign, in the very shot in which Tony died beneath it, reinforces the ironic difference between the storyteller's moral reading of it and Tony's reading of it earlier. Whereas the sign delights Tony, beckoning him with its invitation to possess the world, implying for Tony that it is both possible and desirable to possess the world, the storyteller makes a different moral judgment. It is simply not possible to possess the world (people are, like the world itself, mortal and material), no more than one can sit at the "top of the world" (which has no top). Even to attempt to possess a world that is merely material, devoid of the human qualities of love and friendship, is worthless. Tony's view of the immaterial, spiritual value of friendship, that essential Hawks value, and of the existence of others and the rights of others to exist, is perfectly captured by his very early ironic question about Johnny Lovo, then his associate, boss, and "friend": "Lovo? Who's Lovo?" That identical question returns in a symmetry that is typical of Hawks when Tony bribes the barber to help uncover Lovo as the man who tried to kill him.

Despite this moral condemnation of human betrayal, of preferring material gain to human companionship, the storyteller admires Tony's resolution, his sense of humor, his absolute energy and indomitable commitment to running very fast and hard toward this unattainable and worthless goal. No one in this gangster world is more selfless than Tony (for example, Johnny plotted Tony's death first). Tony just does what everyone else does, does his gangster's job, better than anyone else—quicker, surer, straighter. Because the gangster world is a bit like Wonderland, a topsy-turvy universe, separate from the real one, it also generates its own, opposite laws. But it is only a bit like Wonderland—and hence its collision with the social and moral laws of the real universe that surrounds it. Tony is the epitome of the very ethic of that opposite world, whose laws he articulated for Guino—doing it first, doing it himself, and keeping on doing it better than anyone else. Like Dr. Faustus or Barabas of Christopher Marlowe, Volpone or Mosca of Ben Jonson, or that first gangster hero, Shakespeare's Macbeth, Tony is so defiantly, exuberantly, and completely wrong, that there is something intriguing, engaging, even alluring about him. Hawks admires Tony's energetic means to his end; his vitality is quite the opposite of life at a "dead stop." It is Tony's end that necessarily leads to the "dead stop." Hawks's narrative problem in this film is communicating this paradoxically exuberant wrongness. The only way that Tony can preserve his gangster ethic, or that Hawks can tell his story of that world and that ethic, is by reducing people to objects.

Tony's error, however, is merely an exaggeration, a distortion, of a Hawks attitude toward human vocation that marks most of his films. The commitment to a vocation for Hawks is always a defiant response to the fact of human mortality. To commit oneself to work, to making or doing something (as Hawks commits himself to making films), is to believe that the work has significance and can somehow outlast or defy the finiteness of life and the infinity of time. The "World" can only be "Yours" by adding some *thing,* some material object, to the world that can endure beyond a human's death, simply because it is an "it"—a thing, a material object. The task of building the great pyramid that allows Pharaoh to "live" forever in *Land of the Pharaohs* is not so distant from the other kinds of work in the films of Howard Hawks— and the novels of William Faulkner, who wrote that script. (The Sutpen plantation in *Absalom! Absalom!,* for example, is another Pharaoh's tomb.) The film of *Scarface* is itself one of those things that has endured beyond the death of its maker. The commitment to work is an existential attempt to achieve the impossible, whether of possessing the world, building the great pyramid, flying the mails, acting on a stage, reporting for a newspaper, or devising a formula to make the old young again. But the commitment to work must never become so absolute and so perfect a yearning for the impossible (as it is for Tony Camonte) that it nullifies the possible if finite human attainments of personal, emotional, spiritual fulfillment—love and friendship. The Hawks film that most fully demonstrates that the conflicting claims of vocation, honor, love, and friendship can be balanced is *Only Angels Have Wings.*

Only Angels Have Wings was based on a story fragment that Hawks himself wrote in 1938, "Plane Four from Barranca," about a group of fliers who had migrated to South America because they could not fly elsewhere—outcasts because of troubles with the law, with drinking and smuggling, with accidents.[19] The four-page fragment introduced a location, situation, and collection of characters rather than told a story; very few of its suggestions found their way into the finished film. A man named "Tex" ran the outfit "the only way it could be run—by complete domination." In the film, Geoff Carter (Cary Grant) runs the airline that way, but Tex has become the name of the scout who merely serves as lookout in the mountain pass. In the fragment, Tex has just married Bonnie; in the film her name is still Bonnie (Jean Arthur), but her coming to accept Geoff's life and, by implication, share it with him becomes the basis of the film's narrative. In the fragment a new, inexperienced flier arrives with his wife, but he is not "good enough" so Geoff must do his job. In the film, the new arrival with his wife is an experienced flier who has not been good enough in the past but proves to be good enough now. From these fragments of people Hawks really knew and incidents he really witnessed arose the film of *Only Angels Have Wings*. Hawks went to talk to Frank Capra on the Columbia lot in 1939; Harry Cohn pulled him aside to ask him if he had a story for Cary Grant and Jean Arthur. Hawks sold Cohn on "Plane Four from Barranca" (still called "Plane Number Four" when shooting began).

Despite the fact that so many of the film's incidents are true (just as Hawks asked gangsters to tell him true stories that he could use in *Scarface*), critics have responded to the film as one of the most outlandish, incredible, and farfetched of Hawks's stories—hopelessly romantic, exotic, and fanciful. According to Frank S. Nugent's review of the film in the *New York Times:* "It is all very exciting and juvenile." [20] Like so many other films and filmmakers of the 1930s and 40s, Hawks and his films would prove to be far smarter than the smug reviewers, who originally chided the films for their stupidity.

But there is something about *Only Angels* that serves as a cutting edge in separating those who can and cannot enter the Hawks world with their minds and feelings. To put it simply, if you cannot admire Hawks's achievement in *Only Angels Have Wings,* you probably cannot admire Hawks, period. While *Scarface* is so easy to respect for its violence, its honesty, its humor, its energy (if so disturbing in its collusion with a moral freak), *Only Angels* demands a much greater willingness to suspend disbelief from its viewers, in return for which it rewards them richly. Just as *Scarface* played two opposite tones off against one another—murderous violence and childish glee—*Only Angels* plays two different opposites off against one another—indomitable, courageous defiance of one's mortality by literally flying into the face of mortality itself and warm, compassionate human feeling and sympathy that link all these mortals in their common (and ultimately hopeless) defiance.

While *Scarface* revealed a Hawks who was just discovering the elements of the Hawks world, *Only Angels Have Wings* displays that world fully sprung. Its indoor setting—the combination hotel and restaurant-bar with its communal eating, drinking, and talking area downstairs, more private sleeping and talking area upstairs—would dominate many Hawks films, from *The Dawn Patrol,* Hawks's first sound film, to *Barbary Coast, The Road to Glory, Only Angels Have Wings, To Have and Have Not, Rio Bravo, Hatari!,* and, in a modified form, *Red Line 7000* (a sign of the modern times, this late film's one-story motel and restaurant-bar cannot occupy the same building). The man behind the bar who owns the place is a comic father figure, often with a foreign accent (nicknamed Dutchy in *Only Angels,* Frenchy in *To Have and Have Not,* Carlos in *Rio Bravo*), whose business seems to survive not on his financial acumen but on his kindly conviviality. With the foreign-speaking Dutchy (Sig Rumann) Hawks manages to sneak one of his referential gags to the movie business into the film, the kind of in-group joke that delighted Hawks and those in the know in so many of his films but went totally unremarked by the uninitiated viewer. When Geoff Carter suggests that Dutchy himself will have to learn to fly one of the planes in his airline, Dutchy begs off by using Samuel Goldwyn's classic malapropism, "Include me out." And the character's heavy accent makes him even sound like Goldwyn.

The indoor texture of this restaurant and bar is dominated by the quality of light that illuminates it. Whereas *Scarface* was cloaked in its deliberately shadowed darkness, *Only Angels Have Wings* is bathed with the warm but limited glow of the kerosene hanging lamps, which push into Hawks's frame from the ceiling. Hawks claims that he got the idea for using lamps, visually establishing the source of illumination and the kind of illumination such lamps would produce, from American paintings—particularly those of Frederick Remington.[21] If there is a single formal feature that distinguishes a Hawks film visually from that of any other Hollywood director, it is its sensitivity to the particular sources (and consequent qualities) of light. This conscious reference to the sources, textures, and evocations of light itself is a very interesting choice to make in the cinema, which is dependent on light for its very existence, both as a photograph and as a projected show. These hanging lamps recur in many other Hawks films (*His Girl Friday, Red River,* and *Rio Bravo* use them most memorably); in *Only Angels Have Wings,* the kerosene lamps are responsible for the soft smoky glow of the indoor shots and the strikingly warm, soft beauty of silhouetted figures who stand outdoors, their bodies and faces defined by the smoky light behind them. These soft silhouettes contrast markedly with the stark, sharp shadows of *Scarface.* These hanging lamps define Dutchy's bar as "a clean, well-lighted place" (to use the title of a famous Hemingway story), a bright social and emotional refuge from the darkness and loneliness outdoors.

Dutchy's place (as even his name indicates) is also a society of nicknames—of those who call each other not by the given labels of their parents or the legal labels of society but by the labels which their own actions and mannerisms call forth in the group: Papa (Geoff's nickname), Kid, Dutchy, Sparks (the radio operator), Gent, Tex. The new flier, Bat, a man who killed his copilot (Kid's brother) and betrayed his vocation by bailing out of a damaged airplane, not only has no nickname; he has lost his name altogether, forced to change Kilgallen to MacPherson as a disguise to hide his past betrayal. These nicknames

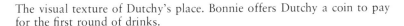

The visual texture of Dutchy's place. Bonnie offers Dutchy a coin to pay for the first round of drinks.

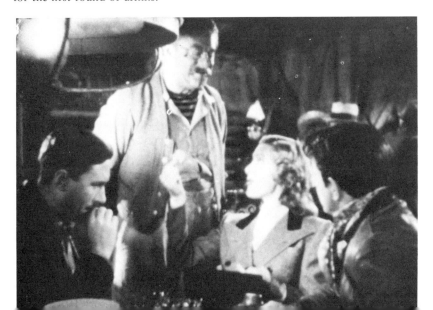

become the social cement that unites the people who work and live together in the films of Howard Hawks: Frenchy, Stumpy, Slim, Steve, Dude, Colorado, Pottsie, Feathers, Chips, Pockets, Cricket, Boofy. The later Hawks films even demonstrate the origins and derivations of these nicknames: the individual men in *Air Force* become a communal team as their societal names—Weinberg, Quincannon—melt into nicknames—Brooklyn, Irish; Alan Bedelian Traherne in *El Dorado* gets clipped to Mississippi; Anna Maria Dallesandro, the woman photographer in *Hatari!*, becomes the simple Dallas.

The social, personal, and professional familiarity between those who use these names in Hawks's films is, of course, mirrored by that same kind of familiarity within the social group making the film. The "Papa" who directs the airline enterprise in *Only Angels Have Wings* parallels the paternal authority figure who directs the filmmaking enterprise, revealing that any large social undertaking to accomplish a task (flying the mail, catching tuna, driving cattle, capturing wild animals) is a metaphor for another similarly large social undertaking—filmmaking. The parallel between flying and filmmaking in *Only Angels* is especially clear in the difference between Dutchy, who owns the airline and pays its bills, and Geoff, who runs the airline and controls its schedule. Dutchy is, in effect, the airline's studio boss (no wonder he sounds like Samuel Goldwyn) and Geoff Carter its director-producer.

This metaphoric link between making a film and undertaking any other vocational task that requires a lot of people, time, and effort, explains the special importance and beauty of those sequences in Hawks films which move outdoors, away from the shelter of the "well-lighted place," to show people brilliantly and thrillingly in the process of actually doing their jobs. In *Only Angels Have Wings*, this section is the spectacular flying sequence—in which the flying and the scenery and the photography are all spectacular—when the new flier with the false name passes the first test of an extremely dangerous and difficult assignment. Like the sequences of catching tuna in *Tiger Shark*, flying missions in *The Dawn Patrol* or *Air Force*, driving cattle in *Red River*, or capturing animals in *Hatari!*, the flying sequence is almost a documentary on the difficulties of the task and the methods of solving them, conveying to the uninformed viewer those difficulties as well as the exhilaration of doing that job well. But there is no way to catch tuna, drive cattle, or capture animals in a movie except actually to catch them, drive them,

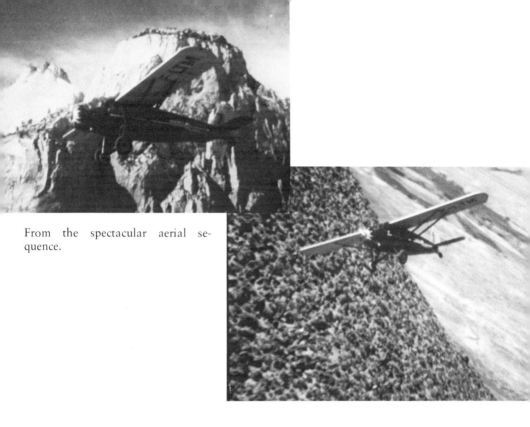

From the spectacular aerial sequence.

and capture them. And there is no way to shoot a dazzling flying sequence in a film except to film an airplane that flies dazzlingly in dazzlingly difficult surroundings. And no way to record this dazzling flight except with a second plane, so the camera itself must fly, observing the "star" performance of its second airplane self.

The authenticity of these vocational sequences in the films of Howard Hawks is one of their major visual beauties as well as one basis of their existential assertion that moving is living is doing. The analogue of the flying sequence in *Scarface* would be the two violent montage sequences, which only suggest the excitement of the gangster vocation metaphorically. While it is possible and acceptable for a camera literally to fly, even movies cannot kill people for the sake of art. The necessary participation of the camera in the vocational actions it records both produces one of the wonders of cinema (our ability to watch people actually doing what we never could actually see them do in reality) and reproduces for us outsiders the excitement and wonder for those people of doing what they do, and love to do, and do well.

Two motifs from *Scarface* return to *Only Angels Have Wings* in a fuller and firmer form. Music, though important in *Scarface* (particularly in defining the relationship of Guino and Cesca), becomes an essential psychological and tonal device of *Only Angels*. Hawks was always uncomfortable with the studio clichés of music, "twenty violins and fifteen cellos and winds, and all of that stuff,"[22] and he tried to avoid unmotivated musical underscoring (the background music that comes from no established source) as much as possible. *Scarface* uses none of this unmotivated music at all, and *Only Angels* uses it only once, during Kid's death scene. But *Only Angels* uses motivated music repeatedly to establish and develop crucial narrative information.

When Bonnie Lee from Brooklyn first drifts into exotic and distant Barranca, a musical number, "Chick-a-chee," defines not only her distance from that culture (she can only watch and listen as the people who live there sing) but also her willingness to appreciate and understand it (she attempts to join in the repetitive words of the song's refrain). When Bonnie feels upset by the death of Joe (Noah Beery, Jr.), the young flier, and even more upset that no one else seems upset about it, the men and musicians in Dutchy's bar drown out her sentimental questions with the overloud and comically derisive singing of the maudlin song, "Send Word to Mother." But when Bonnie comes to understand the men's courage and stoicism in the face of death, she herself leads the musicians in a rousing rendition of "Some of These Days," accompanying herself, like Cesca, at the piano. After this show of bravado, Bonnie begins to think again of the dead Joe, and she almost unconsciously (like Johnny Lovo with his saltshaker) begins to pick out the sorrowful melody of "Send Word to Mother" on the piano, the tune that the men used to razz her earlier, this time played feelingly and mournfully. Roused from this brief return to her mournful revery by a caustic comment from Geoff, Bonnie regains her composure by plunging into an exuberant chorus of "The Peanut Vendor." After a dissolve, however, the tune has melted into the placid "Liebestraum," setting the quiet mood for her first intimate conversation with Geoff. In *The Road to Glory*, Lt. Denet (Fredric March), also plays "Liebestraum"—but as a slimy means of sexual seduction. He self-assuredly tells his intended sexual target, "I'm establishing the mood. That's the only way to do it. Music." Hawks himself regularly uses music just as cunningly and deliberately to establish the mood.

Guino's flipping coin also returns to *Only Angels,* but it serves a much more central narrative function in the later film. The coin again belongs to a best friend, Kid (Thomas Mitchell), who flips it repeatedly throughout the film, not nervously and unconsciously as Guino flips his, but more pointedly and deliberately. The flipping coin does not suggest Guino's nervous energy beneath the cool exterior but Kid's conscious, measured sense of his assurance and control. This is the coin that Kid always uses to decide disputes with Geoff, decisions that always guarantee Kid will take the toughest jobs because the coin is two-headed. Geoff discovers Kid's strategy only late in the film, when Kid volunteers for a difficult mission if the coin comes up heads. As in *Scarface,* the coin continues to live after the friend's death. But after Kid's death, Geoff keeps the coin as the single material reminder of his friend's existence. He then passes the coin to Bonnie (the narrative journey of this material object foreshadows the journey of counterfeit money in *His Girl Friday* and the snake bracelet in *Red River*) at the film's conclusion: Geoff's way of "telling" her that he wants her to stay without using the words to tell her. He only tells her to stay if the coin comes up heads. Though Bonnie takes this flippancy as Geoff's ultimate rejection, his callous inability to respond to her or any woman, she discovers his love—as Geoff discovered Kid's—when she sees that the coin has two heads.

Both the use of music and of the coin reveal that *Only Angels Have Wings* is one of the most perfectly and elegantly symmetrical of Hawks's narrative constructions. Hawks and Jules Furthman use this symmetry to build what could be a wildly improbable and exotic tale into a solid structure of narrative logic. Everything in the film happens twice. There is music after the film's first death (Joe's) and music after the film's second death (Kid's)—except the musical passage there, mirroring Geoff's sorrow for a death that cuts much more deeply, is not "Some of These Days" or "The Peanut Vendor" but mournful singing and the melancholy strumming of a solo guitar. This guitar underscores the delicate "whispering" scene between Bonnie and Sparks, although no one can overhear them; Hawks is still using music "to establish the mood." After the death of Joe, Geoff and Sparks pick through the dead man's material belongings, the mortal remains of his life, from which Bonnie selects the piece of jewelry she will give to Lily, Joe's grieving woman. After the film's second death, Geoff and Sparks pick through Kid's things in the same way, from which Geoff selects the two-headed coin he will give to Bonnie, his woman.

Early in the film Geoff pours water over his head to sober himself up for a flight; late in the film he pours water over the head of a drunken Judy, the woman from his past, now married to Kilgallen, to sober her up. Early in the film Kid interrupts the first intimate scene between Geoff and Bonnie to summon him for a flight; late in the film he interrupts an even more intimate scene between them for the same purpose. Both interruptions are followed by the need for coffee. The two flights that produce the two deaths are both built around the recitation of numbers—calling out the figures that indicate the plane's altitude; in the early scene Joe calls out his altitude as his plane nears the ground, but in the late one Kid calls out his altitude as his plane attempts to fly over the fog in the pass. There are two wagers between men to decide who will fly and who will remain on the ground—between Joe and Les after they first meet Bonnie and between Kid and Geoff in the scene when Geoff discovers that the coin has two heads. There are two conversations between Bonnie and Sparks—early and late—in which he helps put her in touch with Geoff's and her own feelings. And there are two scenes in which Bonnie decides to leave on the next boat—early and late—and both times she changes her mind and stays. Hawks emphasizes the symmetry by Bonnie's wearing the same tight-fitting suit in both—the suit she wore when she first arrived in Barranca—that contrasts with the loose-fitting clothes she has worn since her arrival. When Bonnie Lee initially comes to Dutchy's she produces a coin to pay for the first round of drinks; in the film's final scene at Dutchy's she receives the two-headed coin that will keep her there.

Such careful and deliberate patterning reveals the way that Hawks views narrative construction; one makes a fictional event credible not by its mundane ordinariness but by its preparation, making it grow from what has happened before. The same attitude dictates the shape of the narrative as a whole, which duplicates the four-part structure of *Scarface*. The first section introduces a newcomer from America to the foreign culture of Barranca and the foreign values of flying: Bonnie, who comes to this new world with our values and from our culture, serves as our means to enter it. Bonnie falls for Geoff, the leader of the fliers and the epitome of that world's values, and the difficulty that separates them is precisely the gulf between her world (which is our world) and his.

The second section introduces a second set of newcomers, "Mac-Pherson" and Judy, but neither of them is really a newcomer. Mac-Pherson's real name is Kilgallen, the man responsible for the death of Kid's brother, while Judy is the woman who burned Geoff before and the kind of woman he refuses to be burned by again. The third section settles the tensions between Geoff, Judy, Kid, and "MacPherson" (just as the third section of *Scarface* settles the lesser of the film's two narrative tensions). Like the third section of *Scarface* it ends with a death, but the death of Kid reaffirms the rehabilitation of MacPherson-Kilgallen. And the fourth section must resolve the relationship between Geoff and Bonnie, overseen, in effect, by the spiritual presence of the dead Kid in the material form of his two-headed coin. Even the film's overall narrative pattern is perfectly symmetrical: the end sections, one and four, devoted to Geoff and Bonnie; the middle sections, two and three, devoted to Geoff, Judy, Kid, and "MacPherson" while Bonnie casually hangs around.

As opposed to the newcomers he found for *Scarface,* Hawks began *Only Angels* knowing he was going to make the film with (or "for" as Harry Cohn would have it) Cary Grant and Jean Arthur, two established stars. There is a sense in which both of these stars are "wrong" for the roles—Grant too smooth, suave, and slight for the tough Geoff, Arthur too warm, sweet, and pure for the Bonnie who's been around. Rather than erasing this potential "wrongness," Hawks capitalizes on it, allowing what's wrong about them for the roles to reshape the roles (*i.e.* the characters) so they become right for the stars. In their very first meeting, when Geoff-Grant walks over to Bonnie-Arthur's table and, without asking permission, takes her cigarette to light his own (he never uses his own match to light his cigarette), it is obvious that both of these characters are "queer ducks." Two identical interchanges between them (more patterning), early and late in the film, establish this metaphor explicitly: "You're a queer duck"; "So are you." The casting of Grant and Arthur in these "off-roles" makes these ducks even queerer.

Hawks is quite outspoken about his troubles with Jean Arthur during shooting:

> Jean Arthur was very difficult to work with. She didn't understand until after the film was done what it was I wanted—which was Bacall.[23]

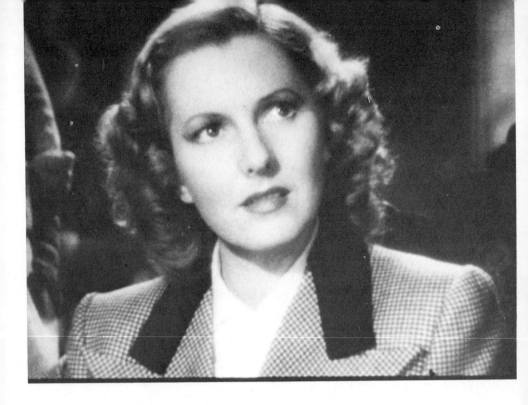

Bonnie and Geoff: The first closeups.

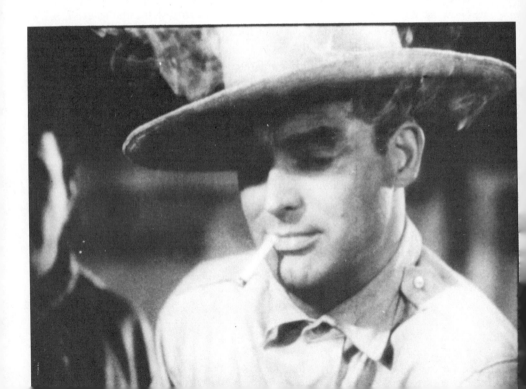

She didn't fit into the kind of girl that I liked and she'd simply
say, "I can't do that kind of stuff." When the picture was over
I said, "Jean, I think you're the only person I've ever worked
with that I don't think I helped a bit." [24]

But then Jean Arthur was difficult for everyone to work with, and no
director (even Capra) felt he could help her much. Part of the Arthur
persona is her sexual purity, her chastity, as opposed to Bacall's sultry
seductiveness. Another is her helplessness, her vulnerability, as opposed
to Bacall's cool and complete control. Jean Arthur seems to be made of
very thin glass that will shatter at the slightest touch; her calm, controlled surface is a desperate disguise that at any moment may dissolve
and melt into a pool of tears. Part of Hawks's gift in wedding a star
persona to a fictional character can be seen in his not forcing Jean Arthur to be Bacall but in letting her be Jean Arthur (but then part of
Jean Arthur's gift was that no one could make her be anything else).

For example, Hawks wanted Bonnie to show her nervousness in
Geoff's presence by unconsciously mishandling her silverware while
eating breakfast. Geoff has just arrived back from a flight to discover
Bonnie Lee calmly eating eggs and drinking coffee; she has not left on
the boat after all. To show that she is flustered and embarrassed (for
there is only one reason why she stayed—Geoff—and he knows it),
Hawks asked her to butter her bread with her spoon, stir her coffee
with her fork, the typical Hawks method of transferring feeling unconsciously to material objects. Jean Arthur would have none of it.

"I can't do that," she said. I said, "Don't you want to try?"
"No. It would just upset me." So what the hell. I just gave up.
And, you know, she's *good*. [25]

Instead of upsetting her (and when Jean Arthur was upset not only the
character melted into tears; the actress took to her dressing room and
refused to come out), Hawks lets her do the scene her way. She starts
chewing her food very slowly, her eyes glance away, the fingers of her
left hand begin to play an invisible arpeggio in the air, and she then
plunges into a long explanation that the Bonnie Lee whom Geoff sees,
the one who stayed, is not really her at all but "must be some other
fella." This is one of the lines that seems as carefully tailored for Jean

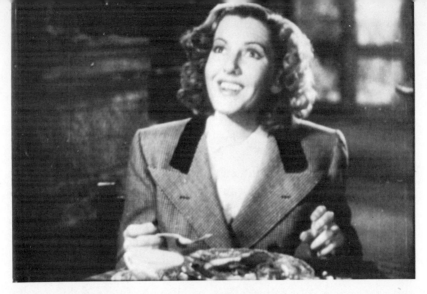

Jean Arthur doing it her way: her cheerful nervousness.

Arthur as her tight-fitting suit. Can you imagine Bacall—or any other female star of the period—referring to herself as a "fella"?

And then, Jean Arthur was not playing against Humphrey Bogart (whom Hawks specifically selected as a sarcastic foil for Bacall's own sultry sarcasm) but Cary Grant, who is far softer, much lighter, and much more obviously vulnerable than Bogart. The casting of the softer, warmer Thomas Mitchell in the friend's role as opposed to the quirky, jerky Walter Brennan of *To Have and Have Not* is another consistent choice in the same key. Thomas Mitchell is always the feeling friend, Brennan the thinking friend. The Grant-Arthur-Mitchell trio simply makes much mellower, sweeter music than the sharper, brasher Bogart–Bacall–Brennan trio. Hawks clearly casts his films not for individual players but for harmonious ensembles of emotional tone, texture, color, and intensity. The characteristic that makes both of these "off-roles" for Arthur and Grant is that the surface traits of the characters (Bonnie as shady drifter, Geoff as indomitably hard) are not congruent with their personas, evocations, and "music" as stars. Ultimately this counterpoint between their personalities as stars and their traits as characters enriches, enlivens, softens, and warms the film, despite a possible Hawks preference for the toughness and hardness of *To Have and Have Not*. The credibility of their ultimate union at the film's climax depends on our sensing of their spiritual unity throughout, their soft feelings beneath the tough surfaces. It is difficult to imagine any Hollywood star

116

of the period other than Jean Arthur who could simultaneously convey her surprise, delight, and consent at the end of this narrative simply by calling out, "Hey!"

After the brief and tense interchange of cigarettes, the first major clash between Geoff and Bonnie establishes the essential emotional gulf that separates them: it reveals itself in their differing reactions to the death of Joe, the major event of the narrative's first section. Hawks's mastery of both storytelling and cinema can be seen in the subtle choice he makes in depicting this essential death—a death that is important (since it provokes the clash of values that divides Geoff and Bonnie, on which their story is built) but not supremely important (since it is a mere starting point of the story, and since Joe is a minor character, and since there will be a far more important second death later in the film). Hawks's narrative strategy, then, becomes to depict Joe's death without actually depicting it, by narrating it verbally, keeping his camera with the people on the ground, not with the flier in the air. The death of Joe seems a terrible mistake on purely visual grounds, since Hawks does not allow us to *see* anything of it; he merely tells us about what is happening off-frame with mere words (as the puttering sounds of the plane's motor invades the visual space). The camera watches Geoff, Kid, and the others as they watch for Joe's plane in the fog. The primary action in the frame for several minutes is talking—Geoff giving Joe advice about the landing, aided by Kid's observations; Joe calling out the numbers, like a litany, of his plane's altitude: "800 . . . 600 . . . 400" and so forth.

But Hawks's choice of telling rather than showing this death is brilliant on two narrative grounds. First, it is a classic demonstration of the power of narrative's appeal to the imagination. We imagine what we cannot see, our minds stimulated by the words. Our inability to see Joe at all parallels the blindness of Geoff and the other characters, who can hear Joe's voice (just as he can hear Geoff's) but cannot see him, separated from his physical presence by the fog. The frame line mirrors the isolation of the man in the air from the community on the ground.

Second, such a parallel again demonstrates Hawks's masterful control of point-of-view, which keeps the narrative focus where it belongs: with the major characters on the ground—Geoff, Kid, and Bonnie—not with the minor character in the air. That focus is sharpened by Hawks's visual arrangement of these major characters into groups: Geoff with

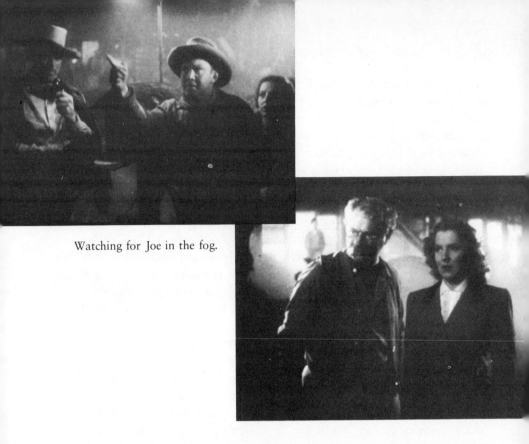

Watching for Joe in the fog.

Kid, who supports his friend by giving him an inevitable cigarette and draping a jacket around his shoulders; Bonnie with another outsider, Dutchy, who does not think as his fliers do; Lily, Joe's woman, wandering unattached between the groups—since she is both so affected by and so irrelevant to the event.[26] Hawks tones the scene visually with the soft silhouettes in the fog, back-lit from the kerosense lamps indoors. And he tones it aurally by eliminating the music altogether (Geoff pointedly tells the piano we hear in the background to stop, and "Turkey in the Straw" abruptly ends), a musical silence that is another example of "establishing the mood" and of concentrating absolute attention on a duet for spoken word and airplane motor.

The reactions to this death define the differences between the values of Geoff and Bonnie. His reaction seems a laconic fatalism. "Joe died flying, didn't he? He just wasn't good enough." The remark parallels a reaction Hawks himself made when hearing that one of the best aerial stuntmen in Hollywood, Paul Mantz, who worked on every Hawks flying film, was killed during the filming of *The Flight of the Phoenix:* "Well, we all get killed sooner or later."[27] But that this fatalism is at least partially a camouflage for Geoff's real feelings becomes clear in several of his actions and reactions that betray his words. First, Kid very meaningfully and shakily lights Geoff another cigarette and hands it to him just after the crash—when Geoff himself seems paralyzed and cannot move. Second, Hawks keeps his camera paralyzed as well; like Geoff and Kid it cannot move for the longest time, savoring the suffused, silhouetted, foggy setting long after the plane has crashed, sustaining the quiet and melancholy mood. Third, there is some truth to Geoff's claim that Joe wasn't good enough, since the young man brashly and rashly disobeyed Geoff's orders to stay up in the air and wait for the fog to clear. Characters usually get into trouble in Hawks's films when they disobey the orders of the wiser leader (for example, de Bursac gets shot in the shoulder in *To Have and Have Not* when he disregards Harry Morgan's order to stay down). Indeed, Kid dies in this film just as Joe does, disregarding Geoff's order to turn back (still more patterning); "MacPherson," however, shows his mettle, after disagreeing with Geoff's decision to dump a load of nitroglycerin, by then doing as he has been instructed. Finally, Geoff betrays his feelings when he tells Dutchy to send Joe's sister the hundred dollars he owes him, which leads Dutchy to remark that Geoff didn't owe Joe any money. Geoff betrays his genuine feelings after a death (as Dunson does in *Red River*

Kid lighting a cigarette for the stricken Geoff.

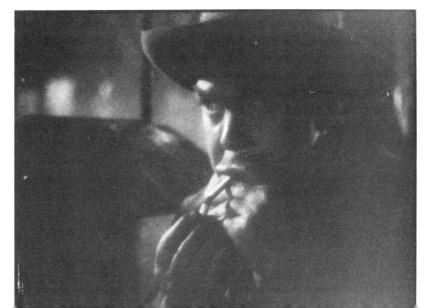

after the death of Dan Lattimer) by wanting to send some material token of appreciation to a survivor.

Bonnie Lee sees only the cold, unfeeling side of Geoff's reaction.
She searches desperately for a reason—for *the* reason: why does anyone
want to fly? Why was this death necessary? She wonders if it has been
her fault; Joe specifically defied Geoff's orders because he wanted to eat
the steak he had ordered for Bonnie and himself. Geoff's response seems
disturbingly cruel in its reduction of her question to the absurd: "Sure
it was your fault. You were gonna have dinner with him, the Dutchman
hired him, I sent him up on schedule, the fog came in, a tree got in the
way. All your fault." Behind this recitation of facts, reasons, and responsibilities lies its existential premise and the very basis of this life of
flying against death to begin with: "we all get killed sooner or later."
Geoff caps his verbal assertion with a pragmatic act: he begins to eat
the very steak Joe ordered. Bonnie asks, "How can you do that?" "Look,
what do you want me to do? Have it stuffed?"

Geoff's response makes a pragmatic sense that attacks Bonnie's
symbolic memorializing of the steak: that it should somehow be treated
with respect as a memorial to the man who is no longer there (which,
of course, is precisely the conventional way society objectifies the ab-
straction of death with commemorative symbols such as tombstones
and cemeteries). There is an immense disparity between the vitality of a
human life and those material objects which can commemorate or symbolize that life (hence the failure of those pathetic trinkets to add up to
the dead Joe). There is no way that a steak can properly symbolize Joe;
might as well keep it a steak and eat it. Bonnie's sentimental symboliz-
ing is therefore drowned out by the razzing rendition of that patheti-
cally sentimental song. But the film makes it quite clear that the men
maintain this pragmatic detachment from the kinds of feelings Bonnie
expresses and the kinds of symbols she respects, not because they lack
those feelings but because to surrender to them would make it impossible for them to continue flying. Geoff, in fact, does surrender to them
after the death of Kid—both by weeping and by keeping a memorial
symbol, which will serve a pragmatic function after all.

The conversation that follows between Bonnie and Sparks (then
joined by Kid) allows her to make more rational sense of her feelings
and her reactions to Geoff's feelings. She admits to Sparks that she
never liked to treat death symbolically and sentimentally, that she never

cared for funerals. "All the fuss and bother never brings anybody back." Sparks makes an admirable confidant because he too is an outsider, the man at the radio, not in the air (just as Groot in *Red River* is the cook on the wagon, not a cowboy on a horse). Sparks never could see "any future" in flying. But when Bonnie tells Sparks and Kid that her own father was a tightrope artist who never used a net, Sparks ironically replies, "Not much future in that either." The conversation allows Bonnie to return to the group inside and join them in song—in effect, accepting their pragmatic rather than symbolic response to the death of a comrade. It also begins Kid's admiration and affection for her (Hawks's typical use of the friend to indicate the value and the future direction of the film's central relationship). And it introduces the thematic conflict between the life of flying—based purely on the immediacy and ephemerality of the present—and the life of permanent human relationships—based on hopes and plans for the future.

This conflict between present and future becomes the basis of Bonnie's subsequent conversation with Geoff. He asks, "Did you ever know a woman who didn't want to make plans?" Her reply is also a question, "What if she were the type who didn't scare so easily?" These two questions become the basis of the narrative that follows. She must come to accept Geoff's values if she wants Geoff, for to change Geoff would be to kill him in a way that would be worse than the death of Joe, who died flying. As Kid asks when she watches Geoff take off, "What do you want to do? Put a net under him?" Again Hawks prefers the subtextual indirectness of questions to the explicitness of statements. The first section closes when she decides to stay and find out the answers to some of these questions.

As in *Scarface* and every carefully built Hawks narrative, the end of this tale is in its beginning. The conflict between Geoff and Bonnie (which is really a surface conflict of social and moral values rather than of internal feelings) dictates the type and the terms of the discovery that each will make. Neither of them needs to discover the values underlying their own lives or the life of the other; they know those by the end of the film's first section. What they must discover is whether their feelings for one another can overcome this conflict of values, whether their feelings are more important than the values. This discovery cannot be made in a flash (like Tony's discovery after the murder of Guino); it can only evolve over a period of time; they must come to feel comfortable enough with one another, get used to being around one another. The process underlying this gradual discovery, which is typical of the best films of Hawks (and especially subtle and complex in the Furthman scripts as opposed to the Hecht scripts), might be called the "Evolution of Trust."

Bonnie must discover that trust by overcoming her squeamishness, by hanging around, just to find out how it feels to see her man take off, not knowing if he will ever return. Geoff must discover that trust by overcoming his stubbornness and growing more comfortable with Bonnie's just being around. As he tells her, "Look, I didn't ask you to stay. I wouldn't ask. . . ." Her response cuts him off, "I know. You wouldn't ask any woman to do anything." This unbending stubbornness will return with Thomas Dunson in *Red River*. Geoff has been burned before because he made the mistake of believing that a woman could come to accept a life with him as a flier. He suspects (and he uses this suspicion to protect himself from being burned again) that flying and women—living in the present and living for the future—are mutually exclusive. Geoff has already decided against using Bonnie as a mere sexual accessory—the only kind of relationship with a woman that is surely bounded by the present. Bonnie must prove to Geoff that she can love him in and for the present. (She had already responded to his sexual proposition with a simple, "Sure.") Only then can Geoff assent to the fact that affections in the present roll inexorably into the future. These evolutions of trust in the films of Howard Hawks, always interdependent and communal, never articulated verbally, usually depict the growth of comfort through the ability to hang around and share jokes.

With the arrival of the newcomers who are not newcomers in the second section we meet two characters who are "dead" in the way that Geoff would also "die" if he were to alter his life and values. That deadness is apparent in Bat Kilgallen's (Richard Barthelmess) loss of his name, the loss of his reputation for being able to do the job he can and wants to do, in his wife Judy's (Rita Hayworth) excessive drinking, and in the fact that neither has told the other about their pasts. He hasn't told her that he is Kilgallen, and she hasn't told him about Geoff. Geoff recognizes Kilgallen right away, but it takes Kid some time. He returns from a flight, asks, "Who's got a match?", and only then recognizes the man who killed his brother. As Kid moves threateningly toward him, Geoff suddenly strikes a match near Kid's face. The simple act of striking the match serves as a kindly warning for Kid to control his emotions, "telling" him to regain his composure without saying anything at all. The match does its job: "I'm all right."

From this point of arrival, the two primary events of the second section are Kilgallen's proving himself worthy of a permanent job and Kid's eyes proving him unworthy of any more flying. Kilgallen in effect replaces Kid as Geoff's most dependable pilot. A mining accident in very rugged terrain requires the emergency use of one of Geoff's planes to fly the injured man, the son of the mine's rich owner, to a hospital. Geoff gives Kilgallen the dangerous job, not willing to risk any of his other men on it. A doctor will accompany him, and when the doctor, who speaks only Spanish, is asked if he is willing to risk the danger, he energetically declaims a stirring speech from *Henry IV, Part 2* in Spanish, which Sparks must translate (Sparks is the interpreter—again the source of communication, not the man of action): "A man can die only once. We owe God a debt. If we pay it today, we don't owe it tomorrow." Kilgallen's response to the translated recitation reveals his own awareness of its application to his own life: "He's no fool."

Although the Shakespearean quote and play are obviously relevant to the values of both Hawks and the fliers of this film, Hawks treats the quotation with a playful irony that softens its blatancy and tempers its explicitness. First, while the doctor declaims loudly in Spanish (converting the speech into a jumble of sounds, of verbal music, as opposed to a series of intelligible words), Geoff goes over a map of the area and terrain with Kilgallen in English. The two languages (English and Spanish) and the two kinds of human speech (pragmatic strategy and de-

Contrapuntal conversations.

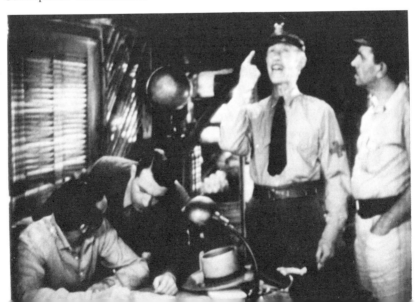

clamatory oration) on opposite sides of the same frame play against one another contrapuntally and cacophonously.

Second, although the quotation mirrors the film's ringing defiance of mortality, a Shakespearean heightening of the more oblique, Hemingwayesque, "We all get killed sooner or later," the line translated by Sparks has been yanked from a highly ironic context. The line is not delivered by a pure character of courage and honor, like Hotspur in *Henry IV, Part 1*, or even by Prince Hal in one of his kingly moments before battle. The line belongs to a minor clown named Feeble (*Henry IV, Part 2*, III, 2, 255), a "woman's tailor" (*i.e.* dress designer), an occupation, then as now, not particularly associated with the stereotypes of masculinity or courage. Feeble has just been forced into service by the play's great clown, Falstaff, and even Feeble's assertion of bluff courage parodies Falstaff's interchange with Hal in *Henry IV, Part I*. "Thou owest God a death," says Hal; "Tis not due yet," Falstaff replies. "I would be loath to pay him before his day." Falstaff, for whom "the better part of valor is discretion," intends to avoid paying his debt to God for as long as he can—just as Kilgallen did when he bailed out of his plane.

When Kilgallen returns successfully from this flight (the sequence in the film that uses the spectacular aerial photography), Geoff offers him a permanent job, though it means his taking all the assignments that are too dangerous for anyone else. Kilgallen's answer: "I don't know any other way I'd want it." Although Geoff is obviously pleased with Kilgallen's performance (he smiles to himself when Kilgallen radios he has landed and taken off again successfully), he refuses to say anything to him on his return other than, "What you want me to do? Pat you on the back?" And although Geoff has a match in his mouth, he pointedly refuses to light Kilgallen's cigarette, as he does Kid's, upon his return from a flight. That act of acceptance can occur only when Kilgallen has thoroughly earned it (just as Matthew Garth must earn the right to add his initial to the Red River D brand).

The encounter with Kilgallen also triggers Geoff's suspicions about Kid's eyes, unable to recognize this marked man immediately. Because Kid has memorized all the charts for eye tests, including the new one that Geoff just received in the mail, he asks Kid to line up two pins in a special box devised for this test. Hawks's control of point-of-view is again masterful at conveying both the information and the emotion of

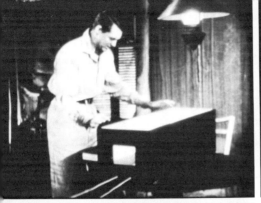
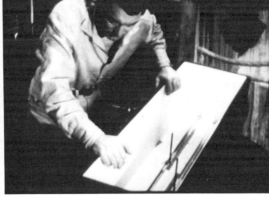

The eye test: metaphor for cinema perception.

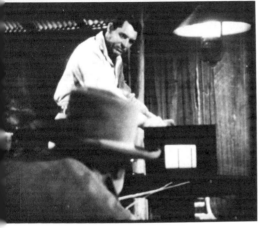

the moment. First, Hawks gives us a shot from a high angle, over Geoff's shoulder, presenting a clear view of the box and its design from Geoff's point-of-view, its two pins obviously far apart. Then Hawks cuts to Kid's point-of-view, over his shoulder, giving us his mistaken visual perception that the two pins are perfectly aligned. By giving us both points-of-view the storyteller not only conveys the different ways that the two men see but engages our sympathies with both ways of seeing, with Geoff's correct perception and Kid's desperate attempt to prove that he can perceive correctly when he cannot.

The two shots also give a clear indication of Hawks's conscious awareness of the cinema's visual processes and potentials. The little box is itself a reference to cinema—illuminated by a single bulb, a monochromatic contrast of black pins within a white setting, a clearly outlined black frame within which space is paradoxically three- and two-dimensional. A shot from Kid's point-of-view, organized in this way, cannot fail to flatten our perception of the actual distance between two such pins in such a box. The monocular cinema eye cannot perceive the subtle gradations of depth that can be perceived by human bifocal vision. Hawks can convey Kid's point-of-view without a predictable blurring of the focus of his lens; even a crisp, deep-focus shot (as this shot is) from this angle, at this distance from the box, could not differentiate the minute gradations of depth between the two pins. This is another of those Hawks shots whose point-of-view is complexly and simultaneously objective and subjective.

Geoff must now give Kid the results of this test, and his method foreshadows the even more terrible result he delivers after the later plane crash. He gives Kid the truth in a simple, four-word declarative sentence: "You're through flying, Kid." Kid's response is one of those Hawks understatements that "says" much more than it says: "Uh huh. After twenty-two years." Geoff explains that he cannot take chances, that he now needs Kilgallen despite the man's past, and that Dutchy's airline will win a necessary and permanent government mail contract if it can continue to keep flying the mail on schedule for one more week (this is the narrative thread on which the later sections of the film hang). The two men stand with their backs to one another; neither can quite bear to look the other in the eyes; their physical positions also "say" more than their words. Kid continues to toss his coin, saying little. And when Kid leaves the room, leaving Geoff alone, he transfers his sorrow for what he has been forced to do to a friend, and his anger at the necessity of doing it, to a simple physical object: he suddenly and violently kicks the chair on which Kid sat during the eye test, knocking it

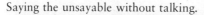

Saying the unsayable without talking.

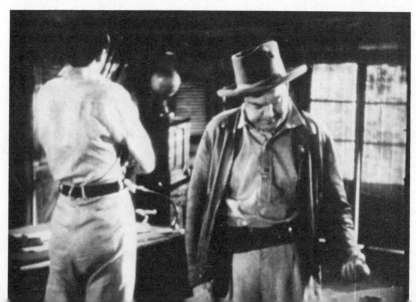

to the ground, as if the chair has been responsible for both Kid's mortal infirmity and Geoff's discovery of it.

The third section of the film weaves these strands more tightly together. Bonnie becomes more comfortable, living with the ever-present danger to Geoff's life, while Geoff becomes more comfortable with her, sharing their moments of humor. As he walks into his room, he sees a coffee pot on the boil. "What's all this? . . . All this cooking?" And there is comic distaste in his use of this most domestic of words. When he burns himself on the coffee pot, Jean Arthur wryly observes, "I thought you never did that." "Did what?" "Got burned twice in the same place." A heel has broken off Bonnie's shoe (just as Susan Vance loses a heel in *Bringing Up Baby*), and she remarks playfully: "Don't I have the darnedest luck? Losing one heel after another." And in this scene in Geoff's room Bonnie makes an open confession of her conversion: "I'm not trying to tie you down. I don't want to plan. I don't want to look ahead. I don't want you to change anything. I love you, Geoff. There's nothing I can do about it. I just love you." (Who else but Jean Arthur could turn this choppy, clipped, halting string of brief declarative sentences into a symphony of sincere emotion?)

The third section concludes when Kid and Kilgallen must share the final flight that will clinch Dutchy's government contract because all the other fliers have been disabled. Les (Allyn Joslyn) broke his arm in a fight, Geoff fired Gent for his refusal to fly a load of nitroglycerin, and Geoff himself has a damaged shoulder because Bonnie accidentally put a bullet in it. (A lot of knots must be tied in this slender narrative thread to get Kid back in the air, one last time, and with the hated Kilgallen.) The two fliers hope to use the power of the new trimotor plane to fly above the fog that chokes the pass. As they climb steadily higher, Kid calls out the numbers for Geoff on the radio, just as Joe did earlier. When the two pilots discover that the plane simply cannot fly high enough, Geoff orders them to return. But Kid presses on—like Joe, claiming to be able to see what he cannot. Kid's claim is never really tested; a huge condor, one of the birds established earlier to be roosting in the pass, crashes into the plane, seriously injuring both Kid and the aircraft, setting two of its three motors afire. When the injured Kid tells "MacPherson" to grab a parachute and jump, this time Kilgallen refuses to abandon his plane and his co-pilot. He stays with the burning ship, brings it safely back to the airfield (where, for a second time in the film, the whole group has poured outdoors to watch for it, just as they did for Joe), and brings it safely down. The injured Kid is carried from the wreckage along with the badly burned Kilgallen.

As Kid lies silhouetted in the darkness, unable to move, he asks "Papa" for a drag on a cigarette, that inevitable object of human communion. Geoff once again gives Kid the hard fact of his physical condition in another simple, four-word declarative sentence: "Your neck's broken, Kid." Kid takes the news as stoically as he did before—but he asks everyone to leave him alone in the darkness. "You want me to go too?" Geoff asks. Kid explains that he isn't afraid; but the experience is like his first "solo"—he's doing something new and he doesn't know how "good" he'll be at it. Geoff discreetly leaves his friend alone with a last cigarette to face the inevitable mortal fact which these fliers devote their lives to defying. Geoff later informs Tex (Donald Barry), the lookout in the pass, over the radio: "Broke his neck. Took off a few minutes ago." Even his euphemism for death is a metaphor for flying (a metaphor which Hawks extends with the death of Quincannon in *Air Force*).

But the flight that led to the death of Kid has led to the rebirth of Kilgallen, the one flier rising from the ashes of the other. (Hawks is aware of the myth of the phoenix; there is a joke based on it in *Monkey Business*.) When Kilgallen returns to Dutchy's bar, his hands bandaged, the men welcome him into the circle of their friendship, and Geoff buys him a drink ordered for him by the dying Kid (a parallel with Joe's steak). One of the men even lights Kilgallen's cigarette for him, since the man with the bandaged hands is unable to light his own. Kilgallen has earned his way back into the society of fliers and into the respect and admiration of that society's "Papa." Further, he and Judy have both expressed their trust in one another by each confessing the past. Those pasts cannot be erased, but they can at least be acknowledged. This acknowledgment is the only way a life in the present and future can be freed from the past.

The film's brief fourth section must concern itself with the present and future of Geoff and Bonnie, to discover if their present and future can acknowledge their pasts. There are two specific narrative issues: will Dutchy's airline get its contract? and will Bonnie Lee leave Geoff or stay with him (an echo of the leaving motif in the death of Kid)? Hawks resolves the two issues simultaneously. Tex radios that the pass is clearing up, an announcement which leads Les and Geoff, with one good arm each, to take the final flight together. The motif of two mutually sustaining cripples returns three decades later with the final comic image of *El Dorado*, the crippled Wayne and Mitchum limping together down the street of the western town. Bonnie Lee must decide, for a second and final time, whether to stay with Geoff or climb back aboard the boat. The fact that she came after Geoff with a pistol to keep him on the ground shows that her trust can evolve no further; she can never accept his life completely. There will always be the worry and the fear. She, like Kid, will "go nuts." Geoff must now move a bit toward her.

She asks him directly: "Do you want me to stay or don't you?" Geoff flippantly tosses Kid's coin: "Tails you go, heads you stay." "I won't stay that way. I'm hard to get, Geoff. All you have to do is ask me." Geoff continues his flipping and his flippancy, bidding her farewell by means of their running joke: "So long, Bonnie. Keep that coffee warm." Left alone, Bonnie nervously plays with the coin Geoff has left in her palm, and then she looks at it (just as Johnny Lovo first plays unconsciously with the saltshaker, then looks at it to make his discovery). This time Bonnie can't find the explicit words for her discovery: "Hey! Hey, Geoff!" And as she stares out the door through the driving rain at Geoff's plane, taxiing down the runway, the very lift of that plane off the ground translates the lift of her spirits (and the rise in our own) into the concrete visual metaphor of flight.

Only Angels Have Wings serves as a critical test of reactions to Hawks's style and work because its many beauties do not disguise, but exist in spite of, its many problems. There is a great geographical vagueness about exactly where the pass is (and how far away it is) in relation to the airstrip. The use of Tex, the radio lookout in the pass, is narratively functional but visually clumsy (his lookout ledge appears to be made of purest *papier mâché*). Hawks apparently found some of the scenes inside Tex's cabin so visually inert that he added an irrelevantly vital and comic touch, a donkey who seems to be Tex's sole companion and who pokes a playful nose into several visually dead frames. And then, of course, there are those condors. True enough, condors do exist in South American mountain passes, and Hawks tries to make their fatal collision with the airplane probable by referring to them when Kilgallen dumps the load of nitroglycerin, an action which has no function other than to make their later destruction of the trimotor more probable. But there is also a sense that these are birdies *ex machina* whom Hawks employs solely so they can bash into that flying *machina* at the worst possible moment. Finally, there is a difficulty with the central narrative problem of nice old Dutchy's needing the permanent contract, or he will go broke and this entire society of aviators, as well as Dutchy's "clean, well-lighted place," will vanish from the earth. Too much seems to hang on this slender thread and too many knots must be tied in it to keep them all hanging there.

What one can ask of a narrative is that if you do grant it its premises and probabilities, does it give you enough back in return. One can see the literal action of *Only Angels Have Wings*—the lookout pass, the condors, the mail contract, and all the disabled fliers—as a mere pretext for the real metaphoric interests of the narrative. The real story of *Only Angels* is the subtextual evolution of trust between Geoff Carter and Bonnie Lee, played against a background of vocational commitment, existential assertion, and male camaraderie. Seen in this manner, the film plays upon such essential human issues as the moral and emotional dynamics of vocational commitment and personal relationships, the existential defiance of mortality when mortality is inevitable and unavoidable, and the expressing of feelings by actions rather than talk. As opposed to Shakespeare's *Henry IV*, which the film deliberately and playfully quotes, *Only Angels Have Wings* reveals that the conflicting claims of love and honor, friendship and vocation can be synthesized. Romantic love and the vocation of honor are not antithetical pursuits—as in Hotspur's farewell to his wife, Kate (*Henry IV, Part I*, II, 3); nor are male companionship and the pursuit of honor (as in Hal's necessary separation from Falstaff to do battle with Hotspur). Not even love and friendship are antithetical—as they are in so many classical dramas that pose the conflict of love and honor. In *Only Angels Have Wings* their compatability is clear in the friend's affection for the lover and the lover's becoming a spiritual extension (and replacement) of the dead friend (with his coin), both friend and lover to the vocational man. Geoff realized the difficulties of being simultaneously a good lover, a good friend, and a good "Papa"—so well that he erected emotional barriers against such a synthesis, which required a partner who could herself be both friend and lover. Geoff Carter and Bonnie Lee transcend these barriers together to achieve that human synthesis.

The shift of the film's title—from the descriptive "Plane Number

Four" to the metaphoric *Only Angels Have Wings*—justifies a metaphoric reading of the film's action. That title sounds very much as if it must be some kind of quote, somewhat Biblical, somewhat Shakespearean, but somewhat modern in its terse obliqueness (like "The Sun Also Rises"). The literal title of the film, as it appears on the film's title card, is "—only angels have wings": in lower case, with both a dash—implying that the four words come at the end of a longer passage—and quotation marks. After a fairly careful search, however, I can find no such passage.[28] Perhaps the phrase derives from some favorite but not very familiar literary source; or perhaps the quotation is a ruse (dash, quotation marks, and all), a deliberate attempt to evoke a literary conceit (like Pope's "Angels fear to tread") but invented totally afresh for the film. As such, the title clearly suggests human limitation and mortality as well as the contrary urge for the impossible; although only angels inherently have wings, human beings still deny their undeniable attachment to the earth by trying to fly. That the impossible can be achieved (however slightly, as indicated by the correlation of numbers in hundreds or thousands with feet from the earth), that human beings can fly for a while with artificial wings, implies the potential to accomplish another impossibility: simultaneously loving and feeling and flying.

6

Comedies of Youth and Age:
Bringing Up Baby and *Monkey Business*

A comedy is virtually the same as an adventure story. The difference is in the situation—dangerous in an adventure story, embarrassing in a comedy.[1]

I like to make comedies because I like to go into a theater and hear people laughing—the more laughter the better I feel. I have no desire to make a picture for my own pleasure. Fortunately, I have found that what I like, most people also like, so I only have to let myself go and do what interests me.[2]

How do you know this is funny? I think it's funny, that's all.[3]

ALTHOUGH HOWARD HAWKS liked to make comedies, and although he invented richly comic dialogue and business for even his most exciting adventure films, only seven of Hawks's sound films are dialogue comedies—tonally and structurally.[4] Two of his best, adaptations of the Ben Hecht-Charles MacArthur stage plays, *Twentieth Century* and *His Girl Friday*, will be the subject of the next chapter. About the other five (*Bringing Up Baby, Ball of Fire, I Was a Male War Bride, Monkey Business*, and *Man's Favorite Sport?*) there is considerable difference of critical opinion. Stanley Cavell, by implication, finds *Bringing Up Baby* the richest of the group;[5] however, Robin Wood finds it Hawks's funniest comedy, not his best.[6] That honor he reserves for the later *Monkey Business*, which Donald Willis finds abysmally dull;[7] Hawks himself, by implication, prefers both *Bringing Up Baby* and *Male War Bride*.[8] Pauline Kael, however, finds *Male War Bride* "not even a good commerical movie."[9] And although both the critics and the filmmaker agree that *Man's Favorite Sport?* lies at the bottom of his comic barrel, there is some dispute as to whether *Ball of Fire*, which bears the scars of Samuel

Goldwyn's production values, sits closer to its bottom or top. *Bringing Up Baby* and *Monkey Business* may not be the two best of the group (I might agree with Hawks about *Male War Bride*),[10] but that the two films speak to one another in one of the most interesting evolving dialogues of comic thought in American sound-film comedy is inescapable.

Made fourteen years later, *Monkey Business* returns to the same issues of the youthful *Bringing Up Baby* in a wiser, older, softer, more wintery way—just as Shakespeare's late romances, written some dozen or fourteen years after his youthful comedies, return more soberly to the world and issues of those earlier plays. In both films, Cary Grant plays a scientist whose life is missing something; in the early film his youth misses life, but in the late one his life misses youth. Both films use animals as metaphors for human behavior—the skeleton of a long-dead brontosaurus as well as two living leopards and a yelping terrier in *Baby*, a laboratory full of chimpanzees in *Monkey Business*. Both films support their animal imagery with the visual imagery of cages: the cell-like pen in which they try to confine Baby (Baby gets out, of course) and the row of cells in the jailhouse where *Bringing Up Baby* reaches its climax; the series of cages for the simians Esther, Rudolph, and the implied others in *Monkey Business*. The use of animals indicates that these are both Darwinian comedies—the evolution of human life from the prehistoric state of the brontosaurus and the primitive state of the ape. This conscious Darwinism is emphasized by the scientist's name, Huxley, in *Baby*, which becomes (with the cockney-ization of a dropped aitch) Oxly, the owner of the chemistry plant, in *Monkey Business*. And the cage imagery implies that a comic use of Freud does not trail far behind the comic use of Darwin in these two comedies, the penning up and letting out of suppressed and submerged animal urges.

The conversation between the two films is emphasized by such other devices as the virtually repeated line at (or near) the beginning of both: in *Baby*—"Shhhhh. Professor Huxley is thinking"; in *Monkey Business*—"Barnaby, are you thinking?" And both references to thinking indicate that the narrative to follow will contrast the human act of thinking with something else—namely, doing (that most central of Hawks concerns) and feeling rather than just thinking. Even the name of the lawyer, Peabody, from *Bringing Up Baby*, returns as the name of the car salesman in *Monkey Business*. These two films, which are obviously companion pieces, erase any doubts about Howard Hawks—and not the writers of his scripts—as the ultimate source of the spirit and the issues of his films, for the two films use two completely different sets of writers (Hagar Wilde and Dudley Nichols for *Baby;* Hecht, Charles Lederer, and I. A. L. Diamond for *Business*), two different cinematographers, art directors, editors, and so forth. Only Hawks remains from the earlier film to converse with himself in the later one—except for a decidedly and deliberately older Cary Grant.

Although the parallel to Shakespeare's evolving comic concerns from youth to age, from the lighter romantic comedies to the darker romances, may seem unwarranted, both these film comedies are clearly (and probably consciously) built on the Shakespearean comic pattern. Stanley Cavell points out the typical Shakespearean contrast between the societally cluttered city and what Northrop Frye calls "the Green World" in *Bringing Up Baby* (where it is named Connecticut).[11] Parallel to *As You Like It*, the lovers of *Bringing Up Baby* manage to intertwine their souls and affections as a result of the salubrious stimulation of this green, forest world. And parallel to *A Midsummer Night's Dream*, they manage to do so after a particularly magical night in a magical forest. As in Shakespearean comedy, there are disguises (produced by the changing of names, clothes, and genders), mistaken identities (produced by the disguises), talking at cross-purposes (produced by the mistaken identities), and low-comic servants who ape and get tangled with their masters. Although *Monkey Business* lacks a magical forest, its parallel is to another motif of *A Midsummer Night's Dream*—Puck's magical flower whose amorous juice transforms human sexual vision. In *Monkey Business* the magical juice is a "gift" of modern science, as opposed to an exotic gift of the gods, but the modern liquid and its effects are just as magical and just as radical in their transformation of amorous human behavior. There is a magician in Hawks's late comedy, just as there is in Shakespeare's *Tempest*, both of whom use art to control or reverse the cycles of nature. In Hawks's film, that magician is merely a monkey.

Like *Only Angels Have Wings*, *Bringing Up Baby* uses its two stars, Cary Grant and Katharine Hepburn, in what were, at the time, off-roles: Grant as the bumbling scientist, Hepburn as the bubbling nincompoop. Neither star felt comfortable with the role at first. But Hawks told Grant:

> You've seen Harold Lloyd in pictures haven't you? . . . Take
> his attitude—How he walks and how he moves, what he's doing,
> how he plays the scene. . . .[12]

The reference to Lloyd (like his references to Chaplin) shows Hawks's
awareness of the world of silent comedy and reveals that his own verbal
comedy is deeply rooted in the physical and visual style of the silent
comics. Even his dependence on highly communicative objects can be
traced to those kinds of objects in that silent world. The parallel with
Harold Lloyd also explains Grant's comic transformation of his star
persona in the film, from the slick, suave, masculine charmer to the
bumbling, bespectacled innocent. In *Monkey Business,* the silent comedy reference shifts from Lloyd to Laurel and Hardy—particularly in
the scene in which husband and wife coolly, calmly, deliberately slop
paint all over the other's body. For Hepburn, however, Hawks had other
advice:

> We had a marvelous little guy on that picture. He was a great
> comedian for Ziegfeld—the fellow who played the sheriff, Wal-
> ter Catlett. . . . One day I said to Katie, "For Christ's sake,
> can't I make it clear what I'm trying to tell you?" "I guess not,
> because I'm not getting it." . . . I said, "Go over and ask him
> how to do that scene." "Now I know what's wrong. Now I can
> do it." She told me, "You've got to keep that guy around." So
> I'd write scenes for him for about three weeks to keep him
> around. Hepburn was perfectly serious being completely zany.
> If she'd tried to be funny or cute, it wouldn't have been any
> good.[13]

The perfect seriousness of his actors' zaniness is one of the remarkable
and essential qualities of *Bringing Up Baby* and the other major Hawks
comedies.

That Hawks's characters are so seriously, so consistently, so perfectly "screwball" reveals his unique contribution to the "screwball
comedy" genre and explains why he is, for many, its absolute master.
In most of the major screwball comedies by other directors the leading
character (particularly the leading *female* character) must at some point
break down, reject her screwball attitudes, and expose them as a mask

which covers her real, warm, and sincere feeling (Claudette Colbert in *It Happened One Night* and *The Palm Beach Story,* Irene Dunne in *The Awful Truth,* Jean Arthur in both *Mr. Deeds Goes to Town* and *Mr. Smith Goes to Washington,* Barbara Stanwyck in *Meet John Doe* and *The Lady Eve*). For Katharine Hepburn in *Bringing Up Baby,* being screwball is not a mask but an essence. She could no more reject her screwball manner than Geoff Carter could verbally ask Bonnie Lee to stay. He expresses his feeling and maintains his psychological integrity by sharing a joke with her about coffee and a two-headed coin. Susan Vance-Hepburn expresses her feeling and maintains her psychological integrity by sharing her jokes and screwiness with another. Hawks himself wondered if he hadn't made *Bringing Up Baby* a bit too perfectly lunatic.[14] But that perfect lunacy redefines "normality" and remakes the world in its own image: the lunatic world itself becomes perfectly normal for those who are perfectly lunatic—more exciting, more vital, and more surprising than the "normal" world, with which these special people want nothing to do. The screwball character remakes the world according to her or his own law—precisely what Tony Camonte, Geoff Carter, Oscar Jaffe, and Walter Burns successfully accomplish in other Hawks films. This alternative private world for Hawks is always more exciting and more interesting than the normal public one where everyone else lives.

Hawks builds this alternative world of *Bringing Up Baby* by modifying the usual four parts of his construction to add a fifth that reaffirms the value of the separate, screwball world—a brief epilogue (or "tag") that returns the film visually and physically full circle to its beginning. *Monkey Business,* consistent with its conception as a companion piece, also uses a brief epilogue that returns us to the beginning. As the Chaplin films indicate, the circle is a particularly effective comic figure for sealing a special world off from the ordinary world surrounding it. Hawks's earlier comedy, *Twentieth Century,* also uses the epilogue to close a comic circle, enclosing the world of the theater upon itself, while the script of *His Girl Friday* originally devised such an enclosing epilogue which Hawks was able to eliminate by implying the circle's spiritual closing without its physical and visual return to the opening setting. With this five-act structure, the ending of these Hawks comedies is literally in their beginning (and literally parallel to Shakespeare's comic structure), whereas it is only figuratively so in the typical four-part construction of the noncomic films, which cannot separate themselves so perfectly from social reality. The reason for the perfect enclosure of Hawks's comic films is their exercising the traditional privilege comedies have enjoyed since Aristophanes: of rejecting all allegiance to normal, pragmatic social behavior.

As in *Only Angels Have Wings,* the careful narrative patterning of *Bringing Up Baby* emphasizes symmetries, and like *Only Angels, Bringing Up Baby* uses these symmetries to imbed a potentially improbable, wildly fanciful tale in the solid probabilities of narrative logic. There are two domesticated animals—Baby, the tame leopard, and George, the monster of a terrier. There are two leopards in Connecticut—Baby and the killer that escapes from the circus truck. There are two night scenes addressed to a second story window of a proper suburban house—to Peabody's in Riverdale and to the psychiatrist's in Connecticut. There are two kinds of cages—the pen for Baby and the jail for humans, although the killer leopard will eventually be incarcerated in this human jail, while the humans and their domestic animals will use the cells not as cages but as places of refuge from the wild beast outside. Susan steals two cars—and the second one, belonging to the psychiatrist, she steals twice. Such patterning allows Hawks's narrative logic to refute the sheriff's sensible observation—everyone knows that there are no leopards in Connecticut—with the astounding yet probable revelation that there are in fact two.

This symmetrical patterning is accompanied by a temporal concentration that carefully alternates day and night sequences in perfect precision. The first section of the film, which establishes the essential conflict between the lives and values of scientist David Huxley and dizzy Susan Vance, uses a daytime sequence followed by a nighttime sequence. The second section, in which Susan carries David off to the Green World of Connecticut, occurs the next day. The third and fourth sequences recount the events of that night, first outdoors, then indoors. And the brief epilogue takes us back to the city, indoors, during the day. The only other Hawks comedy to use the same temporal compression of *Bringing Up Baby* and a similar succession of days and nights (other than *His Girl Friday,* in which there is a single, compressed day followed by night) is its companion film, *Monkey Business,* which almost exactly reverses the day-night succession of *Bringing Up Baby.*

The film's first section, establishing the clash between the scientific order of Dr. David Huxley and the vital disorder of Susan Vance, is itself a microcosm of the whole film's symmetry and balance. It divides nearly into two halves, day and night; and each of those halves divides into further halves, indoors and outdoors. The overwhelming impression of the indoor daytime scene, inside David Huxley's museum where his life is his work and his work his life, is of confined, calcified, and motionless deadness. Even the conventional establishing shots—a large, stolid, carefully framed brick building; a heavy metallic plaque, reading "Stuyvesant Museum of Natural History"—participate in this inert impression. The first indoor shot of the museum is filled with living things that have been petrified into dead things (which for Hawks means motionless things). There are statues of long-dead mammals and reptiles, glass cases filled with the inanimate parts of formerly whole moving animals, and the plaques of frozen, formerly swimming fish hang on the wall. A huge skeleton of a brontosaurus fills the center of the frame, another former living thing of beauty and power converted into a statue—a motionless artifact. The statuesque skeleton seems to press down and engulf the man who sits beneath it, frozen in the classic attitude of another statue—Rodin's "The Thinker" (for, after all, "Dr. Huxley is thinking"). Even the man has become a statue—motionless, inert.[15] And the platform, on which he sits and thinks, surrounds him with its metallic scaffolding, struts, and supports—a perfect visual cage.

Nothing lives in this room—quite ironic since its function is the study of forms of life. The room parallels that huge library in *Ball of Fire*, where the professors compile an encyclopedia that will contain the knowledge of all life in a room that contains no life—until Snow White invades this home of the seven experiential dwarfs. Dr. Huxley is himself under glass—behind those Harold Lloyd glasses. They will come off later in the film (just as they come off in *Monkey Business*). And Dr. Huxley is also emprisoned by his scientist's smock—tightly tied around his body. Similarly bound is his colleague Dr. Latouche, a shrivelled male whose lack of sexual vitality and identity is underscored by Huxley's mistakenly calling him Alice, the first name of his fiancée. That fiancée, Miss Swallow (Virginia Walker), is the ultimate sign of death in this room. Under glass, like Huxley and the exhibits in the display cases, tightly bound by her black clothing, the color of funerals and death, giving her a shape that parallels the constricted rib cage of the brontosaurus itself, Alice Swallow is the ultimate attainment of a life

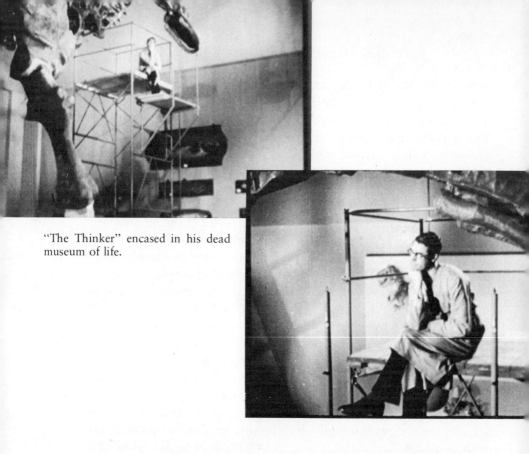

"The Thinker" encased in his dead museum of life.

yearning for death—like all the "life" in this room. Although the noun her name suggests is a delicate bird (not nearly as vital or powerful as a leopard or brontosaurus), even more significant is the verb it suggests—the devouring of another human being, just as Jonah was swallowed by that huge fish. For David Huxley, the brontosaurus seems destined to be his whale. As Swallow tells him, it will be their child, the product of their marriage, the result of their union.

But the scene also contains subtextual suggestions that Huxley knows something is missing from that room. His first utterance, as he stares at the fossilized bone he holds in his hand, is, "This must belong in the tail." Although there is something very harmless about the surfaces of this line, the fact that "tail" is a familiar bit of sexual slang, that the bone sticks up into the frame in an erect position, and that Huxley grasps this erect bone firmly in his hand as he contemplates it, all suggest masturbation. (Recall the falsie in the first shot of *Scarface*. It would be a mistake to bet against the cleverness of the film's maker at being

140

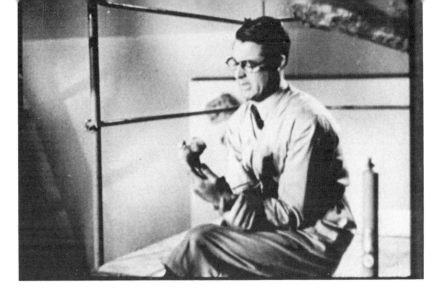

Confusion about the bone.

able to sneak delightfully sexual jokes past the censors and stick them into the most innocent-seeming of scenes, particularly when sexuality is a major issue of the scene and the film.) One might describe the whole narrative to follow as David's education about which bones go where.

Huxley is similarly disappointed when Swallow informs him there will be no honeymoon and that this skeleton will be their child. "You mean, no . . . ?" he begins to ask. No, their marriage will be based purely on their dedication to his work. There is also a hint of Huxley's discomfort in this house of death with his sudden use of slang, describing the impression he intends to make on Mr. Peabody, the lawyer who is supervising a gift to the museum of a million dollars. "I'll knock him for a loop." This use of slang also leads directly to *Ball of Fire*. Finally, there is a sense that David Huxley is himself painfully scattered and disordered in this room that is ordered to death. As he moves to its huge heavy door to make his exit, there is something both scattered and stuttering about his path and his movements—as opposed to the perfectly ordered lines and rectangles of the room. The remainder of the film will work on his subtextual potential for and delight in disorder.

With David Huxley and the brontosaurus Hawks has returned to his familiar concern with human vocation—this time in a comic and critical way. The vocation of David Huxley lacks life. Hawks's satiric disdain for the work of Professor Huxley (and for that of Professors Potts and Fulton in *Ball of Fire* and *Monkey Business*) may seem the

141

typical cliché of Hollywood comic antagonism toward "absent-minded professor-types," an attitude of films that can be traced to the first decade of this century when professor-types were filled with both fear and trembling by the movies. The disdain, however, is also consistent with Hawks's preference for those occupations which put a person closest to life (which are also those which put one closest to death). The work of David Huxley, like his life as a whole (once again for Hawks, one's life is one's work), is too safe, too enclosed, too airless, too tidy. The irony that it is a work devoted to the study of life emphasizes that Huxley is a man who really knows nothing about what he claims to know (the psychiatrist in this film is another of those ignorant sages who presumes to know). In the remainder of the film David will discover what he does not know about life, and the series of madcap events to follow will be his new university.

The outdoor scene of the prologue's day sequence introduces us to the woman who will be the professor's professor. Out on the golf course, bathed in sunlight, surrounded by grass, sky, and trees, David Huxley encounters Susan Vance when she mistakes his golf ball for her own. The visual imagery, the quality of streaming light and shadow, and the evocations of the woman herself all contrast markedly with the strict rectangularity of objects, the stuffy evenness of light, and the restrictive clothing of the people in the previous indoor scene. Susan's hair is free and flowing, her dress white and loose (as opposed to Swallow's, which is black and binding), her walk spirited and sure—mirrored and transmitted by the traveling shot which moves with her in the active direction, from left to right, at her pace and in her rhythm, the typical Hawks method of conveying human spirit, power, and vitality. Susan's talk moves in the same rhythm, at the same pace, with the same energy and speed as her walk. This setting—visually, vocally, and spiritually—is Susan's world. Although she makes the mistake about the golf ball— and the later mistake when she takes David's car—she is the one who seems at ease and in harmony with her environment, while the bumbling David is obviously out of his milieu and his depth. Susan's naturalness in that visual setting is underscored by the shot in which she sinks a twenty-five foot putt—in a very convincing Hawks long shot. There is no editing trickery here; she actually must sink a long putt in order for Hawks to film her sinking a putt—like filming airplanes in the air and cattle crossing a river.

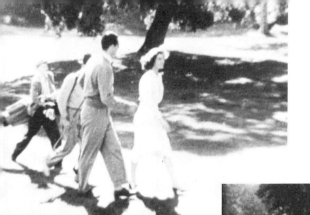

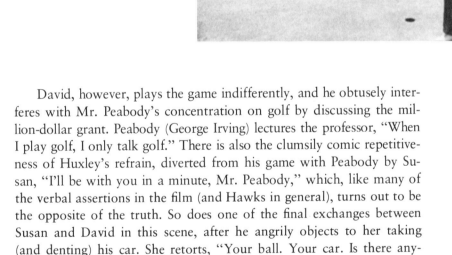

Susan's world: striding across the fairway, sinking a putt.

David, however, plays the game indifferently, and he obtusely interferes with Mr. Peabody's concentration on golf by discussing the million-dollar grant. Peabody (George Irving) lectures the professor, "When I play golf, I only talk golf." There is also the clumsily comic repetitiveness of Huxley's refrain, diverted from his game with Peabody by Susan, "I'll be with you in a minute, Mr. Peabody," which, like many of the verbal assertions in the film (and Hawks in general), turns out to be the opposite of the truth. So does one of the final exchanges between Susan and David in this scene, after he angrily objects to her taking (and denting) his car. She retorts, "Your ball. Your car. Is there anything in the world that doesn't belong to you?" "Yes, thank heaven," he answers, "you."

The night sequence of the prologue first moves back indoors, to a fancy restaurant where a top-hatted-and-tailed Huxley, meeting Peabody for an important dinner to discuss the grant, again makes a physical fool of himself. He clumsily drops his hat, then bumps heads with the hatcheck girl when they both stoop to pick it up. The low-comic business again emphasizes both his social and spiritual clumsiness. His second meeting with Susan appropriately begins and ends with a prat-fall (another perfect Hawks circle). As Susan plays the bizarre physical game of tossing olives into the air to catch with her mouth (conveying both her physical coordination and her spiritual eccentricity), she drops one of these olives on the floor—whereupon David slips on it and slides into the frame on his backside. "First you drop an olive, then I sit on my hat. It all makes perfect sense."

A string of growing comic embarrassments will follow to make even more perfect sense. Susan will mistake another woman's handbag for her own (just as she mistook David's golf ball and car earlier). This mistake leads to the suspicion that David is a thief (he will be mistak-enly suspected later of being both crazy and a peeping tom). She will rip the back seam of David's tail coat (another possible reference to Harold Lloyd and his ripping clothes in *The Freshman*); this rip leads to one of Susan's many comic understatements that fails to fix herself as the cause of David's misery: "Oh, you tore your coat." But David gets even with her when he accidentally steps on the train of her gown, pulling it off without Susan's knowing it, and exposing her vented back-side to the eyes of the world. David's series of spontaneous improvisa-tions (covering her backside with his hat, pressing close to her with his entire body) attempts to protect her modesty and spare her embarrass-ment—the first time that David acts spontaneously and improvisation-ally in the film, and the beginning of his education which will teach him spontaneity and improvisation. The two of them, their bodies pressed together, make a sort of stage exit from the elegant restaurant in perfect unison, two burlesque comics or tap dancers shuffling behind the music-hall's proscenium arch (like the exit of Laurel and Hardy, wearing the same huge pair of pants, in *Leave 'em Laughing*). The comic "stage-exit" will return at the end of *His Girl Friday* and *To Have and Have Not*.

Before her stage-exit, Susan discusses David with—appropriately enough—a psychiatrist she meets in the restaurant. The purse she mis-takenly took belonged to his wife; she will later take the man's car (more symmetry). Twice. A brilliant piece of physical business deflates the doctor's pretensions to know (just as Hawks deflated Dr. Huxley's), implying that his intellectual balloon is filled with hot air. As the psy-

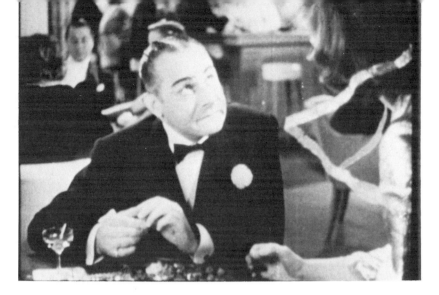

Eruption of the psychiatrist's unconscious.

chiatrist (Fritz Feld) counsels Susan against referring to people as crazy, suggesting she realize that we all have our little oddities, he unconsciously squints his eyes and squeezes his mouth in a comic grimace of which he is totally unaware—unaware both that he is making the grimace and that it looks very silly. The psychiatrist, without knowing it, is an unwitting example of the very oddities he so calmly professes to understand. Ironically, Hawks himself feels similarly about unconscious human tics and the way they can make us all seem a little crazy.[16] But he puts this belief into the mouth of a man he finds ridiculous.

This ironic method also complicates the psychiatrist's explanation of David's relationship with Susan, which seems absurd on its surface but actually explains the underlying psychological basis of the love affair in this (and every other) Hawks film: "The love impulse in man very frequently expresses itself in terms of conflict." By putting this Freudian cliché into the mouth of a psychiatric clown, Hawks simultaneously ridicules the clown and his "science," establishes an essential piece of narrative and psychological information, and softens the blatancy of the information by making us suspect its declarer as a man who knows nothing, but whom we know to be a fool. His psychiatric cliché turns out to be another of the film's verbal predictions which appears to be totally false but will prove to be perfectly true. In the same way, Susan keeps telling David, "Everything's gonna be all right," even when everything appears that it's not gonna be all right at all (for example, when

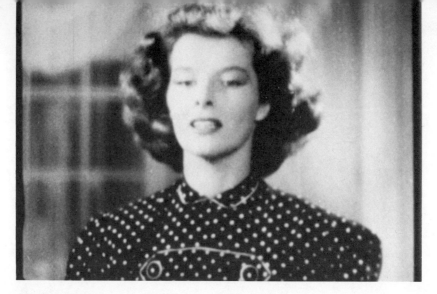

The first closeup.

David mistakenly clouts Peabody in the head with a rock). But, in another of the film's full-circle reversals, the verbal assertion that seems obviously false will turn out to be ironically true, just as their apparent conflict really is love (because it is potentially love from the beginning).

Susan must prove this potential to the man who is too blind to see it. When his glasses come off, he will see much better than he does. As in many amorous comedies, the hero's comic flaw in *Bringing Up Baby* (as in *Monkey Business*) is a defect in vision which the comic action will cure. The "blind" David has told Susan that he is going to be married the next day, at which point Hawks gives Susan a very meaningful close-up—the very first close-up in a film that, as usual for Hawks, uses close-ups very sparingly. After pausing in this close-up to take in David's information with a slight catch of her breath, Susan's overt response is a tinkling laugh (she already sees more than he does). This verbal utterance of David's will also turn out other than as expected. David bids farewell to Susan for what he assumes will be the final time: "In moments of quiet I'm strangely drawn to you. But there haven't been any quiet moments." After he makes this definitive farewell, he takes the pratfall out of the frame that closes the prologue. By the end of this prologue, the pratfall itself has become a comic physical symbol (like Chaplin's kicks in the pants)—the external sign of David's lack of knowledge and control. There will be more unquiet moments to come—for the quiet of Swallow is the quiet of death, and the noise of Susan is the noise of life, fun, and feeling.

146

The film's second section chronicles Susan's strategy to get David to her outdoor world of spontaneous vitality, to get him to Connecticut, to do anything that comes into her head to keep David from being Swallowed on the morrow. The section begins with two phone calls for David—one from Swallow, the other from Susan. Hawks frequently relies on the telephone for significant narrative purposes: in *Scarface* with Angelo; in *His Girl Friday* as Hildy's link to the outside world in general and to Walter in particular; in *The Big Sleep* as part of Marlowe's and Vivian's strategies and counter-strategies; in *Monkey Business* as Edwina's appeals to Hank for help; and the radio in *Only Angels Have Wings* serves as its telephone. The perfect structural balance of these two phone calls not only establishes the two women as antagonists but, in effect, converts them into the two warring sides of David's own soul, the one luring him to a quiet hell that seems like heaven, the other to a spiritual heaven that seems like hell. Hawks intensifies the contrast of these "Good and Bad Angels" with contrasting visual imagery as each speaks on the phone: Swallow is pinched, cramped, and black; Susan free, flowing, and white.

Juxtaposed with each of these phone calls is a new arrival from the animal kingdom (further elegant patterning). While David talks to Swallow a package arrives containing the intercostal clavicle, the final bone needed to complete the brontosaurus. This dead reminder of David's vocation is also a reminder of Swallow herself on the telephone. David will carry the bone with him to Connecticut, but he will lose it there. Susan's phone call is accompanied by the introduction of the tame leopard, Baby, a very much more living organism than that intercostal

Baby's entrance: sharing the frame with Susan.

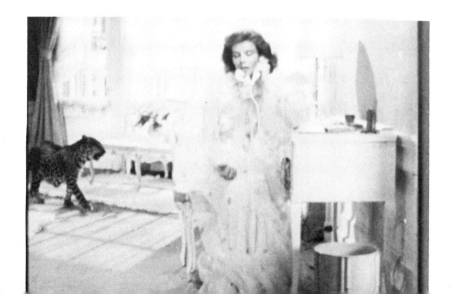

clavicle, which, in Susan's opinion, is "just an old bone." Baby becomes Susan's ally—and in Connecticut they find a third, another animal, the terrier George. These three musketeers manage to get rid of the bone and swallow Swallow. Susan first uses Baby to get David to her apartment, from which it is only a short step to Connecticut, claiming she needs his help since he is a zoologist and understands animals (an irony, since he most certainly does not). When David is incredulous, Susan takes a pratfall—and blames it on an attack by Baby. Hawks's camera drops to the floor with Susan, sympathizing with her energy and strategy, whereas in the opening shots of the film it stared upward at the distant David, disassociating itself from the man, his "thinking," and his world. David, the leopard tamer, then runs off to Susan's—taking his parallel pratfall first—carrying Swallow's bone with him.

When David meets Baby his initial response is fright. He climbs on a chair to avoid the animal's advances, while Baby plays cunningly with his cuff. Late in the film David will use a chair to advance against and control a leopard, getting his chance to play leopard tamer after all.

The low angle sympathizes with both
Susan and Baby.

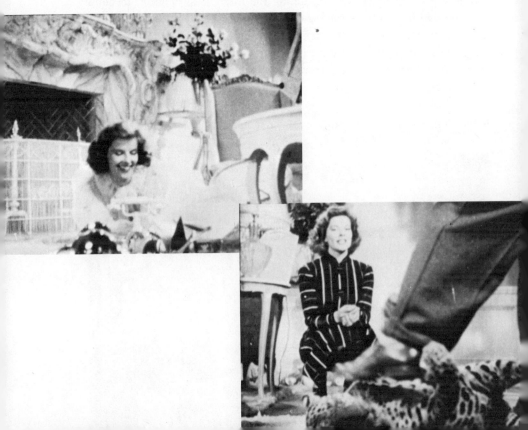

This Baby responds to a piece of music (as so many beings do in Hawks), "I Can't Give You Anything But Love, Baby," and he calmly and gracefully stalks toward the record player that utters his name and purrs in approval. There is an ambiguity about Baby's particular sex, which seems consistent for a film in which so many of the human characters are themselves sexually ambiguous. Although the pronoun "him" gets attached to the beast twice during the film, that diminutive "baby" is more frequently the slang term of endearment that a breezy or tough American male might reserve for his mate. Baby, who first appears in a frame beside Susan and almost seems to emanate from her, becomes the perfect sexual link between Susan and David, sharing the potential sexual characteristics of both or either.

Hawks's method of photographing the animal emphasizes it as such a link; he juxtaposes Baby and the humans in the frame as much as possible, leading to their visual interplay and physical coexistence within the same framed spaces. When Hawks later introduces the terrier George,

Identical triangles with the animal between.

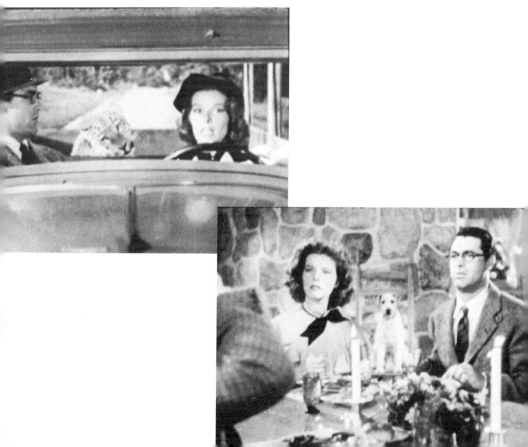

he will photograph him in the same way—sharing the frame with the humans rather than separated from them by the use of editing. Hawks's composition of the ride in the car to Connecticut, which puts David, Baby, and Susan into an isosceles triangle (Baby, like Poppy in *Scarface,* sits squarely between and behind them), is precisely mirrored by his composition at the supper table in Connecticut when Susan, George, and David sit in an identical isosceles triangle. Only in the nighttime sequences with Major Applegate (Charlie Ruggles) will Hawks resort to editing separate shots of the people and the leopard. Whether this other photographic method is intentional (implying that Applegate and the animal cannot share the same emotional space) or unintentional (either the leopard or Ruggles declined the other's company), these edited shots of the animals are far less effective than those which keep the beasts and the people in the same space.

The reason is not simply our belief in the authenticity of shared cinema space as opposed to our suspicion of trickery with montage—a point developed by André Bazin.[17] Shared cinema space in narrative cinema can be used to imply shared emotional space, a spiritual conversation between the beings enclosed by that framed boundary, a sharing which transmits itself not by explicit words but by the evocations of physical proximity. Such subtextual communication and implication is especially important to a director like Hawks who pushes so much of the film's thought and feeling below the surface of words. In *Bringing Up Baby,* people do attempt to converse with the animals who share those spaces—the song David and Susan sing to Baby is one familiar kind of Hawksian conversation. Later in the film, both Susan and David attempt to converse verbally with George; George and the humans talk at cross-purposes, however, as characters inevitably do in such comedies, for his shrill, irritating barks are his sole response to their articulate questions—barks that frequently invade the visual space from off-frame and drown out the human utterances altogether. By implication, these people are not only seeking a conversation with the animals who share the frame but also with the animal within themselves, particularly David's coming to know and express the Susan-Baby-George (as opposed to the Swallow-Bone-Brontosaurus) in himself. Baby, its name implying both conjugal life and conjugal love, must be brought up and brought out in David in order for him to be a whole, live, human animal.

Susan sends Baby to fetch David when he attempts to leave her apartment and go to Swallow. As David walks in the frame, holding the box with the bone in his right arm, Baby walks casually alongside him without his knowing it—a comic visual metaphor for his solid confidence in that dead bone and his conscious ignorance of the Baby in him. When he notices that Baby will not desert him, he knows that he has no choice but to go to Connecticut. When he gets there, the bone will come out of the box—as it lies on top of a bed—and be buried in the earth by the animal accomplice, George. David himself will be called "Mr. Bone" as a pseudonym, a name that is consistent with the film's clever verbal and visual sexual puns—for bone needs only an *r* to become a familiar term of sexual slang, and the bone David held at the beginning of the film looked as if it had an *r,* and Applegate later makes the mistake of adding a letter, a *y* not an *r,* to the name of Bone.

The trip to Connecticut is another series of low-comic embarrassments and disasters, all of which are necessary elements of David's education about Baby and the bone. Most of the embarrassment arises from the fact that Baby, like all animals, must eat—and his healthy appetite contrasts markedly with the inability of humans to consume their supper in a later dinner scene. Baby helps himself to breakfast when Susan's car rams a poultry truck (the second time she rams another car), sending its occupants onto the road and into Baby's gullet. Hawks, of course, does not show Baby devouring any of these creatures—including two swans—since it would decrease our sympathy for him, just as viewing Tony's murders directly would do the same in *Scarface.* We merely watch and hear a befeathered David (the birds' feathers parallel O'Hara's boutonniere) total the contents of Baby's meal. Then David suffers the embarrassment of buying Baby thirty pounds of steak from the butcher in a small Connecticut town. When asked how he's going to cook it, David replies, "It's going to be eaten raw." "Do you grind this up before you eat it?" David answers, "This isn't for me. It's for Baby." The butcher and his customers, who share Hawks's frame with David, find him a very strange daddy. Meanwhile, Baby has leapt from Susan's car to another, like Susan preferring another's car to its own; so Susan takes a second car that is not her own, to avoid arrest. The small-town constable, Slocum (Walter Catlett), who is introduced in this scene, will get the chance to arrest her later. And she will escape that arrest as she does this one—by stealing this very car.

In Connecticut, Susan continues David's education by stripping him of his clothes. Having nothing else to wear, David grabs the first thing hanging in the bathroom—and Hawks uses David's shadow on the wall effectively to build suspense about what exactly he might be doing. When he emerges from the bathroom, he is wearing a woman's white, sheer, and fluffy negligee—exactly the kind of loose and free clothing the film has identified with Susan. David, disguised in Susan's clothes, unknowingly reveals a truth about himself; he has the potential to be a free and vital Susan. The false clothes reveal his true soul's apparel. His putting on those clothes has been a piece of spontaneous improvisation; from this moment forward, his life becomes a series of spontaneous improvisations. For in this embarrassing physical disguise (Cary Grant's first female impersonation in a Hawks film), he meets Susan's aunt, Mrs. Carleton Random (May Robson), the woman who intends to donate the million dollars to David's work. They talk at cross-purposes, for this is Mrs. Random's house (which David does not know), while he is a stranger wearing very strange clothes (and what is he doing in her house and in those clothes?). During this uninformative verbal interchange, Hawks and Grant underscore David's frustration with a spontaneously improvised line that seems so startling for 1938 today's audience might actually wonder if it really heard what it thinks it heard. "But why are you wearing those clothes?" Mrs. Random asks. David answers, as he leaps madly and devilishly in the air, "Because I've gone gay all of a sudden!" The response, like his disguise, not only relates to the film's central issues of sexual fertility and exuberant improvisation; it is a reminder that certain seemingly contemporary terms have a long tradition (particularly among show people). Hawks could probably get this word past the censors because either they did not hear it or could not understand its sexual connotations.

The second section ends when David gets a new (but no less comic) suit of clothes—a ridiculously inappropriate and very binding riding habit. To get this at least masculine outfit, he has had to improvise again, convincing both Mrs. Random and her servant, Mrs. Gogarty, that he is a lunatic who will do something violent without it. Now David must use a disguised name in conversing with the woman who intends to give Dr. Huxley a million dollars, because, as Susan points out in another of those ridiculous understatements which exclude her contribution: "Oh, David, I'm afraid you've made a rather unfavorable

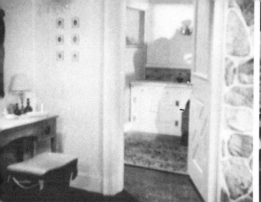
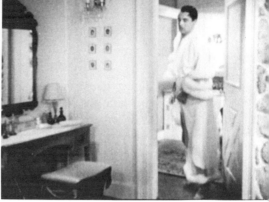

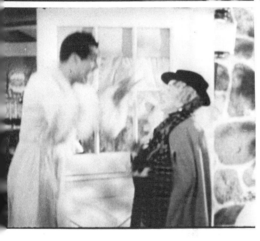

The shadow emerges from the bathroom, wearing a negligee (but no glasses), and goes "gay all of a sudden."

impression on her." Meanwhile, Susan has seen David without his glasses for the first time (when the clothes come off, the glasses do too), and likes what she sees. David not only looks better without his eyeglasses; there is a sense in which he sees better too. It is the same sense in which he is more alive, more truly his potential self, in Susan's clothes than in his own. George, who is far less polite than the supposedly wild leopard and whose yapping presence entered the house with the yapping Mrs. Random, has buried the "old bone," the reminder of David's former unspontaneous self. So Susan and David must follow George everywhere, playing with him, conversing with him, hoping he will lead them to the spot where he buried the thing. "Isn't this fun, David? Just like a game." Once Susan has transported David to her outdoor world, she can reintroduce him to the playful fun of childhood—the spontaneously energetic play that is so missing from his stiff and stilted adulthood.

The childish fun continues in the film's third section, that night, which takes the characters outdoors again—away from the proper, civilized dinner party and into the magical forest. Not coincidentally, the month is June (as Mrs. Random pointedly informs Horace), and the night may even be midsummer eve. In this section we meet the film's final character, Major Applegate, another sexless, lifeless, nonanimal bumbler and stutterer—the typical Ruggles persona. Applegate is so bumblingly ignorant of his own sexual identity that he later tells the constable, when asked who he is: "I'm the niece, er, I'm the aunt, er, I'm Major Horace Applegate." Applegate is also ignorant of animals, though he claims to be a big-game hunter, as ignorant of animal life as the zoologist David. He smugly and falsely identifies the leopard's cry as that of a loon, and then pedantically tells Mrs. Random, "That was a loon, Elizabeth. Loon. *L, Double O, N.*" For Applegate, animals are a matter of letters not of life, just as for David they are matters of skeletal frames, not of whole living, moving bodies. Applegate, like David's older colleague, Latouche, at the museum, is a visual reminder of where David's sexless, animal-less life with Swallow might lead.

Once outdoors, Susan and David have two apparent goals—recapturing Baby, whom a drunken servant, Gogarty (Barry Fitzgerald), has mistakenly let out of its cage; and following George so they can recapture the intercostal clavicle. Hawks is still using these two opposite suggestions of animal life in perfect balance. But beneath these apparent goals is the underlying spiritual union of Susan and David—spending this magical night of childish fun and games, and mistakes, and pratfalls, together. Susan and David are playing together—just as Baby and George play with one another in the sequence. Among the playful pranks is Susan's opening a cage to let a second leopard on the loose—this one a vicious killer on his way to the zoo. Like the people, even leopards wear disguises in this film. When Susan ducks beneath the branches that David inadvertently pushes in her face, he reprimands her, "Susan, this is no time to be playing squat-tag," another reference to a childhood game.

They take pratfalls down ravines, into a river, over the trunks of trees. As opposed to the earlier pratfalls, whose comic clumsiness mirrored the social discomfort and the spiritual blindness of the man who took the pratfalls, these spills, which the two of them take together, fit into their night of playful fun. So does Susan's hippity-hoppity walk, when she breaks the heel of a shoe, or her netting David's head, a comic image of capture, in the spill that separates him permanently from his

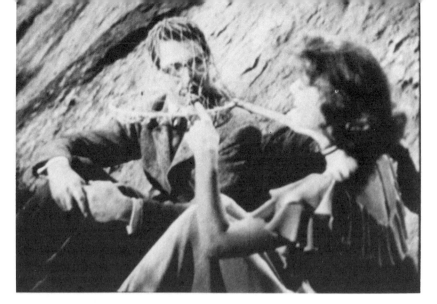
Comic capture.

glasses. When Susan confesses, "I do so like being with you," David is still unconquered; "You do? Well, I like peace and quiet." David's rejection produces Susan's most tearful moment (another childish ploy reminiscent of Stan Laurel), "After all the fun we had." Then Hawks snaps her tearful tenderness with a low-comic gag (a typical Chaplin touch) as Susan takes a pratfall over a tree branch and out of the frame (the film's second pratfall out of the frame). When David lifts her from this fall, the two share their ultimate emotional union with an almost kiss. They will not separate emotionally again.

Hawks celebrates this emotional union with a musical moment of spiritual communion; but this familiar use of music in Hawks fits uniquely into this film's playful ironies. Baby has gotten himself on the roof of a house—the one belonging to the psychiatrist—so Susan and David must improvise together to lure him off it. For the second time, they hold a nighttime conversation with a house. Baby's favorite song, "I Can't Give You Anything But Love," will be their text; Susan and David, holding George in his arms, begin their spontaneous serenade. After the first few bars, George joins in, followed shortly by Baby himself. The result is a very strange rendition of the song in close harmony—in fact, a Barber Shop Quartet arrangement for four voices, two human and two animal. (Hawks may be doing McCarey's duet for Cary Grant and the terrier, Mr. Smith, in *The Awful Truth* two better.) In this synthesis of song and "speech," human and animal, wild and tame, adult action and childhood game, the film reaches its ultimate spiritual synthesis and harmony as well.

But that discovery and its acceptance by David must be demonstrated in action and by action; the film's fourth section gives him the opportunity to demonstrate his new spiritual union with Susan rather than the old and dead one with Swallow (who returns to the film in this section). Because Susan appears to be crazy (singing to a leopard on a roof in Connecticut in the middle of the night!) and David appears to be a peeping tom, the constable and the psychiatrist take both of these suspicious persons to jail. All of the film's characters will eventually get to this jail and into its cells—Susan, David, the battling Gogarty, Mrs. Random and the flustered Applegate, Baby, George, the killer leopard, Peabody, Swallow, Slocum, the psychiatrist, even the two men transporting the killer leopard to the zoo (only Mrs. Gogarty remains at home to answer the telephone). Farce comedies typically end with this gathering of all the personages; the one way to eliminate the ignorance (the disguises, mistaken identities, and talking at cross-purposes) on which farce depends is to bring all the characters face to face to remove the disguises and reveal the mistakes. In indoor farces (like Jonson's *The Alchemist* or Feydeau's *A Flea in Her Ear*), this gathering is usually achieved by opening all the doors, bringing the characters out of the little cells where they have been confined, kept ignorant by their confinement, so they can all see one another. *Bringing Up Baby* ironically achieves this dispelling of ignorance by putting them back inside the separate cells—but because these cells permit their inhabitants to see beyond them, the cells both confine and illumine.

This visual and narrative use of the cells in the fourth section continues the film's paradoxical use of the cage motif—Susan's desire to get David out of one kind of cage (the glass display case for dead things) and into another (the cage for wild living animals). The fourth section also sustains the paradox by making it unclear whether the characters would prefer to get in or out of these cages, depending on whether the cage is perceived as a prison or a refuge. Susan gets out of her cage by improvising, pretending that she is a gangster's moll, that they are all members of "the leopard gang." She transforms herself into "Swinging Door Susie," and her exit from the cell, as she rides its swinging door, is a moment of both childish play and adult grace, another Hawks

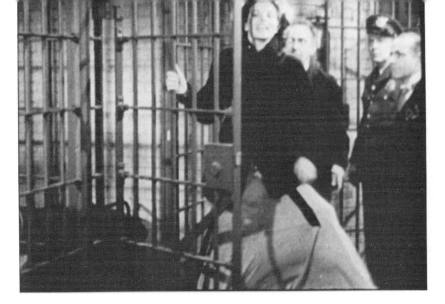

"Swinging Door Susie."

equation of life and motion. In one of those moments of self-reference in a Hawks film, David warns Slocum, "She's making all this up out of motion pictures." (Like, for example, *The Awful Truth,* in which his "sister" calls him "Jerry the Nipper." But then Susan's "society moniker," Vance, also comes from that film.) But David himself refers to movies when he names his associates as "Mickey the Mouse and Donald the Duck." Susan may also refer specifically to *Scarface* when she sniffs one of Slocum's cigars (just as Tony Camonte sniffed Johnny Lovo's cigars) and pronounces it a "two-fer"—"two fer a nickel." The male-like female that Susan impersonates in this scene parallels the female-like male that David impersonated earlier when wearing Susan's negligee, contributing to the film's collapse of apparent opposites—human life and animal life, adulthood and childhood, freedom and confinement, male and female, surfaces and essences.

After Susan's escape, David remains in the jailhouse for his own improvisations with the first leopard, Baby, whom he now approaches with familiarity and pets with fondness (as opposed to his initial fright and reticence in facing this beast). Then Susan returns to the jailhouse, dragging the killer leopard behind her at the end of a rope. Hawks again shows narrative cunning by deliberately omitting the scenes which show precisely how she snares this beast. Susan tells the recalcitrant leopard, "I'm just as determined as you are" (echoing Cesca's determination in *Scarface*), and she is just as determined with this leopard as she has been with David. David then takes over, improvising again, playing Susan's heroic animal tamer, spontaneously addressing the leopard with a chair (another form of human-animal conversation) and prodding him into an empty cell (even the fellow animals, George and Baby, have fled into a cell with the humans to escape this vicious beast). After David's moment of masculine assertion he faints dead away in Susan's arms. Caught and captured.

The fifth section, the film's brief epilogue, returns us to David's museum during the daylight. The black-clad Swallow dismisses David as a potential mate with more animal imagery, "You're just a butterfly." David has again seemingly returned to the calcified pose of Rodin's thinker (and that pose precisely parallels the attitude of the stone dinosaur statue that sits in the frame beside him, whereas the living Baby previously had accompanied David without his knowing it). Just as David seems doomed to the world of puzzlement and death where he began, a black (but loosely) clad Susan enters that world (her dress perhaps a sign of deference to that world). Susan has both the million dollars for David and the intercostal clavicle. (See, everything *is* gonna be all right.) With Susan's entrance, a living force invades that mausoleum; David himself springs to life and into motion, spontaneously scampering up the scaffolding behind the huge brontosaurus. He puts

"The Thinker" again, beside his dinosaur.

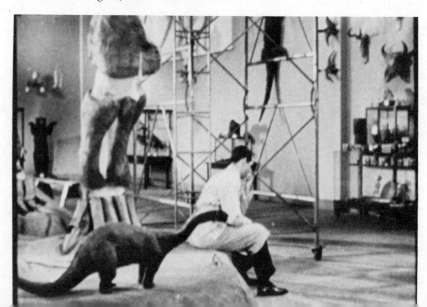

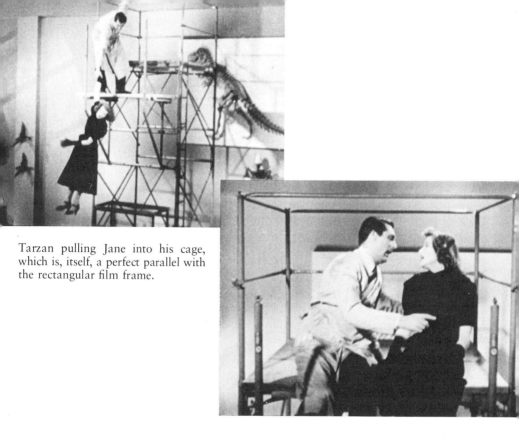

Tarzan pulling Jane into his cage, which is, itself, a perfect parallel with the rectangular film frame.

that skeleton between Susan and himself, using its size, its age, and its deadness to protect him.

But to no avail. Susan improvises too—by scampering up the ladder on the other side of the brontosaurus. As they speak Susan begins to sway on that ladder. Her sway is the one way to bring motion (*i.e.* life) to that room of motionless dead matter, which she fills with her vitality. The rhythm of her motion seems to elicit David's vitality as well, for he begins to sway with her, confessing that he just spent the "best day of his life"; he's never had so much fun (that all-important word of vitality for Hawks and this film). That immense edifice of deadness that separates them must come tumbling down, and down the brontosaurus comes when Susan starts to fall off her ladder and David must take some immediate spontaneous heroic action to save her. He grabs her arm as she dangles in midair, and the visual image to which their bodies refer is not a frozen Rodin sculpture but that familiar synthesis of human and animal life in the movies and American popular culture: he Tarzan, she Jane. As this Tarzan pulls his Jane to safety, he pulls her into the visual

159

cage of his scaffolding, the exact same cage where he began the film alone, grasping his bone. Now, with the closing of another perfect Hawks circle, he will be caged with another—a living human-animal being, not an "old bone."

Bringing Up Baby translates the Evolution of Trust that underlies an adventure film like *Only Angels Have Wings* into comic terms—the evolution and expression of the calcified character's energy, vitality, and spontaneity. David Huxley discovers the value of living limbs (like the arm of Susan Vance that he pulls into his cage) rather than dead bones. This spiritual evolution, in the film's comic view, is every bit as vital to the human species as that Darwinian evolution which has guided the progress of biological life from the Age of the Brontosaurus to the Age of Tarzan. The film's breathless, breakneck pace reinforces and propels its comic evolution, for the driving rhythm of its talk and action is Susan-Hepburn's rhythm, with which David-Grant must keep pace if he wants to stay in the movie—just as he must keep up with her on the golf course if he wants to stay in Hawks's moving frame. While the pace of the opening scene in David's museum is slow and lumbering— in both speech and motion—once Susan strides across the fairway in the second scene the film hitches itself to her walk and talk—and David must grab hold to stay aboard. He can only do so by matching her instantaneous and spontaneous surprises with surprising improvisations of his own. His ability to improvise so quickly is both a sign of his underlying ability to improvise and of his successful development of that necessary talent.

Like so many "screwball comedies" (and so many romantic comedies from Plautus to Shaw) the underlying issues of *Bringing Up Baby* are human wholeness, spiritual vitality, and sexual energy. Unlike so many other "screwball comedies," however, the characters in *Bringing Up Baby* achieve that wholeness not in spite of their screwiness but because of it; to be screwball is itself to be exuberantly alive. Hawks anchors this screwball sequence of potentially wild impossibility (how do you get a leopard on a roof in Connecticut so you can sing, "I Can't Give You Anything But Love"?) in the perfectly probable logic of his carefully patterned, symmetrical fictional construction. The film's consistent verbal and visual motifs (animals, cages, bones), its pratfalls, its breathless pace complexly underscore its essential thematic issues— human spontaneity, animal vitality, sexual fertility, childhood fun. Like

A Midsummer Night's Dream, the film's wildly fanciful and farcical action is the means to improve the amorous vision of its young lovers, so they can achieve a harmony both with nature and with themselves.

Monkey Business looks very differently at the claims of animal vitality and childish spontaneity. While *Bringing Up Baby* affirms that it is somehow natural and necessary for adult humans to behave like animals and children, *Monkey Business* reaffirms that it is somehow natural and necessary for adult humans to act like adults and humans. It is the "somehow," the definition of nature itself, that has shifted from its vital, exuberant, Wordsworthian formulation in the earlier film (which Hawks made at the age of 42) to its savage, subhuman, Hobbesian formulation in the later one (which Hawks made at the age of 56). For Hawks, as for Jean Renoir and François Truffaut, the claims of nature seem less attractive and less simply desirable as a human being gets older. Both *Bringing Up Baby* and *Monkey Business* retreat into the past to formulate their definitions of nature. For David Huxley, his dedication to a brontosaurus and the fossilized remains of other creatures and species who died millions of years ago represents his retreat from life itself. For Barnaby Fulton in *Monkey Business,* his dedication to a drug that will transport people backward into their youth is a rejuvenation that is also a regression—a contrary movement against the natural cycles of life and of natural evolutionary history itself. While *Bringing Up Baby* allows David Huxley to discover what makes life life, *Monkey Business* allows Barnaby Fulton to rediscover what makes human life human and civilized human society civilized. The youth to which Fulton's drug transports its imbibers is, as the film's script describes it, a world where there is "no philosophy, no science, no statesmen, nothing. There'd just be poetry." [18] It is a world of feeling without thought, passion without reflection, simple doing without complex making. It is a world, in short, which nullifies all the complex accomplishments of human history and human civilization, all sciences and arts, not the least of which is this very movie, a complex evolutionary synthesis of both science and art.

The shift of Cary Grant's scientific specialty in the two films from zoology to chemistry plays an integral role in the later work's redefinition of nature. Because his science in *Bringing Up Baby* was the study

of animals, beings about which he himself was ironically and patheti-
cally ignorant, David Huxley's education had to be about animals, about
which he was already supposed to be educated. Although Huxley was
able to use his science to make art (the skeleton of the brontosaurus
and the other artifacts in his museum are very much like films—imitations of life built from lifeless pieces), he was unable to apply it to life—
the essential purpose of that science. But the science of chemistry is
itself a kind of art, combining materials and elements into new compounds that previously did not exist in nature. While David Huxley
betrays the essential principles of zoology when he converts life into art,
Barnaby Fulton fulfills the essential principles of chemistry when he
transforms life into the art of new chemical compounds (just as a filmmaker transforms bits of life into compounds of art).

The art and science of chemistry is uniquely human and uniquely
adult. It requires lengthy and careful study, of which humans alone are
capable. It requires thinking so that one can extend one's study, by
developing new formulas, into regions that have not been entered before. It requires a whole organized, civilized society so that certain
members of it need not worry about their food, safety, or shelter; only
then can they have the leisure to perform the art and science of chemistry. And it requires a vast tradition of previous performing and thinking about that art and that science. Chemistry, like filmmaking, represents a kind of ultimate step on the evolutionary ladder, the evolving of
human thought and accomplishment over the whole course of natural
history to bring humans to the ultimate escape from the tyranny of
nature itself—restructuring, reformulating, and remaking nature in its
own image (another parallel between making drugs and making films).
This process has evolved to such an advanced and civilized state that
Barnaby Fulton can produce the drug, B-4. B-4 (be-fore) what? Before
art and science and *homo sapiens* and evolution itself, a reversal and
negation of the entire process that led to the making of B-4 and to
Monkey Business.

The shift of the film's animals, from the felines and canines of *Baby*
to the simians of *Monkey Business,* is also consistent with its shift of
sciences. The ape occupies that step on the evolutionary ladder that
comes immediately B-4 the final human one, a step that is very close to
human life (for apes can ape human motion and emotion) but very far
from it (for apes cannot think, talk, read, and build). To use Hawks's

terms, one crucial difference between apes and humans is that apes are not capable of any vocation, any professional pursuit or commitment, other than being apes. The proper companion of the ape in *Monkey Business,* just as George is Baby's companion in that film, is the human infant, closer to the human than an ape but still in a sense subhuman in being subverbal, subrational, and subvocational (just as George is both more and less of a domesticated baby than Baby). Once a drug can return an adult to his youth, it is only a short step back to his childhood, then to his infancy, then to the state of animal being B-4 animals became human beings. All of these steps in the evolutionary and biological ladder exist in this film, and those who take the drug progressively descend them. This careful comic study of reverse evolution is the thematic premise on which *Monkey Business* is built.

The aging of Cary Grant (who has admitted his own experimenting with peyote in this period) as Barnaby Fulton fits squarely into the film's contrast of youth and age (just as the aging of Jean Gabin fits deliberately into the conception of Jean Renoir's *French Cancan*). Grant, his voice far slower and lower than in *Bringing Up Baby,* his glasses even thicker, his movement more enervated, less staccato, more vacant, more languid, becomes the film's physical image of middle-aging in deliberate contrast to the exuberant Grant we remember in films like *Bringing Up Baby.* The range and variation in Grant's roles for Hawks (the bumbling Harold Lloydish Huxley; the cool, strong Geoff Carter; the absent Barnaby Fulton) is simply and subtly astounding—to which we will add the outlandishly florid eccentricity of Walter Burns in *His Girl Friday* (his quiet exasperation as Henri Rochard in *I Was a Male War Bride* is closer to the key of Barnaby Fulton). Such range and variation show the subtle changes a director like Hawks could ring on a "personality" (rather than an "actor") he knew so well; they also throw the whole distinction between a personality and an actor into some doubt.

The aging Cary Grant is matched in the film by the aging Ginger Rogers, no longer the Golddigger or Astaire partner but, like Grant himself, an adult with whose past we are familiar from other films and whose past seems clearly past. Together, Grant and Rogers as Barnaby and Edwina Fulton seem a return to Susan Vance and David Huxley, fourteen years later, married, contented, comfortable, domesticated, balancing the demands of love and work. They no longer play together as children—but then how long can married adults remain children?

And they have no baby (all the children in the film belong to others). The lack of a child either reveals the dulled vitality of their married life or the fact that to have given them one would simply interfere with the film's thematic contrast of childhood and adulthood, if the adults who act like children also had children.

Most of Hawks's dissatisfaction with the film can be traced to Ginger Rogers. Cary Grant didn't want a youngish wife, "so everybody I suggested for it was turned down and finally Ginger Rogers was brought up and we had Ginger Rogers." [19] Even directors with the commercial power and artistic ability of Hawks must accede to the power of stars— if they want to use the stars. In the original conception of the story, apparently only Barnaby was to experience the drug, but Ginger Rogers wanted to do the "getting young thing" too: "She wanted to do it and I had to let her do it." [20] More compromises—partially because by the 1950 television era the stars, and not the studios, producers, and directors, had the power. "I thought it was lousy and it made her play badly all through the whole picture." [21] The director may be a bit harsh on her. Only in the gum-chewing, sling-shooting scene of the film's fourth section does Ginger Rogers get too obviously cute for words. At most moments, her quiet deliberateness seems to match the calmly placid playing of Cary Grant.

There is, perhaps, a vague feeling that the film does not quite "take off" as *Bringing Up Baby, Twentieth Century,* and *His Girl Friday* do, does not quite burst, snap, crackle, and pop into surprising life with the brilliantly suited eccentricities of the spirited actors and actors' spirits. But then its theme works against these bursts of brilliance; there must necessarily be something more leaden, more plodding about a film that uses only occasional sequences of giddy youth to contrast with its usual study of placid age. But this sense of heaviness in both tone and rhythm seems to afflict many of the Hawks films after 1950, regardless of their themes (about which more will be said later), and it is this leaden feeling that may interfere with recognizing the subtleties and symmetries of the film. What Hawks perhaps found most wanting about the film is that the spirits and evocations of its stars did not completely carry its wildly outlandish events from the solid rock of credible human behavior to the airy heights of screwball lunacy. "*Monkey Business* went too far, became too fanciful and not funny enough." [22] What could go further or be more fanciful than *Bringing Up Baby*? I think Hawks may have been responding to the fact that the stars themselves, especially Ginger Rogers, could not be as fanciful and could not go as far as the story needed them to be and go. This would not be an uncommon problem in Hawks films after 1950.

For several critics, *Monkey Business* is one of Hawks's most "organic" films.[23] By "organic" they mean that everything is prepared for, everything flows from what precedes it, every event in the film seems to echo or respond to another—the principle of narrative symmetry and logic that distinguishes every major Hawks film. The first section establishes the two halves of Barnaby Fulton's life—his conjugal life at home and his professional life at work. The first half appropriately takes place at night, the second appropriately during the day—the precise mirror image of the opening section of *Bringing Up Baby*. The alternation of day and night in these two comedies reflects the observation of Fen, the woman Thomas Dunson loses in *Red River,* that "the sun only shines half the time; the other half is night." Each of the three remaining sections of the film chronicles one taking of the drug, one "trip" into the character's youth: first by Barnaby alone, during the day, in a spirit of scientific experimentation ("The history of discovery is the history of people who didn't follow rules"); then by Edwina alone, at night, in a spirit of defiance—showing that if he can do it she can do it too; then by the two of them together, in the daylight, accidentally rather than intentionally. In the script, titled "Darling, I Am Growing Younger" when shooting began, Barnaby was to take the drug by himself the first time, then the two of them together the second and third times. The pattern of "tripping" in the film is both more symmetrical and more carefully motivated than it is in the script. The film then concludes with a brief epilogue, back at the Fulton home at night, which is a return to the beginning (like *Bringing Up Baby*) and a reaffirmation of their life together, rediscovered as a result of their "trips." Although Stanley Cavell labels *Bringing Up Baby* one of Hollywood's comedies of *re*marriage,[24] there seems a far greater sense of *re* in *Monkey Business*.

Even before the credits, the film begins with a self-referential gag which sets the comic tone and defines its comic protagonist. Cary Grant opens the front door of a pleasant and respectable-looking bourgeois home, the only such conventional home in all of Howard Hawks, as if to welcome us inside, wearing a tuxedo and black tie. But an off-frame voice (either Hawks's own or one that speaks for the film's storyteller-director)[25] directs him, "Not yet, Cary." Whereupon Cary says "Hm," in mildly puzzled confusion, and closes the door again so the credits can appear in their proper place and the film can then begin. The device (which is not indicated in the script) both allows Hawks to inform us that there is something "absent," puzzled, vacant, confused about the character that Grant plays as well as that this film is surely a comedy (such a gag could precede no other kind of film) and, further, that part of the fun of this comedy, part of the comic game the storyteller will play with his audience, is that we all know this is a Cary Grant comedy, whomever else he may play. The gag also informs us that there is something vacant, something dead, about the life inside that superficially comfortable home, just as there is something dead inside David Huxley's museum of life.

This sense of the character's "absence" and deadness dominates the first part of the film's prologue. After the credits, Grant opens the door once again, permitting an evening-dressed Ginger Rogers to leave the house, after which he remains inside, closes the door, turns off the porch light, and leaves her standing alone outdoors. Not only will Barnaby not go out with her tonight; he is not really with her at all, mentally "absent" while physically present. His body is somehow vacant, uninhabited by the thoughts and feelings that must propel it if it is to act and move sensibly. But the woman is not very surprised by this behavior; she has seen it before. She reenters the house through the front door, and the camera moves into that world with her, sharing the point-of-view of this more normal, more present character (just as it shares Jean Arthur's view as the means to enter the world of Barranca). Instead of going out for the evening, they will stay home; she will cook up an informal supper, for, after all, she knows that Barnaby is "thinking" and is lost in that thought. She helps him get out of his formal evening clothes, revealing her awareness both that Barnaby needs mothering and that he needs help with even the simplest physical tasks since his mind has transported him elsewhere—to his work and his formula and his laboratory.

The strategy of such an opening scene is in one sense precisely opposite that of *Bringing Up Baby* or *Only Angels Have Wings*. While these two earlier films established an essential conflict between two characters who collide with one another upon their first meeting, this kind of beginning establishes the dynamics and dimensions of a stable human relationship that has existed—successfully—for some period of time. Their home is comfortable, their knowledge of one another is comfortable, they are even comfortable with each other's faults—her mothering and his absence. But if comfort is the reward of a stable relationship, boredom, dullness, and the taking of one another for granted are its dangers. The conflict of such a story must necessarily develop between the comfortable surface of their life together and the potential boredom and deadness that lie beneath the surface and of which they are unaware. In another sense, however, the narrative strategy of *Monkey Business* is identical to that of *Bringing Up Baby*—to chronicle an achievement of human synthesis so that "thinking" is not opposed to feeling but somehow balanced with and by it. Their means of achieving this synthesis must be the rediscovery of precisely why they are comfortable with each other, how that comfort evolved, and what it is they have to be comfortable about. They must become conscious of the comfort they take for granted.

The means to this consciousness of feeling will be the very formula about which Barnaby is so absently thinking. As is so often true of Hawks, Barnaby's work, his vocation, provides the final answer for his personal life as well as its initial problem. The source of the tension in this opening sequence—Barnaby's thinking about his formula—will also be the source of the tension's resolution by the film's closing. Barnaby articulates the film's central narrative question, the problem which has stimulated his thought about a new rejuvenating drug: "It's queer about people. Through no fault of their own they get older." This inescapable (and, for Hawks, rather explicitly articulated) existential fact is the comic analogue to that other which underlies the adventure films: we all get killed sooner or later. Barnaby's formula, about which he is thinking, intends to escape this inescapable fact of human existence, just as his preoccupation with thinking has led to an escape from their evening out together. In their youth, Edwina's and Barnaby's evenings out had also been escaped—but their own sexual and emotional intensity, their feelings, kept them at home together. Now his thinking keeps them home. This married couple is itself a perfect example of the existential fact Barnaby noted earlier: through no fault of their own they have gotten older.

In the second half of the prologue, the next day at Barnaby's laboratory, the middle-aged scientist finds himself indeed in the middle of physically luscious youth, the secretary Miss Laurel (Marilyn Monroe), and doddering dirty old age, his employer Mr. Oxly (Charles Coburn). Miss Laurel, like that earlier secretary, Angelo, is another dope, incompetent at the most basic secretarial skills like typing and the use of words. Hecht and Hawks use their familiar method of malapropism to define her "mind" at the outset. "Aren't you early?" Barnaby asks her. "Oh yes," she replies, "Mr. Oxly's been complaining about my punctuation so I'm careful to get here before nine." Although Marilyn Monroe became famous for these dumb-blonde impersonations, directors before Hawks had tended to cast her as a serious siren. But Hawks saw her sexual quality not as real but as fantasy, as silly not serious—and so another star persona emerged from a Hawks conception (in *Monkey Business* and *Gentlemen Prefer Blondes*).

Miss Laurel (perhaps the name is an abbreviation of the Lorelei she becomes in *Gentlemen Prefer Blondes*) becomes Barnaby's sexual lure, the parallel to Edwina's Hank Entwhistle (Hugh Marlowe), her childhood sweetheart. Although Barnaby later tells Edwina that Miss Laurel is "half-infant," Edwina's jealous response is, "Not the half that's visible." But the half that isn't visible, her mind, is indeed infantile—a fact that makes Miss Laurel no more serious a threat to the marriage than Hank, whose mind is still fixed on its infantile childhood object. Laurel-Monroe's half-infant mind is also especially appropriate in a film about "thinking" and reverse evolution. Miss Laurel shows Barnaby another part of her anatomy not usually visible, the legs beneath her skirt, encased in a pair of acetate stockings invented by Barnaby. "Aren't they wonderful?" she asks. Hawks's camera, as well as a peering Oxly in the rearground, admire Laurel's display of her stockinged legs, introduced by this pronoun with no clear grammatical (only a visual) antecedent. Barnaby self-consciously explains his visual interest to Oxly, "Miss Laurel has just been showing me her acetates"—with an obvious pun on the word's similarity to assets (or a briefer noun). In many of the film's mature sequences characters explain or apologize for the public display of their private passions and fancies; that sort of apology makes mature people mature and public society possible. Oxly himself must apologize to Barnaby for employing such a secretary: "anybody can type." Later, the scientists in Oxly's employ must pretend that they keep no liquor in the laboratory. In the childhood sequences of regression, however, no such apologies are ever perceived to be necessary.

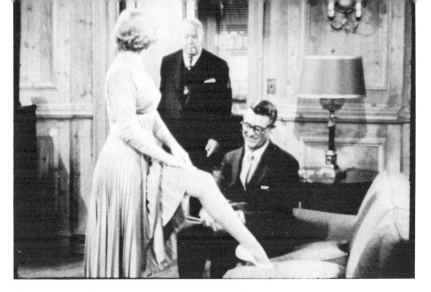

Huxley examining Miss Laurel's acetates while Oxly, like the film viewer, observes.

Oxly, the old ox at the other extreme of the film's chronological spectrum, is most personally interested in the success of Barnaby's experiments. He intends to test the drug personally. It is Oxly who has coined the term B-4 to promote Fulton's neutrally named formula, X-19, a sarcastic swipe at the way American industry glamorizes science in order to market it. The selling of drugs is not very different from the marketing of movies. The script's original coined name for the formula was Cupidone, in comparison to which the film's B-4 is more subtle, more clearly related to the film's reversals of time and evolution, and more clearly related to the postwar popularity of the new B-vitamins. Oxly's advertising logo couples B-4 with the drawing of a bird—"What's the vulture doing?" Fulton asks. Oxly explains that the bird is the mythical phoenix, rising from the ashes of its own spent body. This motif of rebirth is another of the film's *re*-themes that, as opposed to *re*discovery and *re*affirmation of that which already is, runs contrary to natural and human cycles—like *re*juvenation, *re*gression, and *re*incarnation. Indeed, later in the film Barnaby himself will be believed to be reborn and reincarnated in the body of an infant after somehow discarding the ashen one he presently inhabits.

A phone call from the laboratory sends Oxly and Fulton scurrying to witness what has apparently been the success of X-19 or B-4. The aged chimp, Rudolph, the simian equivalent of an 84-year-old human

169

being, has suddenly erupted into frisky play. "Rudolph" swings madly from the hanging lamps of the laboratory, defying the commands of the humans below with his chaotic and exuberant movement. The visual imagery of "Rudolph's" spontaneous play has several interesting relationships to Hawks's work in general and to this specific film. First, the visual image of the chimp swinging in midair recalls one of the final images of *Bringing Up Baby* when the Tarzan-like Huxley grasps the swinging Susan, suspended in midair. But in that film, Huxley's regression to apehood was a sign of his discovering the exuberant animal vitality in himself. Even Susan's rocking on that ladder before her tumble echoes the to and fro motion of "Rudolph." A second Hawks irony is that "Rudolph" uses the room's hanging lamps, a consistent visual motif in Hawks films, as the means of his airborn play. This time the lamps are electric (as they are in *His Girl Friday*) rather than kerosene (as they are in *Only Angels Have Wings* and *Red River*). But for the ape to use hanging lamps as the branches of trees is to use them not as civilization intended and not for the purpose for which they were invented, but as simple natural, physical objects. Electric light, like the science of chemistry, is another of the ways that civilized human society has evolved to escape from the constraints of nature, producing light when nature itself is unable to do so—just as eyeglasses are a civilized invention to escape the natural defects in human vision. For "Rudolph" to use a lamp as a tree is another example of both reverse evolution and a negation of Hawks's definition of human community, since those communities always exist by gathering around and under these lamps.

Civilization as the jungle, electric lamps as trees.

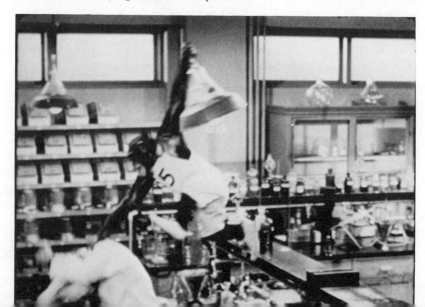

Barnaby discovers, however, that despite this chimp's exuberance, his formula still has not been proven. Unfortunately, this chimp is not Rudolph but Esther, a six-month-old female chimp, who has been mistakenly dressed in Rudolph's clothing (an ironic Hawks use of a familiar motif—putting a chimp, not Cary Grant, into the clothes of the wrong sex). The very idea of putting clothes on chimps is, of course, also part of the film's contrast of nature and civilization. The mistake has occurred because the muttering janitor, Gus (who parallels the muttering Gogarty in *Bringing Up Baby*, a man who also makes a mistake with an animal in a cage), put the wrong clothes on Esther after bathing her; either he then left the cage door open (as both Slocum and Gogarty do in *Bringing Up Baby*), permitting her escape, or Esther was able to let herself out by discovering the secret of the latch. This incident is to be a foreshadowing of several "organic" events that will narratively grow from it. Gus will be the origin of another mistake—when he changes the bottle on the water cooler and leaves the machine exposed. Esther, in a prophetic act, removes Fulton's glasses as he examines her— the first of four times when those glasses, like Huxley's, come off. And they will later come off because either he or Edwina drinks the chemical mixed by this very chimp and dumped in the very water cooler which Gus leaves open. Finally, this case of mistaken identity of a younger animal for an older one will be paralleled by the later mistaken identity of an infant for the adult Barnaby Fulton.

The film's second section, which chronicles Barnaby Fulton's first trip into his youth, begins with the mixing of the chemical that provides the transportation. As Barnaby sits and mixes (Hawks and Grant cleverly add some improvisatory mumbo-jumbo that parodies chemical jargon—2000 milligrams of thus and such), Esther sits in her cage and intently watches. Hawks executes a series of cross-cuts between the working scientist, concentrating mightily on his task, and the watching chimp, concentrating mightily on the man. The photographic method of cross-cutting is precisely opposite the choice Hawks made in *Baby* of keeping the people and the animals in the same frame. Whereas the framing in the earlier film emphasized parallels and similarities, the communion of humans and animals, the montage method of the later film emphasizes contrasts and differences, the opposition of humans and animals. Esther may appear to be concentrating, as Fulton is concentrating, but apes are incapable of concentration in this sense. They are

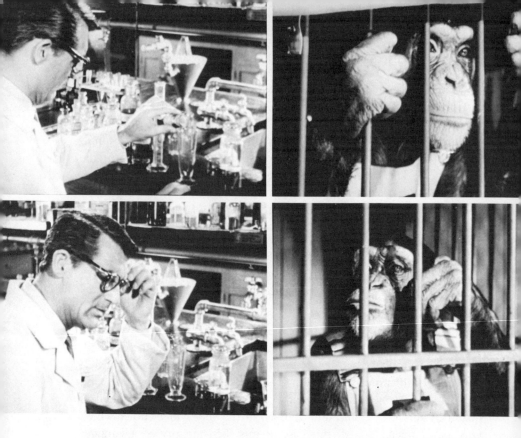

capable only of looking as if they are concentrating and of concentrating on the surface physical gestures and movements of beings, not on abstract issues of quality and quantity. Hawks's handling of point-of-view with this series of cross-cuts is also remarkable because the tight, extreme close-ups mirror the psychological sense of concentration by both Fulton and Esther. Yet by cutting back and forth between them, the storyteller disassociates himself from either figure of concentration and identifies his (and therefore our) interest as the process that differentiates the two types of concentration.

The cross-cutting to develop both parallels and contrasts continues in the next section, in which Esther swings out of her cage on its door—another "Swinging Door Susie"—and Fulton uses the heating, mixing, and incubating machinery in the adjacent laboratory. Both man and chimp are busy at work—or play. Hawks then cuts back to Esther's sitting in the very chair just vacated by Fulton, using a camera position parallel to the one for observing the scientist; the camera watches the chimp mix chemicals exactly as the scientist had done. Her intentness and concentration mirror both her own concentration in the previous

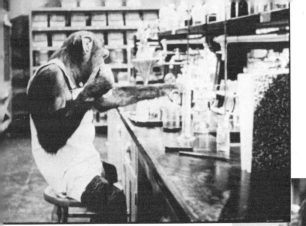

Aping the scientist.

series of cross-cuts as well as Fulton's. Indeed, this intentness and concentration make the wildly impossible premise of the film's remaining action narratively probable. An ape is going to swing out of her cage (a probability established by a previous escape), mix the chemical that will transport humans back to their youth (a probability established by Esther's intense concentration on Barnaby's mixing), and then toss away her chemical discovery, because it tastes bitter, into the water cooler (a probability established by Gus's changing the water bottle), where people will drink it by mistake. This series of probabilities is aided by the fact that the life-reversing purpose for which the drug is intended is an existential impossibility to begin with (like David Huxley, there is something that Barnaby Fulton does not know about his science). So it is as likely that an ape can discover the impossible by accident as it is that a human can discover it by science. Hawks's comedies can credibly sail so far into the sea of impossibility specifically because the narrative vessels have been built with such carefully and complexly fitted planks of probability.

Barnaby drinks the drug which he has carefully mixed and heated,

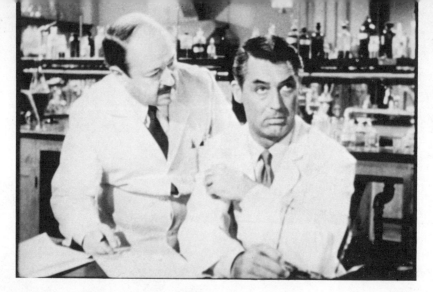

Vision without glasses.

washing it down with Esther's spiked water from the cooler. In scientific terms, his experiment lacks sufficient controls since either the water or the mixture could produce the results to follow. Those results include Barnaby's discovery that he is blind with his glasses but can see perfectly without them; off they come again, just as Esther removed them. His bursitis has disappeared—so Fulton does a cartwheel, paralleling the swinging, circular animal movements of Esther earlier. With these two actions in the lab the man is now aping the ape, whereas previously the ape had aped the man. The man can still speak, however, and his series of adventures begins (as do both others) with a physical gag followed by a self-conscious verbal pun. First the burlesque gag as Fulton walks directly past his colleague—arm extended to shake his hand—to answer the telephone instead. Then, after the telephoning Edwina tells him that they can get a good buy on a car, Barnaby answers, "Good buy? Well, goodbye to you too. (*Hanging up the phone*) Watta joke. A real knee slapper."

He sets off for a haircut (which will be a youthful crew cut), to buy some clothes (which will be a youthful plaid jacket and argyle socks), and to buy that car (which will be a youthful sports car rather than the good buy on a dependable sedan). The film develops one of its consistent visual motifs on this shopping trip when Barnaby approvingly examines both his new haircut and his new clothes in a mirror. The mirror motif relates to the film's examination of human vision, for though

174

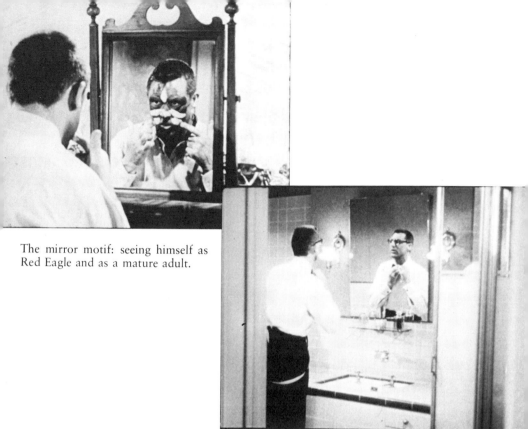

The mirror motif: seeing himself as Red Eagle and as a mature adult.

Barnaby can see how his body looks with the new hair and clothes in the mirror, his brain does not tell him how ridiculous a person of his age and with his body looks in that style of hair and clothes. The story-teller observes the youthified Fulton observing himself, drawing a distinction between what Barnaby can see in the mirror and what we can see of Barnaby, the difference between how he sees and how we see. The film's mirror motif culminates with Barnaby's final descent into his youth as he intently (like Esther) looks in the mirror in order to apply his Indian war paint correctly without his brain's ever wondering if it is correct for a grown man to apply Indian war paint at all.

While buying his sports car, Barnaby meets up with Miss Laurel, who has been sent to fetch him; Barnaby recognizes her instantly by the mere sight of her ankles beneath a large billboard sign. "Is your motor running?" she asks him. "Is yours?" he replies. The two set off motoring together for an afternoon of fun—both indoors, roller skating (he takes a pratfall); and out, swimming (he takes a belly flop). With the pratfalls, the subject and style of the film have deliberately reverted to *Bringing Up Baby* of fourteen years earlier, in which David's physical clumsiness mirrors his social and spiritual inadequacies. Barnaby Fulton's body and grace are simply not up to the youthful tasks his desire asks them to perform. The shooting and visual style of the film in this section also differ markedly from the earlier quiet confinement. The camera and action have moved outdoors, where motion is larger and freer (like Esther swinging on that light fixture) and where the camera itself participates in that motion. As Fulton drives along in his car, the speedy and reckless driving gives the camera an opportunity both to escape from its deliberate constriction in the mature sequences and to regress to the youth of cinema itself, to the automobile gags and stunts of the Mack Sennett silent comedies. Grant links the silent and sound traditions of comedy when he improvises yet another Hawks reference to the movies: he assures Miss Laurel, "I like you, I like you," intoning the words with a childish repetitiveness and patting the top of his head in the manner of Jerry Lewis, whose familiar line at the time was, "I like it, I like it." The trip comes to an end, however, when the drug wears off and Fulton, still driving the car, discovers that he cannot see without his glasses. The car bounces to a halt with a bump into the fence of the Oxly Chemical Plant (actually the Fox parking lot, clearly identifiable by any insider).

The film's third major section, that night, chronicles Edwina's own trip into her youth. Actually, these characters do not exactly travel into their own youths. The sexual aggressiveness that Barnaby displayed with Miss Laurel under the influence of the drug (not to mention the wild clothes and haircut) may not have been a characteristic of the young Fulton at all. His youthful trip may have been a regression to the youth he never was and never had, the suppressed and repressed one. This comic Freudian suggestion is supported by Edwina's retreat to a very pranksterish, aggressive youth after drinking the drug, although Barnaby informed us that she was really a very sweet and retiring young girl. Similarly Freudian, after Edwina's trip Barnaby wonders about her "hidden aversion or subconscious discontent." In its reverse Darwinism, *Monkey Business* also suggests that as humans become more animal and less human, they also become more id and less superego in their escape from civilization and its discontents. Edwina's very decision to take the drug herself in this third section of the film is triggered by an aggressively jealous reaction to Barnaby's afternoon with Miss Laurel, his face covered by lipstick. "Yes, it is unbelievable on roller skates."

After aggressively snatching the drug and drinking it, Edwina, like her husband, washes it down with water from the cooler, the real source of the drug's potency. She observes, as her husband did (careful symmetrical patterning again), "Even the water tastes bitter." Edwina's released libido now takes several aggressive forms. First, a physical gag: she stuffs a live fish down the front of Oxly's pants and plants a pie on a chair for the seat of those pants. This comic attack on those two male areas directly beneath the belt is another juxtaposition of Freud and the burleycue gag. Like her husband's experience with the drug, her altered physical behavior is accompanied by a self-conscious play on words. "Oh, my," says Oxly, as his pants encounter the cream pie. "Oh my, get me piece of pie," chants Edwina in rhythmic response, as she begins to jitterbug through the laboratory, in tempo with her words—like Esther swinging on the chandelier or Barnaby turning a cartwheel. True to her movie past, when Ginger Rogers regresses she becomes a hoofer.

Finally, she drags Barnaby off to the Pickwick Arms Hotel (Edwina drives the sports car this time), to the bridal suite where they spent their wedding night. Ginger Rogers jitterbugs and then dances the last slow dance with her husband—a deliberate echo of her routines with Astaire, in films which were contemporaneous with *Bringing Up Baby*. The slow dance is to their favorite song, "The Whiffenpoof Song," which becomes this film's "I Can't Give You Anything But Love." The script called for "The Music Goes Round and Round," which might have fit better into the film's theme of temporal regression, but "The Whiffenpoof Song" is more childishly sentimental. As they retire for the night to their chamber, Edwina takes an off-frame pratfall in the corridor (the parallel with Barnaby's previous slips). And the camera, though confined indoors in this sequence, still works more freely and actively in this section than it does when the characters act their age. As is typical of Hawks's control of point-of-view, the camera mirrors subjective feelings by acting the same age that the characters feel themselves to be but never obscuring the storyteller's judgment that they either are or are not acting their age.

In their hotel room, Edwina reverts to her blushing, bridal, presexual modesty, changing clothes in the bathroom, emerging all shy and jittery, then using her nervousness to pick deliberate quarrels with her husband—preferring both her mother's and Hank Entwhistle's to his company. In her anger, Edwina knocks off Barnaby's glasses, pushes him into the hall wearing his pajamas, and ties a knot in the belt of the pajama bottoms that has gotten caught in the slamming door. In the film's Freudian terms, she is tying more than a piece of cloth into knotted disuse. Without the protection of the drug to ease his self-consciousness, a blind Barnaby Fulton takes a pratfall, strays into the wrong hotel room, tries to sing his own room's door back open again with "The Whiffenpoof Song" (a parallel to singing Baby off the roof), and strays into the laundry room where he takes a comic fall down the laundry chute. The original script planned a much longer (and very funny) sequence of embarrassments that included his trying to coax Edwina to open the door by using a nickname, Eddie (one can imagine the reaction of people in the hotel corridor to his gender confusion, asking his darling Eddie to forgive him and let him back in the room), and by his wandering into so many strange bedrooms and beds that the police are summoned to apprehend a cat burglar (parallel to the peeping tom in *Baby*). The scene was trimmed either to save money, to avoid the tricky sexual innuendoes, or to keep the focus on the film's central couple rather than indulge in a fairly riotous series of mistakes of a night.

The sober light of day begins the fourth section, in which the previous night's damage must be undone. A shivering Barnaby must wear Edwina's coat for warmth (Cary Grant doesn't wear a dress in this film, but there is this woman's coat). She must tell both her mother and Hank, whom she telephoned the night before, that she does not want a divorce. And Barnaby and Edwina return to the lab for the spare pair of glasses that will restore his adult vision. Barnaby has decided to destroy the formula, because of its danger, and as Edwina and her husband chat calmly, they drink several cups of coffee (she two, he three) made from water out of that same water cooler. All they know is that even the coffee tastes bitter—the same initial response as for the previous two trips.

Hawks's camera strategy for observing Edwina's and Barnaby's sliding off on a trip they do not know they are going to take is a marvel of understated detachment. Barnaby sits conversing on a stool, in the middleground frame right, in the same place where he departed for his first trip, suspended between animal life (the cages to his right) and human civilization (the chemicals to his left). Edwina sits in the foreground frame left, exactly the place from which she departed for her

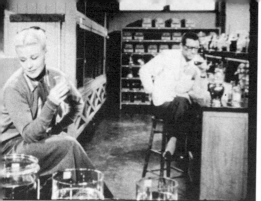
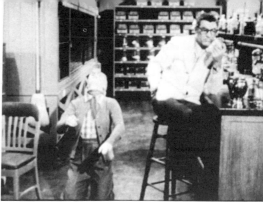

Detached observation of the data in Hawks's carefully balanced frame.

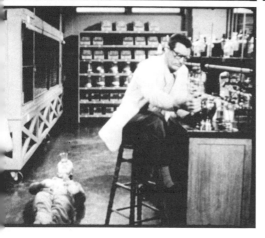

previous trip. The perfectly balanced frame synthesizes both previous journeys. Without making a cut, Hawks will keep us within that perfectly balanced frame, detachedly (indeed scientifically) observing two people gradually become unbalanced together within the same frame. While Barnaby rambles on about the effects of the drug, he gradually becomes so hypnotized by the sound of his words (the typical Hawks use of speech as sound) that he does not even notice the strange behavior of his wife, directly to his right. She first becomes hypnotized by the swimming fish in the bowl in front of her, just as she did on her previous trip before dumping the fish down Oxly's pants. Then she starts to move away from the camera, into the mid-ground beside her husband, and as she walks she suddenly shuffles into a little tap-dance step, an unconscious, improvised (and unscripted) little shuffle which comes so easily she doesn't even notice she did it (a wonderful use of Ginger Rogers's particular abilities). Edwina then unconsciously puts a glass of water on her forehead while Barnaby hypnotically recites the diminishing ages to which the drug might transport the taker (a comic parallel with Joe's calling out his altitudes in *Only Angels Have Wings*). As Barnaby intones the declining figures, "12 . . . 10 . . . 5," Edwina starts to dip toward the floor, backwards, bending her knees, the glass still perfectly poised on her forehead, sinking lower and lower with each lower number of decreasing age. At the end of the speech, Barnaby is still hypnotically chattering, with no visual awareness of Edwina's strange actions at all, while she lies flat on her back on the floor beside him, the glass still balanced on her forehead (another superb and improvisational use by Hawks of her unique physical gifts).

The perfect coordination of words and movement in the shot, echoed by the perfect balance of right and left in the frame, while the camera mutely and motionlessly observes the physical data, allows this point-of-view shot to achieve a multiplicity of views and attitudes. We are aware of both causes and effects in this detached shot that neither figure in the frame knows anything about. We know what both the left and right halves of the frame contain, while the occupant of each half is ignorant of the other—and ignorant of the reason they are ignorant of the other half. When Edwina arises, without ever knowing she has been on the floor, Barnaby observes that taking an overdose of the drug might turn a person into an infant (a necessary bit of preparation for the action to follow). He naturally and unconsciously takes off his glasses, not even noting he no longer needs them. Although unconscious of these physical facts, the two share a self-conscious gag (to parallel the beginnings of the previous two regression sequences): she pulls away the chair on which he is about to sit (the same one on which she set Mr. Oxly's pie); he catches himself and turns to her: "Ha, ha."

The final trip the two take together will be the longest of the three in the film (they drank the most water for it, and it is, after all, the climactic one) and it will take them back even further than their previous regressions—to childhood (by implication even infancy) rather than postadolescence. This regression also has several parts—indoors and outdoors, the couple together, then each of them separately. First, Barnaby, Edwina, and their new friend, Esther, enter the boardroom of the Oxly Chemical Plant; the Board of Directors has assembled to make Fulton, who has just been described as "one of the great scientific minds of the age," an offer for his formula. A now tomboyish, eight-year-oldish Edwina, chomps on a wad of gum, shoots rubber bands (mostly in the aggressive direction of Miss Laurel's derrière), and scrawls a huge

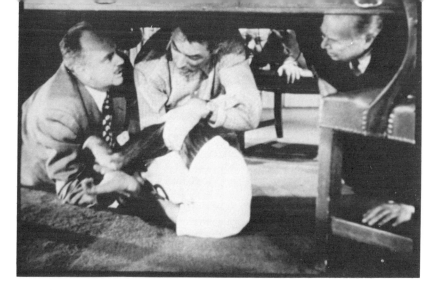

Doing business with a monkey under the table.

heart, containing the inscription, "Barnaby loves Edwina," with chalk on the blackboard—as if the boardroom were a schoolroom. When the directors ask Barnaby how much money he wants, he confers with Esther, his business associate (an appropriate companion in this tale of reverse Darwinism), and announces, "A zillion dollars," which he later amends, "and a nickel." This childish conception of money parallels the psychiatrist's lure in *Bringing Up Baby,* coaxing what he thinks to be a mad Susan into his house by offering her "a million dollars—all in one dollar bills." Most striking in the boardroom scene is its defiance of the usual procedures of adult business. Rather than sitting down at the huge and impressive conference table, Barnaby, Edwina, and Esther both stroll on top of that table and duck beneath it when Barnaby drags Oxly and the other directors to the floor for their financial dickering (as a delightful Esther tumbles circularly in and out of Hawks's frame). And the scene ends with Esther swinging on another chandelier, flying above the table, pelting the adults below with lightbulbs (another transformation of invented human artifact into simple natural object—the fruit of a chandelier tree).

Barnaby and Edwina escape outdoors, into the sunlight, as he kicks a can and she tags along behind him. The sight of a housepainter, with his many alluring buckets of paint, leads to their Laurel and Hardyish paint fight, complete with Stan and Ollie's use of the monosyllable "hmmm," driving Edwina home to the telephone again and a call to

Hank. As opposed to the childhood play of David and Susan in *Bringing Up Baby,* which brings them together, the childhood play in *Monkey Business* is based on savage aggression and drives Barnaby and Edwina apart. While Edwina falls asleep (as in *A Midsummer Night's Dream,* sleep is the means to alter or restore human vision), Barnaby joins a group of neighborhood children, playing cowboys and Indians (more aggression), with a plan to ambush Hank upon the rival's arrival (still more aggression). Barnaby, now in the war paint of "Red Eagle," urges burning him at the stake, but one of the children (George "Foghorn" Winslow) sensibly observes that you can't do that. "Somebody'll stop us the minute we light a fire. They always do." Winslow, with his deep adult voice and cautious adult reasoning imprisoned inside a child's body and behind a child's face, fits perfectly into the film's contrast of youth and age. In a film in which adults behave like children, Winslow reveals the potential for children to behave like adults—a contrary (and more natural) collapse of apparent opposites.

Winslow's sensible argument wins the day; they decide to scalp Hank instead. But, as Winslow soberly counsels, "You can't scalp anybody unless you do a war dance first . . . You gotta sing when you do it." "Red Eagle" Fulton then leads the kiddies in a Hawks musical number of communal celebration and solidarity—except this is a childishly savage song, with no articulate lyrics ("ugga bugga wug glug") and no coherent melody (a pure chanting rhythm rather than a coherent melodic pattern). The song celebrates a reverse Darwinian "community" of child-animal irrationality, savagery, and inhuman inarticulateness. This "community" ties Hank to the stake when he arrives and "Red Eagle" Fulton dances around him, waving a pair of garden shears—supposedly for the scalping, but a wonderfully comic Freudian image of aggression and castration.

Meanwhile, a now adultly rational Edwina awakes to touch the bare buttocks of an infant sleeping beside her. A series of carefully built interlocking probabilities produces what will be an astounding conclusion—Edwina's belief that the infant beside her is her own husband, Barnaby. First, a neighborhood cleaning lady has been assigned the task of watching the infant, but as she hangs the laundry out to dry, the infant toddles off into Edwina's bedroom. Second, Barnaby has changed his paint-soaked clothes (he has put the paint on his face instead) in order to impersonate "Red Eagle." When Edwina awakens to feel a naked body beside her in her husband's usual sleeping place, when she sees her husband's clothes on a nearby chair, and when she remembers the possible effect her husband described of the regenerative drug's making one an infant, it makes perfect sense to her that this infant is her husband. The storyteller himself seems to comment on this uncanny series of probabilities. Just before Edwina's mistake of identities, the cleaning lady has observed Barnaby's behavior as "Red Eagle" and mutters, "The things some people think of."

Edwina scoops the infant up and takes him, by taxi, to the Oxly Plant, where she hopes the scientists can find an antidote. The brief scene in the taxicab, which does not exist in the script, is the film's comic culmination and produces perhaps the funniest single moment in the work of Howard Hawks. Its humor arises from Hawks's subtle and thorough control of point-of-view, another single shot, without a cut or a camera movement. The shot keeps Edwina, who sits in the back seat with the infant, frame left, and the cabbie, who sits in the front seat, frame right, in the frame together for its duration, and creates a counterpoint between these two spaces and these two halves of the frame. The principle of this shot is precisely the same as that of the shot which began this final "trip," the balanced framing of Edwina and Barnaby together in the lab after they drink their spiked coffee. Edwina talks to the infant on the left while the cabbie watches the road on the right. At first, he makes no visible reaction to her chatter at all; after all, he is a cabbie and has seen and heard plenty. He finds the subject of her conversation a bit odd, but it is not so strange for parents to baby-talk with their children. But when Edwina says, "Barnaby, I'm your wife," the cabbie can restrain his facial muscles no longer, and we observe (but without a cut or a close-up, in this same continuous balanced frame) his visible take of astonishment, which releases the comic tension of the shot to produce the loud laugh.

Hawks's handling of point-of-view produces this loud laugh by simultaneously giving us three differing points of view. We understand the process, the sequence of probabilities, that has led to Edwina's conclusion about the identity of this infant, so we understand precisely why she talks to him as she does and how she feels about him and his, in her mind, transformation. But the cab driver in the right foreground is a total innocent to this series of bizarre events and interlocked probabilities. He simply reacts to a stranger talking to an infant (a little odd)

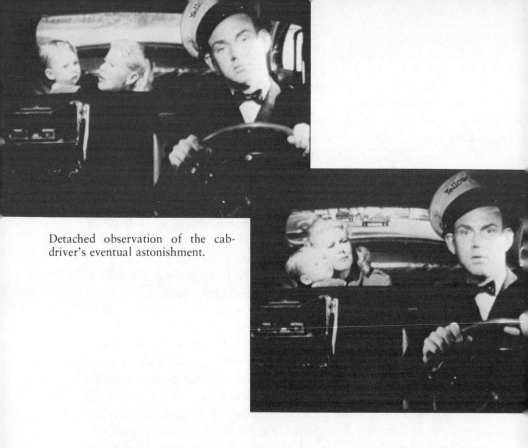

Detached observation of the cab-driver's eventual astonishment.

and calling him her husband (very odd, since babies cannot be husbands). We can understand precisely how the cab driver must view this conversation and its participants, how it and they must seem to him—just as in *Bringing Up Baby* we can understand how strange it must seem to strangers to hear a man order thirty pounds of raw meat for baby. In his comedies, Hawks delights in revealing the distance his story has traveled from everyday probability with a scene that juxtaposes those observers who are innocent of the comic circumstances with those participants who are entangled in them.

The third point-of-view in the shot is precisely this juxtaposition, the audience's sharing the joke and the scene with the storyteller, for we know more than either of these two figures in the frame. For example, we know precisely why they are both sharing this frame at this time—the process that has brought them together at this point in the story. In this framing, we share the ironic realization that those who inhabit the same physical space do not inhabit the same mental space at all. The way we can best share this ironic realization with the story-teller is simply to watch it with him from the detached position of the observing camera, whose distance and triangular position in this scene (as in the coffee scene earlier) creates a third "character" who is a synthesis of the perceptions of the camera, storyteller, and audience.

After arriving at the plant, Oxly tries to converse with the infant, just as Huxley tried to converse with the subverbal George—again without success ("He's being evasive again"). All the directors and employees then join to serenade the baby to sleep, using "The Whiffenpoof Song" as a lullaby, a parallel to serenading Baby in the earlier film. And as in that earlier film, the serenade represents a climactic triumph of bizarre narrative probabilities. It seems perfectly credible for a group of adult scientists and businessmen to sing a lullaby to an infant so that when he awakes he will become the adult he really is. Ironically, the strategy works, for the adult Barnaby crawls through the window into the room where the infant lies asleep, just as he initially departed through this very window for his first "trip" in the film—the closing of another perfect Hawks circle. To use a window as a door is a further sign of nature at war with civilization, child's play in conflict with adult vocation, just as "Swinging Door Susie" in *Bringing Up Baby* escaped Slocum's jail through its window. Barnaby lies down beside the infant, with a wonderfully sly, improvisatory, sexual directive to the playful baby: "Please. No familiarities. Just go to sleep." And Edwina walks into the back office to discover her husband's return, although she suffers some confusion: "Now there are two of you." Barnaby is no less confused: "What do you mean you thought it was me?" innocent of the strange series of narrative probabilities from which he was absent.

When the two now sober adults walk back into the laboratory, drawn there by the eruption of off-frame noise (as is typical of Hawks), they discover that the entire staff of the Chemical Plant has regressed to childhood hysteria. Just as the climax of *Bringing Up Baby* gathers all its characters for its narrative and thematic culmination in the jailhouse, the climax of *Monkey Business* reduces all its assembled human adults to the childishly savage monkey business in the laboratory. They spray each other with bottles of seltzer, accompanied by Esther, who also holds a hose; a scientist swings from a hanging lamp—just as Esther did earlier; Oxly himself chases Miss Laurel with a seltzer bottle, another comic Freudian object that probably performs more energeti-

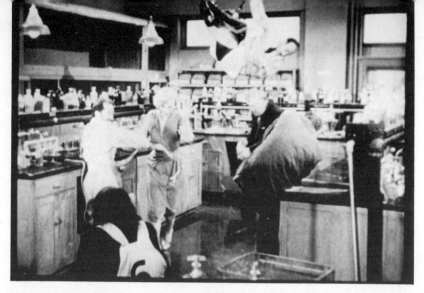

The ultimate reduction to the chaotic absurd.

cally than the organ for which it is a subtle surrogate. Oxly also indulges his aggression when he sprays Barnaby full-face with that watery weapon, whose liquid spray visually evokes the memory of that other comically vulgar liquid stream in *Scarface*. All of those adults have partaken of the water cooler, washing down a nip of whiskey with the spiked water. One remaining rational employee quickly and simply explains they now know that the source of the drug is the water cooler (a quick and effortless way to tie off this narrative thread, as opposed to a rather lengthy, uninteresting scene of discovery and explanation in the script). The fourth section of the film ends with this chaotic and climactic reduction of adult scientists to the absurdity of childhood animality and aggression.

The epilogue returns us to the civilized, adult Fulton home at night, where, as they did at the film's beginning, Barnaby and Edwina dress for an evening out. There is another mirror in the scene, and this time when Barnaby uses a mirror to attire himself, he sees the adult he ought to see; he sees Barnaby Fulton, not "Red Eagle." Edwina wears another dark evening dress, just as she did at the film's beginning. But as opposed to Barnaby's emotional absence and vacancy in the film's first scene, he is now aware of the meaning and value of his home, his wife, and his life. He announces that he has a "new formula": "It doesn't come in packages or bottles. You're old only when you forget you're young. It's a word you keep in your heart, a light you keep in your eyes." This very explicit discovery represents a rediscovery of his human feelings, and a resynthesis of thought and feeling—those two human functions which must be synthesized but whose initial conflict began both *Monkey Business* and *Bringing Up Baby*. The strains of "The Whiffenpoof Song" seep into the frame from the sound track, a soft reminder of the emotions and experiences they share and have shared. Barnaby wonders, "What time did you order the table?" Perhaps they will stay home again this evening instead of going out. This time it will be Barnaby's feeling, not his thinking, that will keep them home—just as it did in their youth. While Susan Vance and David Huxley in *Bringing Up Baby* find each other, Barnaby and Edwina Fulton in *Monkey Business* find each other again.

7

Two Hecht-MacArthur Plays
into Howard Hawks Films:
Twentieth Century and His Girl Friday

I can tell you a story on Lombard. . . . she was one of the most attractive girls that you could find. And she acted like a schoolgirl. And she was stiff. . . . We were rehearsing the first day and John Barrymore began to hold his nose. I made him promise that he wouldn't say anything until 3 o'clock in the afternoon, but I could see him getting very worried over her stiffness, and obviously nothing was happening with this girl. Well, I took Lombard for a walk around the stage and I said you've been working hard on the script. She said I'm glad it shows. And I said yes you know every word of it. And I said how much do you get paid for the picture? She told me. I said that's pretty good. I said what do you get paid for? She said, well, acting. And I said well what if I would tell you that you had earned all your money and you don't owe a nickel, and you don't have to act anymore. And she just stared at me, and I said what would you do if a man said such and such a thing to you? And she said I'd kick him right in the balls. And I said, well Barrymore said that to you, why didn't you kick him? And I said, what would you say if a man said such and such to you and she went Whnnnnnah—snarled, you know, with one of those Lombard gestures. And I said, well he said that to you when he said such and such a line. Now we're going back in and make this scene and you kick him, and you do any damn thing that comes into your mind that's natural, and quit acting. If you don't quit, I'm going to fire you this afternoon.[1]

That happens to be the kind of woman that I like—I don't see why they have to sit around and wash dishes.[2]

Howard Hawks did not fire Carole Lombard from *Twentieth Century*, and the verbal-mental-physical sparring of that film's kicking and "Whnnnnnahing" became the first of two battles of wits and words originally written by Ben Hecht and Charles MacArthur for the stage that Howard Hawks turned into moving (and talking) pictures. Despite their stage origins, the two properties fit very well into the Hawks canon and the Hawks concerns—not surprising since Hecht, with and without MacArthur, worked very well with Hawks on such other films as *Scarface, Viva Villa!, Barbary Coast,* and *Monkey Business.* The central issue of both plays, *Twentieth Century* and *The Front Page,* is the familiar Hawksian theme of vocation, the potential conflict of professional and personal life. In *Twentieth Century,* the commitment to acting conflicts with other more sincere forms of human feeling and expression. And in *The Front Page,* the commitment to newspaper reporting conflicts with such other human pursuits as love, home, and family. Both plays pose these conflicts as unresolvable tensions: Lily Garland must choose between her professional liaison with Oscar Jaffe and her personal longings for a George Smith; Hildy Johnson must choose between work with Walter Burns and marriage with his girl Peggy. Hawks's two films, however, resolve these dramatic conflicts, consistently with both his own beliefs and his deeper and subtler perception of human psychology. The conflict between vocation and personal expression is merely apparent, merely a superficial self-deception by one of the central characters (in both, it is the woman's self-deception). In both, the only way that the two central characters can achieve a true personal fulfillment is through a complete vocational fulfillment, for these people *are* actors and newspapermen. For them to deny what they do well and love to do is to deny what they are.

The shift to two erring female characters in the two films reveals a key difference from both *Bringing Up Baby* and *Monkey Business,* in which the male is out of touch with his own feelings and must be guided to his internal discovery by the more knowing female. Both Susan Vance and Edwina Fulton know more than their supposedly knowledgeable mates, whose vocation is a kind of knowledge that must be supplemented by another, spiritual knowledge of which they are ignorant. In *Ball of Fire* and *I Was a Male War Bride* both the male and female characters come to a knowledge of themselves and of one another, for

190

they both suffer from some kind of ignorance. However, both Oscar Jaffe of *Twentieth Century* and Walter Burns of *His Girl Friday* know something that Lily Garland and Hildy Johnson do not (Walter knows it a lot more consciously than Oscar does, and the whole strategy of that film's structure is his proving it to Hildy). Lily dreams of a home "with a cookie jar and little feet pattering up and down the stairs," while Hildy longs to be a woman rather than a newspaperman. But both of these dreams are mere dreams and longings, illusions, abstract cultural clichés of happiness that may suit some people but simply will not do for those who are essentially actors and newspapermen.

Oscar Jaffe and Lily Garland are a matched set, a complementary spiritual pair, professionally and personally. So are Walter Burns and Hildy Johnson (revealing the psychologically perceptive brilliance of Hawks's shifting Hildy's sex from the Hecht-MacArthur male to a Hawks woman). The strategy of both narratives is to lead these two women to discover this inescapable and essential spiritual union, without which neither their personal nor professional lives can thrive. In the two plays on which the films are based, the underlying and subtextual issue of spiritual union and human complementarity is much fuzzier in Hecht-MacArthur's *Twentieth Century* and almost embarrassingly absent from their *Front Page*. The question, does Walter Burns want Hildy Johnson for any reason other than his reportorial skill, is not (and cannot be) raised by the play.

Hawks structures these two adaptations almost identically—to one another and to all his other narratives regardless of their sources. He adds a lengthy initial section, a prologue, to both these three-act plays, converting them into the four-part construction of all Hawks stories. He also pins a brief epilogue on the tail of *Twentieth Century* which closes the comic circle; an epilogue originally conceived for the script of *His Girl Friday,* which returns Walter and Hildy to the newspaper office, was eliminated by the implied spiritual reunion of the pair as they set off together—simultaneously to cover a news story and to get married. The opening prologues of the two films, which do not exist in the two original plays, occupy at least one third of the films' running times. Given the importance of Hawks's beginnings at establishing the moral and psychological issues of the narratives which follow, to create these new and lengthy beginnings is, in effect, to create two new narrative works altogether out of the previously existing plays.

The prologue of Hawks's *Twentieth Century* establishes the initial

clash, then growing closeness, then disruptive separation of two characters who come to know one another (like David and Susan in *Bringing Up Baby*). The prologue of *His Girl Friday* establishes the existing
relationship of a previously married couple (like Barnaby and Edwina
in *Monkey Business*). Both of these film prologues force our narrative
attention on the central couple—their clashes and harmonies, conflicts
and similarities—who are themselves ignorant (especially the women)
of the psychological dynamics which underlie their relationships. The
openings of the two plays, however, force our attention on the physical
milieu and the varied assortment of bizarre character types who inhabit
it (the train's passengers in *Twentieth Century,* the reporters in *The
Front Page*), rather than the central couple and their feelings for one
another. In both plays, the central pair never comes face to face (or
mouth to mouth) with one another for their verbal thrusts and parries
until near the end of the second act. Both films bring them face to face,
body to body, and word to word from the beginning. The subject of
both films is the mind, spirit and feeling beneath those faces, bodies,
and words, while the subject of both plays is the particular social world
that contains those faces, bodies, and kinds of words.

The teaming of the established Barrymore and the newcomer Lombard in *Twentieth Century* was the first of Hawks's casting master-
strokes—to be followed by Bogart-Bacall in *To Have and Have Not*
and Wayne-Clift in *Red River*. "I believe it's terribly interesting for the
audience to see a new girl playing with a man who's well established."[3]
Barrymore had been well established at parodying himself for years before *Twentieth Century* (for example, his impersonation of the fallen,
once-great actor in *Dinner at Eight*) and would continue to parody himself until his death (for example, *The Great Profile* in 1941). When
Barrymore asked Hawks why he wanted him for the role, Hawks replied, "Well, it's the story of the greatest ham in the world, and God
knows you fit that."[4] The outrageousness and exuberance of Barrymore's hamminess give *Twentieth Century* much of its life. There are
his outrageous physical poses—stretched out on the floor with his quill
pen; the Byronically statuesque, black-caped suicidal stare at the lights
of the city beneath him; the balletic toe dance to impersonate Sagittar-
ius, the archer; the curled up, self-contained, hunch-backed retreat to
the inner self as he sits alone on a spiral staircase during Lily Garland's
triumphant opening night; the flamboyant expansiveness of his hands

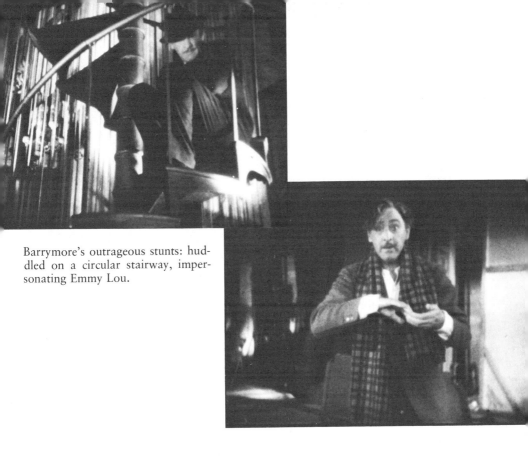

Barrymore's outrageous stunts: huddled on a circular stairway, impersonating Emmy Lou.

and arms during his "mad scene" after Lily leaves him, hurling buckets of paint across her pictures and posters to efface her from both the world and his memory. Barrymore matches this physical outrageousness with his verbal stunts—the high, wispy impersonation of a doorbell during rehearsals, "Ting-a-ling-a-ling-a-ling"; his campy impersonations of all the play's ridiculous roles, from the twittering girlfriend, Emmy Lou, to the shuffling old Uncle Remus; his saccharine address to the cast at the opening rehearsal that no matter what he may say or do, "I love you all"; the instantaneous transition from his cackling impersonation of a soothsayer, "cackle, cackle," to the shrewdly economic footnote, "forty dollars a week."

Barrymore accompanies these physical and verbal stunts with bits of in-group humor which, as is typical of Hawks, refer to the actual making of the film itself. In his greeting to the cast, Barrymore-Jaffe tells them how much he loves the theater and "all the charming people in it." This film is about two of those "charming" people—and they are

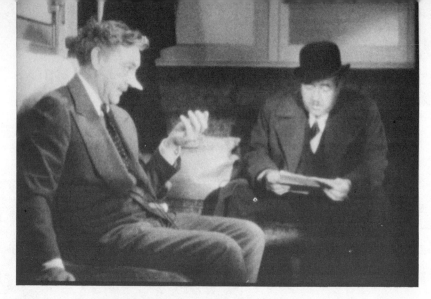

"The Great Profile" as Pinocchio.

both monsters, as is Barrymore himself, both on- and off-screen. When Jaffe dreams up his Passion Play, whose dramatis personae include a hundred camels and an ibis, he decides to house these beasts in a small zoo, which he will construct next to the green room. Since the green room is theatrical jargon for the actors' lounge, Barrymore implies that the human lounge is also a zoo, but for human rather than bestial monsters. There is Barrymore's lordly contempt for the disguise he employed to evade the Chicago sheriff: "I never thought I should sink so low. To be an actor." As the actor who despises acting removes his costume for this disguise, he begins to play with his putty nose. Barrymore and Hawks then execute the film's most outrageously funny piece of self-reference when Barrymore pulls the putty into a hawkishly pointed beak, then turns his head to the side so Hawks can photograph "The Great Profile" in profile. That profile has become Pinocchio's, a monstrous beak that is a parody of the face which is Barrymore's trademark and meal ticket. Hawks and Barrymore then top this parodic nose-play with an outrageous gag: Barrymore sticks his finger up that putty nose to pick it.

The "new girl" in the film, Carole Lombard, was Hawks's second cousin, with roots in the same Wisconsin town as his own family. Although he thought she was "the worst actress in the world," she was also a "marvellous gal, crazy as a bedbug. . . . If she could just be herself, she'd be great for the part."[5] So the task that Hawks undertook

194

on the film, to make an unknown girl into a comic star, precisely paralleled the action of the film itself, Oscar Jaffe's making the unknown Mildred Plotka into the star Lily Garland. The film of *Twentieth Century* becomes a comic version of the Svengali-Trilby melodrama, the master singing teacher who molds a shapeless female vessel into a great vocal talent; he then becomes possessed by that voice and wishes to possess her body and soul as well. Hawks's film twice refers specifically to the Svengali story (itself a 19th-century melodramatic retelling of the Pygmalion myth), when Lily refuses to accept its applicability to herself, "I'm no Trilby," and when she derogates her master, Oscar, "That fake Svengali." And the Svengali story will also underlie *His Girl Friday;* in the opening scene, Hildy tells Walter, "Scram, Svengali." Ironically, Barrymore had made a serious version of the Svengali tale in 1931,[6] to which *Twentieth Century* is the comic reply. And in Howard Hawks's quest to create new stars we can see his own Svengali tendencies, a parallel and a sense of possession which Lauren Bacall specifically felt and described in her dealings with her master.[7] Like Svengali, Hawks remade Bacall's voice.

These levels of irony, conscious self-reference, and unconscious applicability enrich and complicate the film's remaking of the Hecht-MacArthur play—particularly the opening section which details the Svengali-Trilby relationship of Oscar and Lily.[8] The psychological core that Hawks-Hecht-MacArthur retained from the play was that Oscar Jaffe and Lily Garland were not real people but theater people—which means they are "actors," not people at all. There is no emotion in the play that is not feigned, not "acted"—love, hate, suicide, the sorrow of death itself. And there is no emotional scene that is not a carefully managed "scene"—including Oscar's arranging the furniture, setting the lights, and directing the reactions for his own death. The two central players of Hecht-MacArthur's play cannot separate playing from living, emoting from feeling, the fake from the real. Indeed, Hecht and MacArthur find these clear oppositions rather blurry in general—and not only in their ironic application to theater people. The play's spokesman for purity, piety, and abstinence, Matthew J. Clark, the man who reads the Bible and the *Saturday Evening Post,* who refuses to buy a Sunday newspaper, and who spreads the word of goodness and Godness (by pasting religious stickers on everything in the train), is himself insane. Although the theater people seem nuts, it is the pious man who is nuts. Later in the play Jaffe himself will be accused of being crazy, merely because he is reading the Bible. This reversal of accepted social values (who is good or bad, sane or insane, nice or nasty) and the corollary collapse of the clear distinction between the fake and the real are hallmarks of the Ben Hecht style; the reversal also indicates Hecht's spiritual link with Hawks, who similarly liked to reverse social expectations (like Bonnie Lee's) and to collapse apparent opposites (like the differences between a David Huxley and a Susan Vance).

Two lines in the Hecht-MacArthur play provide the source for the film's lengthy and complex prologue: (1) Oscar reminds Lily of his changing her name from Mildred Plotka to Lily Garland and (2) Lily accuses Oscar of telling everyone that he chalked lines on the stage floor to teach her how to walk. The process of Mildred's conversion to Lily by her following the chalk lines on the floor to stardom becomes the basis of the film prologue's first sequence. Its second sequence chronicles Oscar's and Lily's possessive love affair—also suggested by a line in the play when Lily confesses to her new lover that Oscar was her only previous love. And the prologue's final sequence chronicles Lily's escape to Hollywood and the consequent Learlike rage of Jaffe after her departure. This three-part invented prologue, with a beginning, a middle, and an end, is a complete (and new) little story in itself as well as the preparation and the foundation for the action of the whole narrative to follow.

The effect of the prologue is not only to deepen the psychological and emotional history of the play's central pair, not only to use the Svengali-Trilby legend in a series of complex applications to the film and its makers, and not only to open the film up spatially and temporally by freeing the narrative from the single train car and the single 16-hour journey of the play. The prologue also recasts the original dramatized story into the "narrative mode,"[9] the way that narrated stories are told (the use of temporal and spatial disjunctions; the sense of a historical chronicle of the past; the use of a narrator—a storyteller—with an attitude about the events and characters in that chronicle) as opposed to the way that dramatized stories are told (spatial and temporal concentration—at least in realist plays; the use of past history only in so far as it can be brought into the present; the presentation in that present of the characters by the characters themselves rather than by a storyteller). The prologues of *Twentieth Century* and of *His Girl Friday* accomplish precisely this narrative restructuring—hence the similarity of these two structures to the other stories by this storyteller.

Oscar and Mildred-Lily come together (a pun probably intended by Hawks's visual imagery) with the aid of a Hawks object, a concrete piece of physical matter. Mildred Plotka sits on the stage waiting for the first rehearsal to begin, not even knowing who she is. Like Bat Kilgallen, she is going to lose her name. Owen O'Malley, the hard-drinking, wise-cracking, word-weaving press agent (Roscoe Karns), a prototypical citizen of the Ben Hecht universe, can find no one who answers to the name of Garland. His puzzled phone call to the master, upstairs lounging on the floor of his office, brings Jaffe to the stage to conduct the play's rehearsal himself. That play, *The Heart of Kentucky,* a predictable piece of melodramatic hokum, is a saga of the antebellum South complete with women in blonde ringlets and faithful family retainers. With such a work the storyteller subtly distances himself from the values and assumptions of Oscar Jaffe, just as he does in that first shot of the reclining Jaffe on the floor of his office. The storyteller implies that the supposed "art" of the "legitimate" theater is much less real, less serious, and less significant than is assumed by its grandiose delusions of superiority to the trashy movies. The rehearsal and the play—its title, characters, and incidents—were all created specially for the film, allowing Hawks, who had never worked in the theater, never even been backstage, a comic and subtle nip at the very aesthetic values that would lead the *New York Times* to find his films "juvenile" but such plays mature.

From the film's first shot of Jaffe, what the storyteller finds remarkable about him is not what he does. His plays, and his poses, and his patronizing treatment of everyone else as his children, are terrible—and terribly silly. But the storyteller admires Jaffe's sheer energy, his devotion, and his unquestioning commitment: Jaffe can take his plays, poses, and patronizing so seriously and carry them off with such uncompromisingly blind energy. Jaffe becomes a purely comic Tony Camonte—admired by the storyteller for the very energy of his wrongness. But he is comic because at least he does not kill anyone (he remakes them); and because his deeds do not take place within civilized society but in a totally enclosed world (bound by the four walls of the theater or the enclosed space of a train); and because all those who come to that world wish to attain precisely what he has attained and what he can help them attain. Actors are not so different from gangsters in Hawks's world.

Jaffe assures Mildred, "Don't be nervous, child. You're not Lily

Garland; you're Mary Jo Calhoun." But of course she is not Lily Garland; she is Mildred Plotka. By the end of the film's prologue she will be Lily Garland, who is no more real, no less fictional, no less a character than Mary Jo Calhoun. Or Oscar Jaffe. Or John Barrymore. Mildred cannot become Lily until she talks better ("You're in America now; the Old South doesn't yodel") and until she walks better (hence the intricate maze of chalk marks on the floor). But when all seems hopeless (Mildred breaks down, feels she can never fulfill Jaffe's demands—her last sincere expression of emotion in the film), Jaffe seizes upon the crucial physical object: a pearl-headed pin, which Jaffe detaches from a flower on Mildred's jacket (a very sly, sexually comic symbol of "deflowering"). In order to provoke a sincere cry of anguish from Mildred, to release her soul, Jaffe decides that, like David Huxley's bone, this pin belongs in the tail. He unexpectedly jabs Mildred from behind, and the believable shriek that results is the yelp with which Lily Garland is born from the cocoon of Mildred Plotka.

This pin, like Kid's two-headed coin in *Only Angels Have Wings* and Dunson's snake bracelet in *Red River,* becomes an ironic token of love and affection—preserved and enshrined as such by Lily as a memento of that momentous cry. Even after she has left Oscar, she preserves the pin in a little shrine—a concrete sign that she preserves her feelings for him as well. This enshrined pin (no such physical object exists in the original play, of course) becomes one subtextual source of the story's psychological credibility and probability—that Lily will indeed go back to Oscar in the end because she really wants to be with him (not to mention the fact that she belongs with him).

That she does belong with him becomes the business of the prologue's second sequence. Oscar visits Lily's dressing room on her (and his) night of triumph to enact another scene of mannered poses and theatricalized emotions. He kneels to kiss the hem of "the artist's" gown; he points out the shiny star he has just affixed to her door—"the golden mark that sets her apart from the world—from any one man." After which he embraces her and (in a close-up of his foot, Hawks's variation on a "Lubitsch touch") closes the door of that dressing room, setting her apart from the world indeed—but with one man: himself. The apartment this unmarried couple shares (although the film was released in 1934, its release preceded the enforcement of the Hollywood Production Code by several months) is also a stage set, and the most theatrical

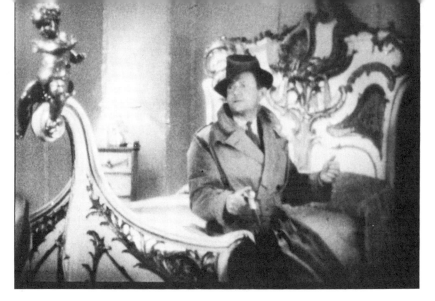

O'Malley (Karns) trying out the outrageous bed for rowing.

piece of furniture of all is, appropriately, their bed, a sort of Louis XIV contraption in the shape of a gondola, surmounted by a golden cherub. The wise-cracking O'Malley quips that the bed seems very well suited for "rowing."

That stage-set apartment becomes, appropriately enough, the backdrop for the playing of theatrical scenes posing as genuine human emotions. Lily plays the "I Want To Get Out into the World" scene: "I'm going out to the Ritz . . . to have a look at some plain human beings for once and act like one." Plain human beings at the Ritz? Oscar has kept her to himself for three years—during which period there have been three hit productions; now she wants to see the world in the form of the Ritz. Oscar plays the "Go If You Must Do Something So Dreary" scene: "Go and dance in that lovely dress in that awful place." He follows this ruse with the ultimate scene, which he will play three times in the film, the "Suicide Ploy," as he stares at the lights of the city beneath him. The indignity of indignities to a theater person, however, is for the audience to walk out on a scene in the middle—which is precisely what Lily tries to do to Oscar. As he intones his funereal dirge in the rearground of the frame, Lily sneaks quietly, on tiptoe, past the camera in the foreground, prompting Oscar to whirl toward her (and us), stopping his obituary with "I'm not finished yet!"

This argument ends with a tearful Lily (her second flood of tears in the film) returning to Oscar's embrace. Their shot of reunion is the

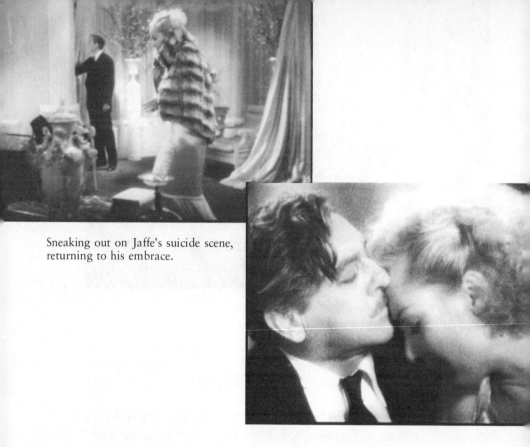

Sneaking out on Jaffe's suicide scene, returning to his embrace.

tightest two-shot, indeed the tightest close-up, in the entire film—the two theatrical faces pressed to each other in needy union, Lily's head slightly below Oscar's, near his shoulder. This scene of argument—revealing how perfectly they play scenes with one another—followed by this tight close-up—revealing how intensely they need one another—provides the psychological basis for Lily's return to Oscar's professional and, presumably, personal embrace at the end of the narrative journey. As O'Malley quips to the other Jaffe associate, the "gray rat" book-keeper, Oliver Webb (Walter Connolly), "In some humpty dumpty way, that was true love" (a line which does not exist in the original play).

Even in this intimate embrace Oscar plays yet another scene—the "I Promise To Give You More Freedom" scene. Immediately after he plays it, he hires a private detective to follow her and to tap her telephone. Lily's discovery of this duplicity drives her away to Hollywood and drives Oscar to his mad scene, raging at Lily's picture, "Anathema. Child of Satan!", an outrageous parody of Lear on the heath. The prologue ends as Oscar selects another anybody, Valerie Whitehouse, to be his new discovery. "Oliver, give me some chalk." The film's first section is a microcosm of the whole—another perfect Hawks circle.

The beginning of the film's second section reveals, however, that Valerie Whitehouse is not Lily Garland and that Oscar Jaffe without Lily Garland is not Oscar Jaffe. His fifth turkey in two years, "Joan of Arc," has just closed in Chicago, leaving Jaffe broke, beaten, and in danger of losing his theater in New York, the center and capital of Jaffe's universe. In some humpty-dumpty way it must have been love between Jaffe and Lily because without her his spirit, talent, energy, luck—whatever made those awful shows into hits—have departed. The remaining three major sections of the film mirror the three acts of the original stage play—the reunion with Lily on the train; Oscar's series of strategies for getting her back; and the ultimate and successful strategy: the staging of Oscar's own death. In these three sections Hawks faces a serious and challenging visual problem: how do you confine the action for an hour within the cramped visual space of a train without the film's grinding to a visual halt? One obvious solution would be to shoot a lot of interesting footage of the varied outdoor scenery one might see from the windows of the train; another would be to intercut visually cramped scenes on the train with visually freer scenes that take place elsewhere. Hawks, of course, does not see such mechanical "solutions" as solutions. As a result, he never cuts away from the train once it leaves Chicago; he cuts briefly, three times, to exciting outdoor shots of the train's churning wheels—only as punctuation between the major structural sequences of the narrative.

Hawks keeps the film alive inside the train by filling it with as much human energy as possible and photographing that energy as interestingly as he can. He moves the characters and the camera around the tiny compartments as much as possible, particularly in his use of low-angle shots which magnify the size and stature of the train's human occupants. As the human figures move in the cramped compartments, they move into differing visual relationships with the camera, which prefers to keep itself cramped as well, from very close (as in Oliver Webb's attempting to wrestle Jaffe to his senses) to medium (as in the calmer scenes of discussion and strategy). Hawks also uses a familiar ally—the shadows of the human figures on the train compartment's walls—to enliven and deepen his visual texture. Mostly, however, Hawks

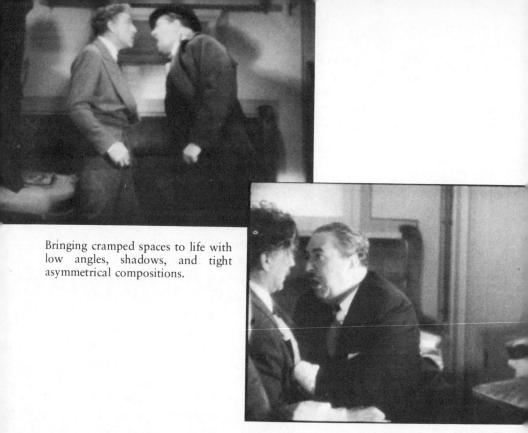

Bringing cramped spaces to life with low angles, shadows, and tight asymmetrical compositions.

depends on his characters—their thought, talk, and feelings—to sustain our interest and his film's energy: Jaffe's outrageous impersonations, O'Malley's verbal salads of vowels and consonants, Webb's exasperation at being the team's only member with common sense (what is anyone with common sense doing on such a team?), Lily's even more Jaffe-like screams, rages, and abrupt transitions (after a long fit of screeching, she claims, "I despise temperament"), and little Matthew J. Clark's (Etienne Girardot) fussy, prissy Puritanism. Those who do not believe that star performances and crackling talk are properly cinematic subjects will never be able to appreciate Hawks's brilliantly "cinematic" solution to his visual problem.

Another of Hawks's clever methods is to use the sound track, particularly the train's whistle, to provide the story teller's off-frame commentary on the action. Jaffe describes the role of the Magdalene in the Passion Play which he has conceived for Lily: "Just her memory has kept the world weeping for centuries." Precisely then, the train adds its opinion of Jaffe's conception and description with a hoot (rather than a weep). A later hoot of the train prompts O'Malley's ironic observation, "It's a dark night, full of unfortunate sounds," after which we immediately hear another unfortunate sound—the off-frame crack of Jaffe's pistol.

The primary opposition in the three sections of Hawks's story that reconstruct the three acts of the original play is between acting and living, playing scenes and feeling emotion, the theatrical and the real—the opposition Hawks carefully establishes in his prologue. When Oscar makes his familiar suicidal promise, this time threatening to cut his throat, Lily retorts, "If you did, greasepaint would run out of it." Lily later observes, "We're not people, we're lithographs," and "We're only real in between curtains." So both Lily and Oscar convert the real train car into a theatrical world "between curtains" for their playing of scenes. Like the four-walled theater, the train is a separate world, cut off from contact with any other, permitting its occupants to structure that world as they wish.

Oscar plays the "Get Rid of the Boyfriend Rival" scene, his arm in a prop sling to protect him from a strange man's blows. He deliberately sets out "to break a human heart" with an apparently broken arm. And Oscar cannot avoid describing the boyfriend's behavior in that "real" scene in purely theatrical terms: "What an exit; not a word." Jaffe finds this smug, cold, unfeeling silence to be "like the Reverend Henry Davidson in *Rain*" (a perhaps deliberate self-reference to the *Rain* scene in Hecht-Hawks's *Scarface*). Then Jaffe plays his "Apologize for the Terrible Wrongs I Done You" scene (the train's whistle again adds its hoots to this one), his "Farewell to the Boys Cause I Gotta Go" scene, in which he "just happens" to drop the pistol in his pocket to the floor (he has carefully wrapped the prop in his handkerchief for precisely this purpose), and, finally, Oscar plays his "Grant Me My Last Request" death scene, in which his last request is merely Lily's affixing her name to the contract which will secure Jaffe's theatrical future.

Meanwhile Lily plays her own scenes: the "Farewell to the Departing Lover" scene—but he refuses to go, and tells her, "Stop acting"; the "Temperamental Artist Who Is So Far Above the Common Crowd" scene ("Who cares about your respect; I'm too big to worry about respect"). Finally, Lily has her own part to play in Oscar's death scene, and it is because she knows what that role is, what is expected from

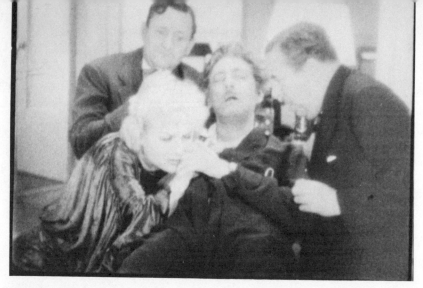

Jaffe's staging of the Crucifixion.

the "Woman at the Side of Her Dying Lover," that she signs that fatal and fateful contract. How can the "Grieving Mistress" deny that "Last Request" in any well-constructed theater piece?

In this reduction of life (and even death) to mere theater (or is it an elevation rather than a reduction? That question will return anon), even the Bible becomes a profane rather than a sacred text, a mere theatrical script. As Jaffe observes, "No one's writing dialogue like this any more." This deflation of the culture's supreme religious text to a profane theater text is at the heart of the film's collapsing the apparent opposites of acting and living; it also indicates the ebullient iconoclasm of Hecht-MacArthur-Hawks, the same iconoclastic energy that produced *Scarface* and would produce *His Girl Friday*. Jaffe's fake death scene is visually littered with crosses, deliberately suggesting the crucifixion: a bunko Christ surrounded by his drunken, carefully coached disciples, with a weeping ham of a Mary Magdalene at his feet. Lily Garland gets to play the Magdalene after all.

The film's brief epilogue returns us to the stage of the Jaffe Theater, where the master begins to conduct a rehearsal of a new play, addressing the new cast with the same old sanctimonious, saccharine opening speech that he used for *The Heart of Kentucky*. Indeed, this new play, like everything else in the epilogue, is not new at all. This time, Lily Garland is not Mary Jo Calhoun, but the same character with a new name, Betty Ann, "this ragged little thing they found walking in the cotton fields." Again Oscar impersonates a ringing doorbell, "Ting-a-ling-a-ling-a-ling." And again Oscar Jaffe asks for some chalk to chart Lily's course of movement. Lily is not quite the same—she is more assured, more self-consciously the star, more capable of screaming back at Oscar. And as the film fades out on her screaming while Oscar chalks the floor, we understand that the characters have indeed come full circle. They are back where they began—a little different but still the same—doing what they did and (given the cyclical sense of the film's construction) what they always will. That maze of tracks on the floor becomes a concrete metaphor (paralleling the tracks of the Twentieth Century Limited) for the film's complicated journey, which, despite the detours and digressions, brings the characters back to where they began and where they belong. Despite its sharp points and angles, the maze of tracks is a circle. Oscar and Lily have not only made a physical journey, a return to the same physical setting as at the beginning, and by means of a train, a mode of physical transportation. They have made a spiritual circle as well, back to where they spiritually were and where they presumably belong.

It is this presumption that leads to the film's most complex moral issue (a moral problem pointedly raised by the fuller spiritual history of these two characters). As opposed to the Lily Garland in full bloom whom we meet in the Hecht-MacArthur play, the Hawks film chronicles the birth, growth, and evolution of Lily Garland as well as the spark of creation which brought forth Lily Garland from the will of Oscar Jaffe: "Let there be Lily Garland." The narrative has been a cir-

The maze of chalkmarks which is a kind of track.

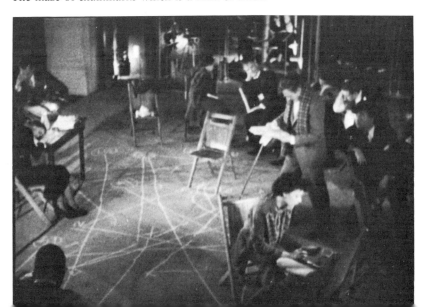

cle, a return to the beginning, rather than a line in some progressive, purposeful direction. Has the evolution of Lily Garland from Mildred Plotka been an evolution or a regressive devolution? To put the film's conclusion in its worst moral light, Lily Garland has returned to become the mere object and instrument of egomaniacal Oscar Jaffe's will, imprisoned in an endless series of dreadful melodramas, forever. This is the conclusion, however, which the film's narrative finds satisfyingly comic, somehow a fertile, happy, positive culmination of the film's narrative journey (like the union of Susan Vance and David Huxley, of Barnaby and Edwina Fulton). How can this be?

The viewer can never find the ending of *Twentieth Century* satisfyingly comic without accepting (at least for the purpose of playing this narrative's game) the storyteller's moral attitudes and premises, which have generated the tale and provided the basis for our understanding it. These moral attitudes take us directly to Howard Hawks's views of life, work, people, and the world. First, the film's storyteller assumes it is better, more interesting, more exciting, to be Lily Garland than Mildred Plotka. Mildred is the name of an ordinary, sober, and sane millinery saleslady, three qualities for which the film (here Hecht and Hawks join hands) has little respect. The model of apparent ordinariness, sobriety, and sanity in the film is little Matthew J. Clark—who is a nut. Clearly, the film says, it is better to be crazy like Oscar Jaffe than crazy like Matthew J. Clark. The storyteller (in this film and others) likes people who are a little crazy—and is not so certain that everyone is not a little crazy anyway. Unlike ordinary crazy people (like Matthew J. Clark and the psychiatrist in *Bringing Up Baby*), the extraordinary Jaffe (like Susan Vance) draws energy, passion, and power from his absolutely surprising and singleminded craziness. His remaking Mildred Plotka into Lily Garland allows her to be and do the same.

Second, Lily Garland really is Lily Garland and not Mildred Plotka. She has the soul of Lily Garland in the body of Mildred Plotka. And Jaffe releases that soul. The storyteller implies that Mildred's body really imprisons Lily's soul, an implication arising from the ease, success, and completeness of Mildred's becoming Lily—unlike Valerie Whitehouse, who never became a Lily because she apparently was not and could not. So for the storyteller, Lily is by implication more herself, more free and less a prisoner, when she is Lily Garland, not Mildred Plotka. This attitude is a reversal of the classic Trilby story, in which the woman's art is an unnatural imposition, forced upon her by the hypnotic magician. Trilby prefers love to her vocation; she'd rather "wash dishes." Hawks believes that if Trilby is so good at her vocation it must be because it comes naturally to her—it is the essence of her being. If she thinks she wants to "wash dishes" it is only because she doesn't know what she really wants, doesn't know what she really is.

Third, the fact that Lily seems sentenced to perform in the same kind of banal play, over and over again, is not itself a sign of spiritual imprisonment or artistic decay. That is what actors do—plays—over and over again, one play after another. The circularity of the film's structure reveals another observation of the storyteller about human vocation. A person with a vocation necessarily repeats it; to be good at a vocation is to have the energy, the will, and the love to do it over and over again, always a little bit different but always the same. There is always another rival gangster to kill, a mail delivery to be flown, a race to be driven, fish to be caught, cattle to be herded. And there is always another film to be made. Hawks, the filmmaker, knows about the repeatability of a vocation, having made 39-plus films, each a little different but each more of the same—just like Jaffe's plays. Despite the familiar American myths of progress and development, of change and evolution, Hawks's films (emphasized by their circular structures) admire those persons with the energy and the creativity to do the same thing again (quite literally with Hawks's two late westerns, *Rio Bravo* and *El Dorado,* which are variations on one another). Despite Jaffe's comic egomania, both his ability to make stars and his will to make stories over and over again speak directly for the filmmaker-storyteller himself, who also made both stars and stories over and over again.

Finally, to sentence Lily Garland to a lifetime of Oscar Jaffe is not to imprison her but to allow her to be most fully and most completely what she is. Lily Garland is a monster—just as Jaffe is himself. These two monsters (like Dr. Frankenstein and his creation) belong most naturally together, the spiritual complements of one another's monstrosity. Were Lily Garland not Lily Garland, things might be otherwise; she might have other more desirable options. But Lily Garland she is. And Lily Garland without Oscar Jaffe would not be truly and fully herself.

This essence and this complementarity relate to a feminist issue which lurks behind this film. While feminist film critics admire Hawks for giving his women as much energy, brains, talent, and spunk as his men (they don't sit around and wash dishes),[10] there may be something sexist about the storyteller's sympathizing, indeed his covert collusion, with Jaffe's attempt to get Lily back into his power. But Lily Garland is not so much a woman as a monster—a parody of a human being, just as Jaffe is. They are not people, but actors (indeed ham actors), and the only way that such monsters can achieve a meaningful spiritual life is to live together in a ham world of their own hammy making (Tony Camonte's problem was that no other monster could live there with him).

The storyteller asks us to see the ending of *Twentieth Century* as satisfyingly comic on the basis of these moral distinctions and definitions developed by implication within the film—not on the basis of our own socially responsible beliefs about human sincerity, social progress, or sexual independence. Hecht and Hawks don't care overmuch for the reigning cultural myths, the ordinary, proper social responsibilities, and the uplifting moral beatitudes. Those who cannot share these attitudes will not find the film fun, will not find the film's ending satisfyingly comic but either morally vicious (such a resolution to such a narrative represents a terrible, even tragic, human defeat) or incoherent (Is the ending and this entire narrative supposed to be comic or tragic? Has the filmmaker made himself clear?). Both these reactions arise either from an inability to observe or a refusal to accept the specific moral values assumed and implied by the storyteller in building this tale.

Precisely the same is true of many other Hawks films—particularly the Hecht-MacArthur companion piece, *His Girl Friday,* which poses identical moral and psychological problems.

Howard Hawks thought *The Front Page* had the "finest modern dialogue that had been written."

> I asked a girl to read Hildy's part and I read the editor and I stopped and I said, "Hell, it's better between a girl and a man than between two men," and I called Ben Hecht and I said, "What would you think of changing it so that Hildy is a girl?" And he said, "I think it's a great idea," and he came out and we did it.[11]

From this little accident arose a film that transformed and transcended the play which Hawks so admired. For one thing, the film threw out more than half of that "finest modern dialogue that had been written" to replace it with even finer dialogue. For another, the film's psychological entanglement of Walter's and Hildy's personal and professional lives makes it, like *Twentieth Century,* a very curious and complex romantic comedy in which love is expressed through work and work is expressed as love.

The Front Page draws a clear distinction between the world of work, of the newspaper game (which is exclusively a world of men), and the world of home and family (which is a world of men with women). One of the reporters in the play worries about his wife in the hospital; another laments he never gets to spend the holidays at home. The wife of one reporter comes looking for her husband who has disappeared, worried more about his drinking up the monthly paycheck than about his health and safety. And Walter Burns himself has been married three times (implying his total failure at private, domestic life), the last marriage ending when he caught his wife in bed with another newspaperman. It is in the context of this opposition between home and work that the male Hildy Johnson of the play decides to get out of the newspaper business, to marry a nice girl (Peggy Grant), and to go to New York City (not Albany) to work for an advertising company (not to sell insurance). But this clear opposition between work and home in the play raises several questions which the play chooses not to answer, hiding behind the schematic opposition itself.

Why do the men play the newspaper game at all if it is so unrewarding? The play implies that somehow newspaper work is "fun," but the sense of fun never comes through as vitally or as clearly as it does in the exuberant teamwork of Walter and Hildy in the film. The play also implies that the nice, domestic cliché of a home life isn't worth much, but this is the merest of suggestions in the play, made explicit in and essential to the film's moral system (1) by the shift of the play's neutral Peggy to the film's comically sexless Bruce Baldwin; (2) by the shift of the new domestic site from the play's big city, New York, to the film's provincial backwater, Albany; and (3) by the shift of Bruce's occupation to selling life insurance, making money from the fear of death. In *The Front Page* Peggy is merely a simple, sweet, pretty, nice person—recalling Hecht's observation in his autobiography, *A Child of the Century,* that the only characters to have any fun in movies were the ones who weren't nice; he decided to write exclusively for these not nice ones.[12] Peggy, however, in his play of *The Front Page* (like her mother, Mrs. Grant) is one of the nice people, and Hecht-MacArthur demonstrate how poorly they could write for these nice characters. Peggy is a very ordinary ingenue, the kind of role that actors themselves describe as "thankless." To sustain the play's schematic opposition of work and home, Peggy must be nice, period.

How good is Hildy Johnson as a reporter in the play and how much does the job mean to him? These questions also have fuzzy answers. Only Walter's insistence on keeping Hildy with the *Examiner* convinces us that he must be valuable to the paper, good at what he does. Hildy spends little time in the play actually doing that job. Hawks, however, adds a scene of Hildy's interviewing the condemned man, Earl Williams, which shows how well, how sensitively, how perceptively she does her job. He also adds Hildy's visual energy at virtually filling the spaces she inhabits with her movement and energy—both the office of the *Morning Post* and the pressroom at the Criminal Courts building—revealing how well she fits into that world, that she is both a source and a partaker of the vitality of that world.

Why does Walter want to keep Hildy with the paper in *The Front Page?* Why does he engage in so many shifty strategies to keep Hildy from getting away? The play's answer is simply that Hildy is *that* valuable to the paper (never very convincingly established) and that Walter is *that* unscrupulous and selfish (never really very convincingly established either). Walter is unscrupulous just as Peggy is nice, a conventional moral opposition which the play has established and which the audience is supposed to accept on faith.

The shift of Hildy Johnson's gender is not merely an interesting new twist on an old tale; it is a strategic twist that remakes the tale altogether. The Walter-Hildy relationship in *His Girl Friday* becomes, like the Oscar-Lily relationship of *Twentieth Century,* a synthesis of love and work, a union of harmonious complements. But in *His Girl Friday* neither Walter nor Hildy is the monster that Oscar or Lily is: Hildy is a sensitive and sincere woman, one of the advantages of using Rosalind Russell, who combines sharp talk, a quick brain, solid sense, and a casual, friendly intimacy. Walter is much softer, more ironic, and more sensitive than both Oscar Jaffe and Walter Burns in the Hecht-

MacArthur play—one of the advantages of using Cary Grant. As a result, the emotional relationship of Walter and Hildy in the film is much richer, more playful, less maniacal, more sensitive to the feelings of one another than that of Oscar and Lily. *His Girl Friday* stands between *Twentieth Century,* a reuniting of a dynamic professional team, and *Monkey Business,* a remarriage of a loving (strange love, but loving nonetheless) human couple.

Like the male Hildy Johnson of the Hecht-MacArthur play, the female Hildy Johnson of *His Girl Friday* feels there is something missing from her life—namely, its femaleness. She wants to be "a woman," not "a newspaperman." In this initial longing (understandable, perhaps, for she is a woman, and sensitive, and intelligent) she commits several psychological and moral sins. She herself is guilty of a sexist differentiation, a schematic oversimplification, between the abstract qualities, urges, and needs of the two sexes. The film's Hildy, who accepts the original play's schematic and conventional opposition of home and work, allows the film to perform its critique of the play's simple dichotomy. Hildy has accepted the kind of cultural myth and stereotype which the play assumes by convention—the proper kind of normal, adult, female American life a woman ought to live. And she has failed to realize how much "fun" she has with the newspaper game, the "fun" which keeps her alive—in body, mind, and spirit. Although the suburban grass of being an Albany housewife looks a lot greener to this woman who takes the newspaper game for granted (just as Barnaby takes Edwina for granted in *Monkey Business*), the narrative of *His Girl Friday* educates Hildy about what she will lose when she walks on that apparently greener grass. Like *Bringing Up Baby* and *Monkey Business, His Girl Friday* is a comedy of romantic education (*Twentieth Century* is much more mutedly so since both its protagonists are so maniacally uneducable).

The shift of Hildy's gender also makes a very great change (if a much more subtle one) in the character of Walter Burns, who, in the context of this narrative and in the guise of Cary Grant, is simply not the egomaniacal monster of Hecht-MacArthur's play (Burns is the Oscar Jaffe of *The Front Page*). For this Walter Burns, Hildy Johnson *is* the newspaper game. His ability to play that game well (here there is a parallel with Jaffe) and his enjoyment, his "fun," in playing it depends on playing it with her. When they play the newspaper game together they are both most alive, most energetic, most in touch with themselves and with each other, most spiritedly human. Now none of this psychological information and motivation comes to the viewer explicitly, by means of the verbal text. It is not in the nature of either of these characters (or any Hawks characters) to verbalize such feelings. We must perceive this psychological complexity subtextually, from the oblique things they say or do, from the way they move, from the way the camera records their motion, from the sounds and rhythms of their voices rather than just their articulate speech.

As is typical with Hawks, all this essential subtextual information comes to the viewer in the narrative's initial section—which, for *His Girl Friday* as for *Twentieth Century,* was invented afresh for the film. The film's opening shot evokes both the long traveling shot that opens *Scarface* and that film's second shot in the newspaper office. Like the first shot of *Scarface, His Girl Friday* opens with an analytic traveling shot, moving parallel with the world it records and surveys; but like the second shot of *Scarface,* it moves from right to left (rather than from left to right) and the world it depicts is another newspaper office—the life, excitement, and intensity of its day-to-day business. The camera tracks to the left, past the working reporters seated at their desks, the copyboys moving between them, the telephone operators at the switchboard, coming to rest on the elevator at the far end of its leftward journey. The moving camera, the melange of sounds, and the human movement in varying planes of depth as the camera tracks past, all convey a world—busy, rich, and alive—as opposed to the emptiness and litter of the world in the first shot of *Scarface.* When Hildy Johnson and Bruce Baldwin emerge from that elevator, the camera begins to track back in the opposite direction with these two focal human figures (just as it retraced its steps in *Scarface* after reaching its limit). And like the opening shot of *Scarface,* the first sequence of *His Girl Friday* is a perfect circle, concluding when Hildy and Bruce—and Walter—return to that elevator. Despite the different cameramen for the two films (*His Girl Friday* shot by the solid Joseph Walker rather than the extraordinary Lee Garmes), the opening camera strategies are strikingly similar—inviting us into a world, established, surveyed, and enclosed by horizontal camera movement.

As Hildy and Bruce journey in the contrary direction, from left to right, the two characters and the camera suddenly come to a "dead stop." Hildy tells Bruce to wait for her; he is not a member of this newspaper world, and he will not be allowed to enter it. Hildy and Bruce are literally separated by the wooden railing and the swinging gate that divide the world of the working press from that of the outsiders in the waiting room. A sign on the gate reads, "No Admittance," and Bruce never will be admitted to that other side of the barrier where Hildy so obviously belongs. The camera cuts to a close-up of Bruce as he slowly drawls, "Even ten minutes is a long time to be away from you." Hildy likes the sentiment so much that she asks him to repeat it (and Hawks also gives her a close-up for her reaction). Although Hildy is touched by Bruce's thoughtfulness, the storyteller warns us to keep our distance—even while giving us close-ups which underline the importance of this interchange. First, the movement—both of the camera and the people—has ground to a halt, a dead stop. There is something interruptive about this stasis after the camera's establishing its vital rhythm at the beginning of the film. After this caesura the camera will return to its movement when Hildy herself starts to move again. Bruce's

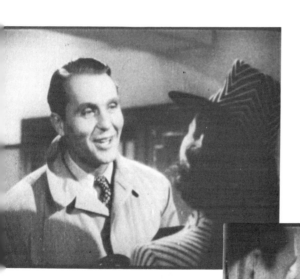

The first two closeups of Bruce and Hildy.

line is an interruption of rhythm, of motion—and in a Hawks film that means an interruption of life and of vitality.

Second, there is something slow and lumbering about Bruce's delivery of the line. Its slowness, emphasized by his repeating it, word for word, participates in our sense of interruption, of pause, of deadness about this brief exchange. The rhythm of Bruce's speech throughout the film is in complete contrast to the rhythm, the melody, of Hildy's and Walter's crackling speech, which accompanies the rhythm and pace of their loping walk. The change of the last name (like the softness of the sound of "Bruce"—with its soft "oo" vowel and soft "s" consonant) from the play's monosyllabic Grant (harsh diphthongal vowel, crisp "t" consonant) to Baldwin (soft vowels and consonants) conveys the slow, shambling softness of a lumbering teddy bear. Hildy is charmed by this endearing slowness. Even the storyteller agrees there is something charming about this teddy bear, the kind of cuddly oaf that Ralph Bellamy made a career of playing. This close-up of Bellamy, though a rhythmic interruption, allows that bearish-boyish charm and warmth to be felt. But the storyteller reveals that Hildy unknowingly returns to her much more natural and vital condition when she starts to move again.

As she strides through the newspaper office from left to right (like Susan Vance striding across the golf course), the camera strides with her, mirroring her motion, rhythm, and energy. As she moves she gracefully, effortlessly tosses greetings, exchanges information with the others who work in the office, showing how naturally she fits in there, how comfortable they are with her and her with them, all of them moving and talking to the same rhythm. But the camera, in conveying her ease and vitality within that space, also disassociates itself slightly from her attitudes. The storyteller both sympathizes with her vital naturalness in this space and judges her lack of awareness of that naturalness. Rather than the camera's conveying the point-of-view of each specific person who addresses Hildy as she walks, which it would and could have done by each addressing the camera lens directly as if it were Hildy herself, the camera describes a triangular relationship between Hildy and her interlocutors. The camera walks slightly ahead of where the off-frame Hildy would be; her questioners speak to the camera's left, where Hildy is implied to be. This triangular shooting

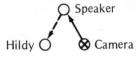

214

perspective implies that the camera, the storyteller, is somehow "ahead of" Hildy, revealing more than she knows or sees. When Hildy reaches the end of this walk at the inner office of Walter Burns, the camera will identify itself with his perceptions of her actions. Indeed, the endpoint, the final destination of the camera's track to the right, is Walter's office (on the far right, as usual), and in walking ahead of Hildy the camera is consistently closer to that office and that presence on the right.

Once inside that office, we receive a lot of narrative information from the dialogue. Hildy and Walter were previously married; the divorce has just become final; she has returned from Bermuda with a new beau, Bruce Baldwin, whom she intends to marry on the morrow (parallel with David and Swallow in *Bringing Up Baby*); the domestic tranquility of the Hildy-Walter marriage was perpetually interrupted by the newspaper game ("I intended to be with you on our honeymoon; honest I did"). Just as Susan Vance never allowed David Huxley any quiet moments in *Bringing Up Baby,* so Walter Burns and the newspaper game never allowed any for Mrs. Hildy Burns. If Susan managed to snare David because she was so "surprising," Walter has apparently been too surprising for Hildy.

Walter and Hildy appear to be very much talking at cross-purposes. He does not extend her even the most ordinary courtesies: she must ask to be seated ("Would you mind if I sat down?"); she must ask for a cigarette ("May I have one of those?"); and a light for it (he merely tosses her the matches, to which she ironically replies, "Thank ya"). As usual Hawks uses matches and cigarettes to convey essential psychological, narrative information. Although Walter assumes she has returned to work for the paper, she has come there to tell him that she is leaving the newspaper business forever, that she is going to marry Bruce Baldwin. The talking at cross-purposes culminates in a duet of overlapping lines, Walter jabbering on about the paper and Hildy, as a pencilled note in Hawks's script indicates, imitating an "auctioneer for Lucky Strike ending with 'Sold American!' " [13]

Despite the surface argument conveyed by the crackling energy of what is said, this opening scene is striking for the implications of that energy about what is not explicitly said. The two apparent antagonists speak in an identical rhythm, in identical cadences, singing perfect verbal duets—which reveal that the two are spiritually and truly one. Their minds click away at the same pace and in the same rhythm (as opposed to the slow Bruce), just as their words do. They rove about the office in

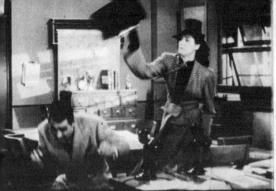
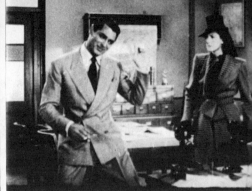

Moving, talking, and ducking in tempo.

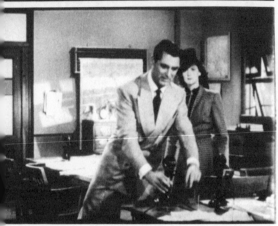

the same rhythm as they speak, including a masterful moment when Hildy, without missing a verbal beat, tosses her purse at Walter's head from behind, and he, without either seeing it or missing a verbal beat, ducks the throw perfectly and tells her that her aim used to be better, then answers his telephone without losing a beat. When they sit down, they sit close to one another on a desk, shoulder to shoulder, in precisely the same attitudes, their bodies touching slightly but chummily, captured by a symmetrical framing which makes them perfect physical (and hence spiritual) halves of the same visual frame. Everything over which Hildy has no control—the pace and inflections of her voice, the movements of her body, her posture, her physical position in the frame—refutes the surface claims of her words. The storyteller and Walter both know what she does not, and the two of them will be narrative allies to bring her to this knowledge. The underlying probability of this narrative—that Hildy, regardless of what she says, really wants Walter and really wants to be a newspaperman despite the fact that she thinks she wants to be "a woman" (whatever that schematic opposition means and is worth)—will grow out of this opening scene's rhythm, pace, verbal music, and visual symmetry, not out of her explicit and conscious talk.

This method reveals Hawks's awareness and deliberate translation of the original play's most interesting stylistic device. The most striking quality of *The Front Page* is its verbal polyphony, its deliberate verbal counterpoint of more than a single conversation or kind of conversation occurring on stage at the same time. The play begins with such counterpoint—the reporters play cards on one side of the stage while McCue uses the telephone to pry into possible stories on the other. Hecht-MacArthur continue the method in such scenes as Hildy's trying to hold two conversations at once (with Walter on one telephone, Peggy on another) or Hildy's making one phone call (to hospitals inquiring about an automobile accident) while Walter makes another at the same time (to his newspaper office). Hawks decided to preserve this verbal polyphony in the film—but not by using montage, the typical visual method of film counterpoint, of which there are only two very energetic uses in the film. Instead, Hawks translates the play's verbal counterpoint, the polyphonal conversations which bounce back and forth within the same theatrical space from left to right, into a visual counterpoint within the same cinema frame, either between left and right, or between foreground and rearground, or both.

But this verbal and visual counterpoint is more than a mere cinema technique. It is a use of articulate speech as a kind of rhapsodic music. Except for the very final upbeat moments of *His Girl Friday,* there is no music of any kind in the film—except for this "verbal music"—just as there is no music other than verbal music in *Twentieth Century.* While the primary verbal music of the earlier film was a series of conflicting duets—Oscar-Barrymore's mellifluous incantations answered by Lily-Lombard's yelps and shrieks—the music of *His Girl Friday* is a series of harmonious, patter-song duets, in which the "singers" share the same visual frame just as they share the same spiritual and musical key. Another of the advantages of using Rosalind Russell (and perhaps the primary reason Hawks chose her above several other star candidates) is that she talks in almost the same key as Cary Grant. Though a woman, she "sings" baritone (a perfect synthesis of the film's male-female paradoxes).* Hawks makes *His Girl Friday* into a kind of "word-

* This quality of Russell's voice became literally true when she sang in musical comedies. For example, in the "Ohio" duet of *Wonderful Town* she sings the baritone harmonic line underneath her sister Eileen's melodic line.

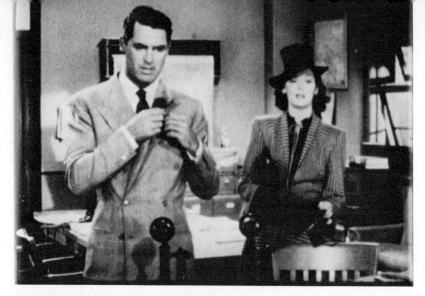

Playing for time as he plays with a flower (note the symmetrical echo of the two telephones).

opera" in which the "music" conveys (as it does in any opera) far more than the words alone. Walter and Hildy sing well together and sing alike, while Bruce's slow dirges simply do not harmonize with Hildy's rhythmic vitality.

Hildy's announcement that she is marrying Bruce tomorrow brings Walter's song to a halt (just as it stopped Susan short in *Bringing Up Baby*). Walter begins to think spontaneously on his feet, fingering the mouthpiece of the telephone in front of him, then the boutonniere which he sticks in his lapel (like Tony Camonte fingering O'Hara's boutonniere to reveal his thoughts and reactions), wondering what he can do to prevent this marriage; his strategy will parallel Susan Vance's—a series of spontaneous improvisations to keep Hildy with him and away from the intended. The newspaper job and the hanging of Earl Williams (the central material of the Hecht-MacArthur play) will serve as Walter's pretext for keeping Hildy with the paper, with him, and with life. When Walter discovers that his rival sells insurance, his ironic response (an improvisation written into the script, longhand) is, "It's adventurous; it's romantic." He will use this ironic perception, that the man who sells insurance lacks adventure, romance, color, and life, as his means of doing battle with Bruce.

Unlike Susan Vance, who battles Swallow by separating David from her and from the old bone, which represents the fiancée, Walter Burns

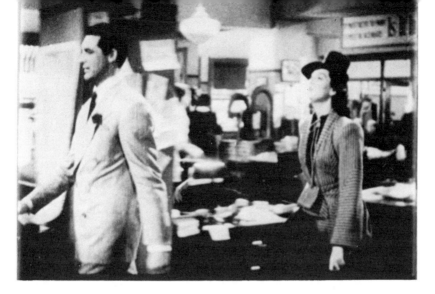

Walter walking firmly in front.

charges out of his inner office directly to confront the foe. He strides out of the room, failing to hold the door open for Hildy in a gentlemanly fashion; he walks ahead of her, failing to let her walk in front as a gentleman should. Despite this ungentlemanly lack of consciousness that she is "a woman," the vitality and rhythm of his walking precisely matches hers and that of the camera—which is now tracking back with them from right to left. Obviously, Hildy is not "a woman" to Walter but an equal, a pal, a "newspaperman." It is Bruce who treats her like "a woman." Walter wants to expose the less attractive characteristic of Bruce's chivalry: its insipid deadness. When first meeting Bruce, he makes a little mistake in identities which is both intentional and metaphoric for Walter's and the storyteller's opinion of Bruce: he assumes that a little, old, shrivelled man waiting outside the office is Bruce Baldwin. When Hildy introduces Walter to the real Bruce Baldwin, (and she sees through Walter's ruse at the start—and enjoys it), Walter shakes the wooden umbrella handle, rather than the fleshy hand of this younger but wooden male. Bruce's umbrella, raincoat, and rubbers (although the day is bright and fine) reveal that his "life," like his vocation, is a perpetual preparation for the worst.

Walter's exposing the lack of adventure and romance in Bruce's being continues in the second half of the prologue, a luncheon scene totally invented for the film, in which Walter improvises strategies for keeping Hildy from leaving immediately with Bruce. Bruce explains the

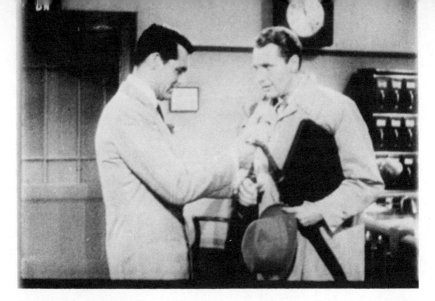

Greeting Bruce's umbrella.

value of insurance: "We don't help you much when you're alive. But afterwards. That's what counts." Walter replies blankly, "I don't get it." After which Hildy administers one of the kicks beneath the table that recur frequently in the scene—although this kick catches the waiter's shins rather than Walter's. (These unseen kicks beneath the restaurant table parallel Tony's playing with Poppy's legs beneath the restaurant table in *Scarface*.) Bruce also explains why he likes Hildy—she's so surprising, a quality that also suggests Susan Vance. Unfortunately for Bruce, Walter and Hildy are able to be surprising together, and that shared ability will reunite them before the narrative's end.

Hawks's framing allows Walter Burns to dominate this luncheon scene visually and narratively; sitting between Bruce and Hildy, Walter dominates both the shot which favors Bruce and the one which favors Hildy. Hawks breaks the scene down exclusively into these intercut shots, which separate Bruce and Hildy spatially, allowing Walter to serve as the visual and spiritual center of the scene's force and interest. Two improvisations allow Walter to buy a little time, for Bruce and Hildy plan to leave for Albany on the four o'clock train. First, he claims that only Hildy can get an interview with the condemned Earl Williams that might spare the man's life; his only other ace reporter, Sweeney, is supposedly at the hospital where his wife has just given birth to twins. This story touches Bruce's sentimental soul; surely they can spare a few hours

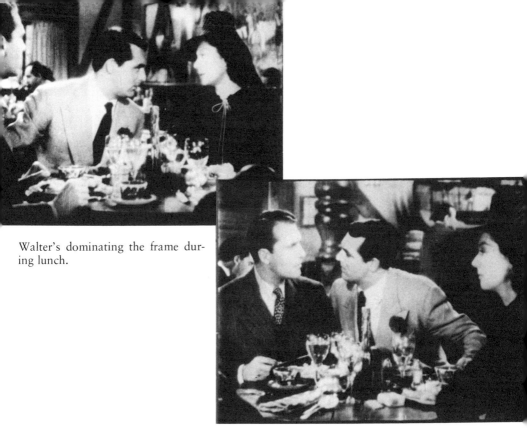

Walter's dominating the frame during lunch.

to save a man's life. They would not want to build their marriage on
another person's dead body (of course, what does his insurance do?).
But Hildy remembers that Sweeney has been married for only four
months; she exposes Walter's sentimental appeal as a fabrication (the
same kind of emotional manipulation that Oscar Jaffe uses to get his
way in *Twentieth Century*). So Walter then appeals to Bruce's professional interests by offering to buy some life insurance. This pragmatic
appeal does not move Bruce at all (who is not moved by self-interest).
But it does move Hildy, who is perfectly happy to take Walter's money.
She agrees to trade an interview with Earl Williams for Walter's pur-
chase of a very expensive policy. Her pragmatism and her immunity to
sentimentality also suggest that she is truly a Walter, not a Bruce. Walter has bought a few hours with this strategy; once he has got Hildy to
the pressroom, he can improvise upon the events that follow to win her
back permanently (just as Susan must first get David to her apartment,
then to Connecticut).

As in the film of *Twentieth Century,* the final three major sections of *His Girl Friday* mirror the three acts of the original Hecht-Mac-Arthur play. The second section trims the Hecht-MacArthur first act—beginning with our introduction to the pressroom and its occupants (the reporters), who await the hanging of Earl Williams; and ending with Williams's escape from prison. The third section follows the play's second act—from Hildy's discovering Williams's means of escape to Walter's joining Hildy in an attempt to aid the condemned man, who is hiding in the rolltop desk. And the fourth section is the play's third act—the discovery of Williams in the desk, the arrival of Williams's reprieve, and the resolution of the conflict between Walter and Hildy. As in his handling of the final three sections of *Twentieth Century,* Hawks accepts—with some modifications—the temporal and spatial confinement of the original play once he plunges into it. Temporally, Hawks brings us to the pressroom during the afternoon (since Hildy arrives there in the afternoon), rather than at night (as in the play). The shift allows the film to journey from daylight into darkness—and allows Hawks to shift the key of the lighting in the room by turning on those electric hanging lamps. The low-hanging lamps complicate the room's visual texture by magnifying shadows, particularly those that cut off the upper reaches of the room and even sliver off the very tops of the human foreheads, emphasizing the eyes and talking mouths beneath them.

Hawks's pressroom, organized in depth: telephones and reporters in the foreground (Frank Jenks, Regis Toomey, Cliff Edwards), Hildy in the midground, McCue (Roscoe Karns) in the rearground staring even deeper at the legs ascending the stairway.

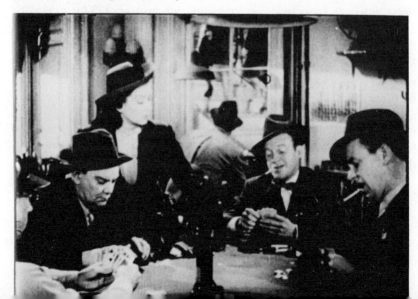

There are spatial differences, of course, between a train and a press-room: while a train is a self-contained world, a pressroom exists within a city and permits both entrance from and exit to the outside world. These differences allow Hawks a bit more freedom in cutting away from the single, confined setting of the play. He deserts the pressroom briefly for Walter's medical examination by the insurance doctor, Hildy's interview with Earl Williams, Williams's psychiatric interview with Dr. Egelhofer, Hildy's pursuing (and tackling) Jacobi to get her scoop on Williams's escape, the mayor's and sheriff's attempt to bribe Pettibone, and Bruce's various trips to the jailhouse. Significantly, each of these visual escapes from the pressroom is extremely and deliberately brief, and all but one escape to an action that did not exist in the original play. Hawks seemed to realize that those scenes which Hecht and MacArthur wrote to take place in the pressroom properly belonged there. Metaphorically, that pressroom is the private world of energy and enterprise in which Walter and Hildy "belong" together, and as long as Walter can keep her in that world he can keep her away from Bruce— who has no place in that world. And by remaining inside the press-room, the storyteller defines both his physical and emotional point-of-view as being allied with that world and with those people on this side of the pressroom door.

Hawks eliminates most of the atmospheric Hecht-MacArthur dialogue that brings us into that world. He also curtails the careful distinctions between the attitudes and abilities of the various members of the press corps—injecting the focal Hildy into that world as soon as possible. While Hecht and MacArthur explore the newspaper world for its own sake, Howard Hawks examines the impact of a woman on such a world. Like her earlier entrance into the newspaper office, Hildy effortlessly turns this world into her world, revealing the harmony of the rhythms of her walk and talk with its rhythms. With Hildy safely tucked inside this world, Walter can take advantage of the lamb who has been left in the other, outside world—usually by locking him safely away in jail. Walter sends a blonde floozie (the "albino") to vamp him (Bruce goes to jail for "mashing"). When the floozie asks for a description of her target, Walter answers (in a line pencilled in longhand in the script) that he resembles "that guy in the movies—Ralph Bellamy." The line is not only a typical Hawks piece of self-reference (for this is a movie and he is Ralph Bellamy playing a Ralph Bellamy type of role); it also reveals the collusion of the storyteller with the spontaneous strategies of Walter Burns. Cary Grant as Walter Burns (or Walter Burns as Cary Grant—it matters not), the storyteller, and the audience participate in this little joke together. Another of Walter's strategies to land Bruce behind bars will be the passing of counterfeit money, and this money (like Kid's coin in *Only Angels*) evolves into a very ironic kind of love token by the film's climax.

The shift of Hildy's gender from male to female makes possible two film scenes in this second section that are in a very different key and tone from those in the play. The first is Hildy's interview with Earl Williams (John Qualen), a scene written especially for the film, which both shows how well Hildy does her job (an ability which gives her equality in the male newspaper world) and shows that because she is a woman she can do it even more sensitively and sympathetically than a male. As Hildy talks flutteringly with Jacobi, who is in charge of guarding Williams and sequestering him from reporters, a twenty-dollar bill just happens to fall out of Hildy's purse to the floor (like Jaffe's pistol which just happens to fall out of his pocket in *Twentieth Century*). Hildy, in all apparent innocence, asks Jacobi if that bill on the floor just happens to be his. The artful bribe (it foreshadows the larger bribe Jacobi requires to reveal the method of Williams's escape) gains Hildy admission to Earl's cell. Hawks shoots this cell from an extremely high angle, emphasizing the inhuman isolation of an animal in a cage (more cage imagery, as in *Baby* and *Business*). As Hildy settles down next to Earl for the chat, Hawks's camera leaves its perch, settling down beside the two of them, framing the pair in an intimate, quiet two-shot. Neither the camera nor the characters move during the remainder of the conversation. The camera's judicious intimacy and delicacy mirrors Hildy's own sensitive response to this condemned man whom she is going to use (she wants her story) but not abuse or make feel used.

Both Hildy and the camera sit quietly without moving: her voice has become quiet—slowed, softened, mellowed. That voice—in rhythm, tone, and pace—now precisely echoes Bruce's, for she is able to appreciate and respond to Bruce's softness and sensitivity, and she demonstrates that ability with Earl. She quietly formulates the economic theory, "production for use," which becomes the psychological mania that "explains" Earl's impulsive killing of a black policeman. This psychiatric hogwash is no more absurd than any other in a Hawks film; his

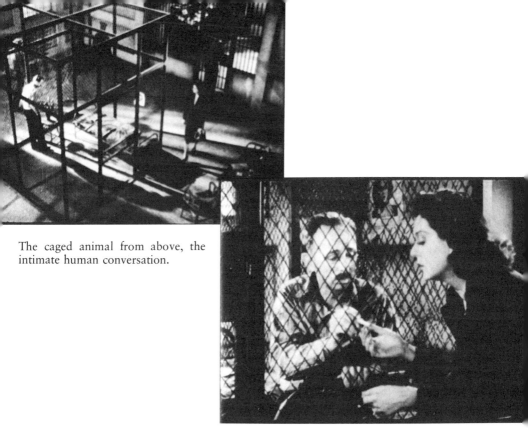

The caged animal from above, the intimate human conversation.

consistent burlesque of psychiatrists and others who pretend to knowledge shows little sympathy or respect for that "knowledge." Hawks's
point is not so much the validity of Hildy's explanation as the fact that
it sounds precisely like the kind of explanation that newspaper readers—and juries—accept as valid. Hildy is a good "newspaperman." While
she speaks she hands Earl the cigarette she has lit for him (that essential
token of intimacy in a Hawks film), but she must apologize for its physical reminder that she is a woman when she asks him to excuse the
lipstick. Earl, however, hands it back to her; he doesn't smoke. Hildy
won't smoke it either, fiddling with it thoughtfully before tossing it away.
This little touch casts an ironic glance at her "production for use" theory. Nobody puts that cigarette to the use for which it was produced.

   The intimate interview with Earl serves several essential narrative
functions in the film. It later allows Hildy to become his very sympathetic captor at the end of this second section. Whereas in the film's
script, the escaped Earl was actually going to shoot at Hildy—with an

unloaded gun—this intimate scene made such an attempted shooting both unnecessary and improbable. This interview between Hildy and Earl, which reveals Hildy's ability to be a woman, a newspaperman, and a sensitive human being at the same time, contrasts markedly with the later inhuman interview between the official psychiatrist, Professor Egelhofer, and Earl, an interview from which Earl is essentially excluded while the professor and Sheriff Hartman haggle over who will get his picture in the papers. The sensitive human focus of the interview also contrasts markedly with the scene originally conceived for the film's script: a lengthy discussion of abstract political issues rather than Hildy's perceptive revealing of both Earl's quirky gentleness and his lunatic lack of self-awareness and self-control.

The shift of Hildy's gender also contributes to the greater depth and feeling of the Mollie Molloy scene, which immediately follows in the film's second section. In the play, the Mollie Molloy scene contrasts the human sensitivity of Mollie, the Clark Street "tart" who befriended Earl Williams, and the callousness of the male reporters, who converted Mollie's sympathetic responsiveness to Earl's feelings into salacious stories for their readers. This contrast is consistent with the play's dichotomy between the hard male newspaper world and the more loving female world of feeling and affection. But in the film, during Mollie's (Helen Mack) tirade about the callousness of the reporters, the now female Hildy hovers in the rearground of many shots of Mollie, saying nothing, just typing her interview with Earl. But her frequent glances in the speaker's direction show her awareness of Mollie's feelings and her sympathy with Mollie's opinions. When the male reporters finally razz Mollie out of the pressroom for weighing them down with her sob stories (this razzing parallels the razzing song in *Only Angels Have Wings*), Hildy accompanies Mollie out the door, escorting her out of the pressroom, and closing the door behind them. The door separates Mollie (like Bruce) from that world in which she does not belong. After the door closes, leaving the men alone in the pressroom, Hawks executes an immense tonal shift, revealing that the men are aware of their callousness, that their callousness (like that of the razzing men in *Only Angels Have Wings*) is the camouflage that allows them to do their job. When that door closes, the action, talk, and movement in the pressroom simply stop: absolute silence and stillness for fifteen seconds. Even the card game goes flat for them. Then Hawks breaks the silence (and em-

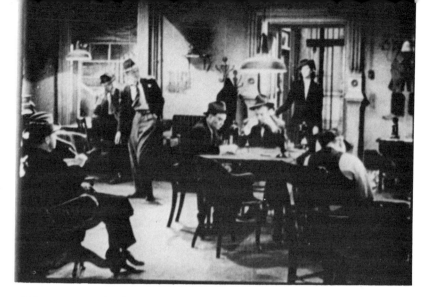

Hildy's power at the doorway, condemning these "gentlemen" of the press.

phasizes the sense of its absolute stillness) with the ring of the telephone; the call is for Hildy, and even the reporter who tells the caller
(Bruce) to hang on does so quietly, as if the telephone had rung during
a funeral. The absolute silence continues for ten more seconds until
Hildy returns, swinging the door open with deliberate slowness (Hawks
emphasizes its slowness by extending the door's opening over two shots
that do not match), standing powerfully erect in the archway as she faces
the male group, and attacking them with the most ironic criticism of
their callousness she can formulate: "Gentlemen of the Press." The power
of her condemnation arises not simply from the irony that the reporters
are not gentlemen at all (one of the film's consistent motifs, as in the
contrast between Walter's ungentlemanly behavior and Bruce's gentlemanly courteousness); it also arises from the fact that although they are
not gentle, they certainly are men, while she and Mollie can be gentle
women.

The scene which closes this second section poses a dilemma for
Hildy, a conflict between her conscious intentions to be "a woman" and
her unconscious instincts as "a newspaperman." Not surprisingly, the
instincts triumph, foreshadowing the film's conclusion in the same way
that her instinctual methods of talking, walking, and reacting do in the
opening scene with Walter. Bruce has telephoned her from jail; his wallet has mysteriously disappeared (stolen, of course, by Walter's personal
thug, Louie). After Hildy leaves to bail Bruce out, the reporters read the

227

interview with Earl which still sits in the typewriter. Not only does their admiration for her writing convince us of her ability as a newspaperman, but they also refuse to believe that anyone with that ability would ever give it up: as one remarks, "Now I give that marriage three months." Hildy returns to the pressroom, telephones Walter, and lets him listen to the sound of her tearing up that very interview (perhaps she *can* give that profession up)—since he double-crossed her with Bruce. That, she claims, is her farewell to the newspaper business. "I'm gonna be a woman, and have babies. . . ."

But as she tries to leave that world of the pressroom, the storyteller again refutes her verbal assertions with her physical actions, over which she has no control. To leave that world she needs her hat and coat. She searches desperately for her hat—which is merely on top of her head. And as she asserts her farewell to the newspaper game, she is unable to put on her coat properly because she has unknowingly stuck her right arm in its left sleeve, and, rather than calmly and rationally extricate this errant arm, she irrationally continues jamming the arm down the wrong sleeve. The coat sleeve, like Johnny Lovo's saltshaker, is a simple Hawks object that conveys more about Hildy's mind and feelings—the fact that she is literally at war with herself—than all her words. This coat has played a role in the film previously; after lunch at the restaurant, Walter, in his typical ungentlemanly way, does not help her with the coat, but Bruce does. And it will play a role later; after Earl's escape, Hildy reveals the triumph of her newspaperman's instincts when, her back to the camera, she slowly takes the coat off. This physical

The battle with the coat sleeve.

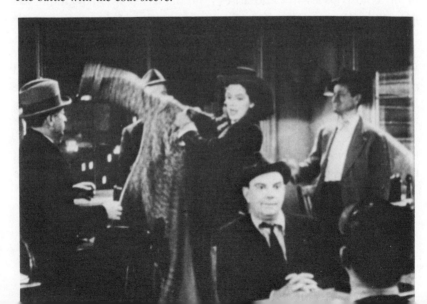

gesture conveys her decision to stay, just as Lovo's manipulation of the saltshaker conveys his decision about Tony. And, like the evolution of consciousness with Lovo's saltshaker, Hildy later uses the coat more consciously than she did when she first could not jam her arm into its sleeve.

The third and fourth sections of the film must allow Hildy to discover consciously what she has already revealed unconsciously: that she belongs in that world of the pressroom. These final sections of the film are built around a series of polyphonal conversations (Hildy's duets with Walter and trios with Walter and Bruce) and around modern machines (either the telephone, the typewriter, or both), conversations which essentially allow her to talk to herself and thus bring her to her eventual discovery. These polyphonal conversations combine the verbal counterpoint of the original play (all of these conversations come directly from *The Front Page*) with the implications of Hawks's framing, which deliberately keeps the duets and trios within the same framed space. Hawks's framing is an external, physical means of depicting the internal conflicts which Hildy feels, the "objective correlative" of her abstract, subtextual emotion. At the center of these carefully framed, internal conversations are those two modern machines of conversation and communication— the telephone and the typewriter. The telephone is Hildy's essential link to Walter, personally and professionally, a connection Hawks establishes in their first scene together in Walter's office where two symmetrically placed telephones on his desk echo the symmetry of Walter's and Hildy's bodies in Hawks's frame, standing directly behind them. The telephone becomes increasingly important in the film's third section, announced by the tracking shot of ringing telephones which begins the section (there is no one to answer them while the reporters are all away, searching for Earl Williams). Hildy, like the other reporters, will phone in her story to Walter—except that she has the "exclusive": how Earl shot Professor Egelhofer "right in the classified ads . . . No, ads" (an improvised line that exists in neither the play nor the film's script).[14]

In the first of these polyphonal conversations, Hildy races back and forth between two telephones: one that links her with Bruce (in jail again) and the other that links her with Walter (in his office). Hawks's stable camera (it pans slightly) simply follows her race from the one phone in the rearground to the other in the foreground, as she, in effect, juggles the two commitments and relationships, the perpetual motion

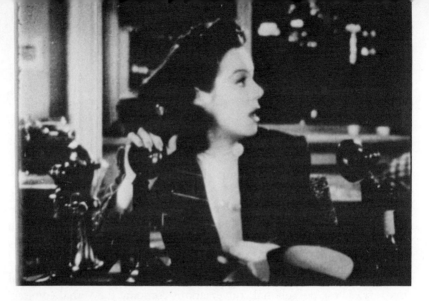

Hildy between two telephones.

of her scurrying body conveying the emotional balancing act she is attempting to perform. The second polyphonal conversation, also between Hildy and Walter on one telephone, between Hildy and Bruce on the other, is tenser, tighter, less active, more still. This time Hildy sits still during the duet, one telephone to her left (Walter), the other to her right (Bruce), addressing one and then the other without moving. Hawks's camera also sits still, again simply observing Hildy juggle two phones, which share the same frame with her and with each other. Significantly, after Hildy hangs up Bruce's phone to continue speaking solely with Walter, Bruce's phone topples over, implying the beginning of his collapse in her affections. This fallen phone may well have been an accident; it occurs so inadvertently, without Rosalind Russell's giving it any thought or plan, that it does not seem to have been deliberate. But would Hawks have kept the take if Walter's phone had been the one to fall?

The third polyphonal number, a trio, brings both Walter and Bruce into the same visual frame as Hildy. She sits at the typewriter, working furiously on the story of Earl Williams's capture. Walter sits to her right, talking to Duffy, his managing editor, on the telephone. We get another busy duet of each doing his/her particular job, separate yet together—"singing" in the same rhythm, tone, and tempo—conveying the energetic harmony of their collaboration. Their work is play, of course, and Hildy-Russell as straight "man" hands Walter-Grant the opportunity to improvise yet another Hawks "tail" joke. "What's the name of the mayor's first wife?" Hildy asks. Then Walter, "The one with the wart on her? (*pause*) Fanny." Without the pause Hawks would never get this "tail" gag past the censors. Nor an earlier one if Walter-Grant did not just "accidentally" mispronounce the name of the effete *Tribune* reporter as Bunzinger, which Hildy must correct to Benzinger. The sharing of spontaneous jokes in a Hawks film conveys the same spiritual harmonies as the sharing of verbal rhythm or vocal pitch.

Bruce, however, has entered the pressroom (where he does not belong) to enter their verbal duet (with which he cannot keep pace or pitch) with his own droning plea. He stands in the frame between Hildy and Walter (both of whom are busy at work), with nothing at all to do (no task, no business) except talk. He literally has no business in the pressroom, and Hawks gives him no physical business there—nor in any other scene of the film except to hold onto that ridiculous umbrella—other than his plodding verbal pleading with Hildy to join him on the nine o'clock train. But Bruce's personal plea interferes with Hildy's professional work—she mistakenly types, "I'm leaving on the nine o'clock train" into her story. His talk also interferes with Walter's concentration and conversation—each of Walter's remarks to Duffy seems pointedly aimed at silencing or commenting upon Bruce's disruptive drivel. And in the midst of this rhythmic counterpoint of singing talk, Hildy unconsciously tells Bruce, "I'm no suburban bridge player. I'm a newspaperman" (another unconscious refutation of her conscious goals, which she is powerless to conceal). Only later, after Bruce's exit, does she return to consciousness: "Where's Bruce?"

Bruce intruding in Hildy and Walter's duet.

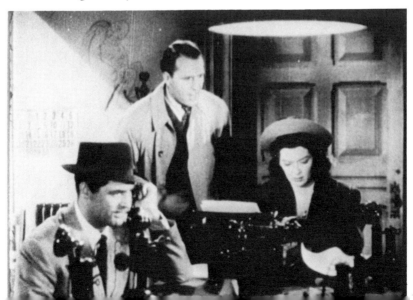

The final polyphonal conversation is a duet between Hildy and Walter on two different telephones; they occupy the same visual frame but two apparently different emotional and psychological frames. Walter has telephoned Butch, one of his employees, seeking help in removing the rolltop desk from the pressroom, the desk in which the escaped Earl Williams is hiding. Hildy, however, uses her telephone to call the city's various hospitals, seeking information about Bruce's mother, whom she fears has been injured in an automobile accident. The sequence uses occasional cutting back and forth between Walter's conversation and Hildy's, but most frequently juxtaposes the two of them within the same frame—Hildy's pacing nervously in the rearground left of the frame, Walter's pacing nervously in the foreground right. Though their goals differ (the purpose of Walter's telephone call is purely professional, Hildy's purely personal—those two conflicting commitments) their vocal, physical, and visual rhythms are identical. So are their postures and positions in Hawks's balanced frame: each of them occupies an identical amount of space beneath an identical hanging lamp.

Bruce's mother, still very much alive, becomes the force that prevents Hildy from going to her son. She bursts into the pressroom, accompanied by a horde of reporters and policemen, to prevent Hildy (who has put that coat on again) from leaving it. Mrs. Baldwin reveals that "some murderer" has been caught and concealed in the pressroom. Walter's floridly emphatic denial (including the suggestion that Mrs. Baldwin is a drunk who has been out "joyriding"), pounded vocifer-

Hildy and Walter on two telephones, symmetrically framed, symmetrical body posture, each of them beneath a hanging lamp.

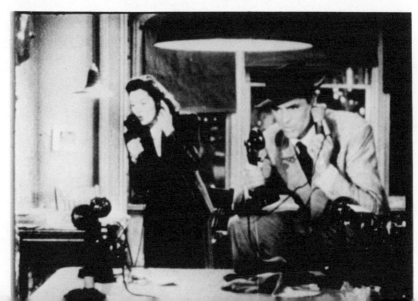

ously on the rolltop desk, leads Earl to answer the coded knock with the three taps that expose his hiding place.

Hawks's handling of the recapture of Earl Williams displays a narrative sensitivity that draws a major emotional distinction between the moments just before and just after the capture. To heighten the suspense before Earl emerges from the desk, Hawks uses one of the film's two major montage sequences. As the sheriff (Gene Lockhart) counts to three before opening the desk's top (this counting will return at the climax of *The Big Sleep*), Hawks cuts away to a close-up of a reporter on the telephone to his paper, alternating both the visual imagery and the verbal information (from Hartman's counting "one" to the reporter's telling his office to "hold on," then from "two" to "right away now," and so forth). As the desk's top rolls back and the tiny Earl pleads, "Go on—shoot me," Hawks's camera tracks in quickly toward Earl's face—the storyteller's method of continuing to sympathize with the plight of a pathetic little man caught between various societal forces and mechanisms.

But as the police lead Earl out of the pressroom and back to his cell, Hawks accomplishes a dazzling synthesis of physical motion, visual

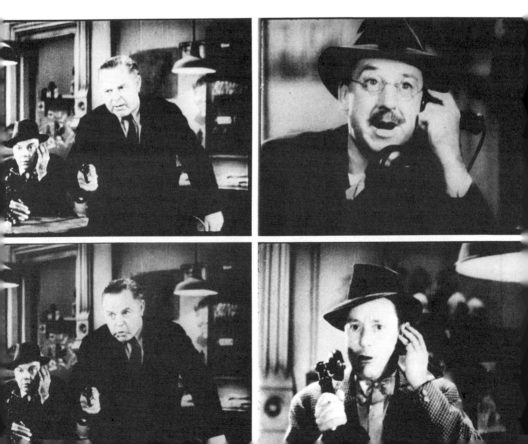

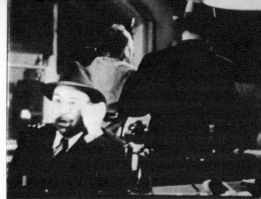

The choreography of space, movement, and dialogue after Williams's capture.

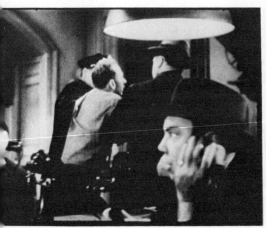

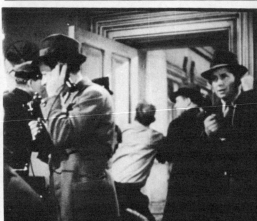

continuity, and verbal commentary. As Earl walks from left to right, the camera tracks with him. Rather than cutting back and forth between the departing Earl and the reporters' descriptions of Earl's capture (a principle of montage that would have been consistent with the method before the capture), Earl "just happens" to walk past the very reporter who, at that moment, "just happens" to be phoning in his particular description to his paper. Earl's walk, accompanied by the camera's track from left to right, manages to put each of the successive descriptions by the reporters into the same frame with the retiring prisoner. There is nothing accidental about this particular verbal-visual choreography. In order to achieve it, Hawks wrote the dialogue continuity for the shot on the set (pencilled in longhand in the film's script), making sure that Earl, the camera, and the line of dialogue all reached the appropriate speaker at the same precise moment. As is typical of Hawks, the shot never proclaims its dazzling choreographing of space because he handles its movement and rhythms so effortlessly and artlessly that the complex choreography just seems to have happened by itself.

Hawks prepares for this dazzling shot with an essential piece of movement and physical business that seems as effortless and natural as everything else in the complicated shot. Just before Earl emerges from the desk, Mrs. Baldwin (Alma Kruger) rushes out of the pressroom to embrace her son, who has appeared (with umbrella) in the hallway, just on the other side of the arch of the pressroom's doorway. As the two outsiders, the two Baldwins, embrace, a policeman "just happens" to swing that door closed, shutting the Baldwins out of the place where they (like Mollie Molloy) do not belong. Bruce will not return again to the pressroom (and will return to the film in only one brief shot—in jail, with his umbrella). The storyteller, in the manner of an Oscar Jaffe, has "closed the iron door" on Bruce, implying that Hildy has done or will do the same. The two "nice" people belong in their world of personal embraces while those who remain inside the pressroom, on the storyteller's side of the door, belong in this world.

By closing the door on Bruce in the same sequence, with the same kind of motion, and in the same rhythm with which Earl himself would be led from the pressroom, the storyteller makes two essential implications. First, that the very excitement of covering the Earl Williams story is itself responsible for the banning of these unexciting people from this exciting world. Like the swinging gate in the film's opening sequence, the pressroom door encloses a world to which there is "No Admittance" for those who do not belong there. Second, that the two peripheral narrative issues (Earl and Bruce) have both been expelled fron

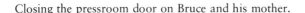

Closing the pressroom door on Bruce and his mother.

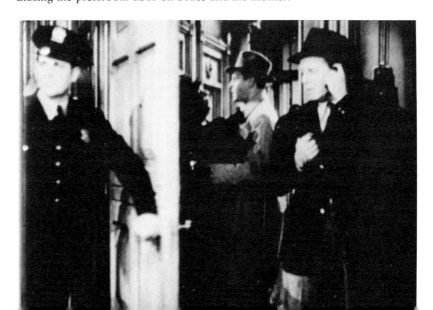

the pressroom, leaving Walter and Hildy to face directly the central narrative issue: each other—their complex feelings for one another that have provided the underlying psychological energy of the narrative from its beginning.

Appropriately enough, our return to the couple still inside the pressroom reveals them physically chained together—handcuffed—a linking that even the corrupt mayor (Clarence Kolb) believes makes them "look natural." Although both the handcuffs and the comment originate in the play, the switch of Hildy's sex in the film converts this image of captivity into an image of natural expression and selection (similar to the images of captivity in *Bringing Up Baby*). The handcuffed man and woman, standing side by side before the mayor, visually resemble a bride and bridegroom at the altar. Despite his bondage, Walter continues to display his defiance with another improvised and surprising piece of cinema self-reference, which links the storyteller's admiration for Walter's assertive energy with the director's admiration for Cary Grant's eccentric ability. When the mayor tells Walter that he's all through, Walter-Grant responds, "Oh yeah? The last person to tell me that was Archie Leach." Archie Leach is Grant's own real name, and that name certainly was "all through"—to be replaced by Cary Grant. Grant spontaneously substituted his own real name for the one in the script, Eddie Kane, producing yet another parallel in the Hawks world between the eccentricities, energies, and surprises of doing any job well and of making films (or of making Hawks's films).

The arrival of Pettibone, the process server, with Earl Williams's reprieve, and his revelation of the previous bribery attempt by the mayor and sheriff, release Walter and Hildy from the handcuffs. Pettibone (the character's name unethnicized from Pincus in both the Hecht-MacArthur play and even the final draft of the film's script), synthesizes many of the film's issues. Like Bruce, he carries an umbrella—upside down and indoors, emphasizing his and its comic ridiculousness. Like Bruce, he puts personal concerns over professional advancement: the mayor's bribery attempt fails primarily because Pettibone does not want to displease his wife. But Pettibone's offbeat humor and surprising spontaneity (aided by the comic playing of Billy Gilbert) link him spiritually with Walter and Hildy. He can talk to them and "sing" with them in the same key; his words, like his mind, move quickly and effortlessly. For example, in the play (and the film's script), after "Pincus" accuses the mayor and sheriff of trying to bribe him, the mayor retorts, "That's absurd on the face of it, Mr. Burns. He's talking like a child." To this assertion in the film, Walter-Grant improvises (pencilled in Hawks's script), "Out of the mouths of babes." Then Pettibone adds (also pencilled) "Hi babe." And Walter-Grant answers (pencilled) "Hiya, toots." In the same spirit, Hildy-Russell later responds improvisationally to the mayor's florid rhetoric of being spared the terrible pain of shedding human blood with a simple, "that's awful." The narrative's characters and the film's players are again inextricable in this scene. They are playing the scene and playing with one another and playing with the script and playing with the director. Work has again become play.

The final scene of the narrative must leave Hildy and Walter alone for her final discovery, which begins with the two of them together, smiling, in a two-shot which again links them visually and spiritually. In the scene that follows, however, Walter and Hildy have switched sides in their argument about the values of a professional life as opposed to a personal home life. Now Hildy wants to remain "a newspaperman" and Walter says he wants her to be "a woman," to go off with Bruce. He talks about his doing something noble for a change. He even hands her that communicative coat. Their reversal mirrors the same switch in the Hecht-MacArthur play when Burns suddenly tells his ace reporter to go off with his Peggy. The motivation for this shift, for Burns's apparent sincerity and sensitivity to Hildy's feelings, is unclear in the Hecht-MacArthur play. Has Walter suddenly been touched with an unselfish human feeling? Or is this scene simply another ruse? Burns gives Hildy his watch as a memento when he sends him away, then telegrams the sheriff of a town on the train's route to arrest Hildy because (as he roars in the play's famous final line), "The son of a bitch stole my watch." If he knew he was going to use the watch to get him back, why did Walter go through the whole touching farewell scene of letting him go in the first place?

The final scene of *The Front Page* becomes a great theatrical stunt with curiously little psychological underpinning (like much of the play as a whole). The final scene resolves the Walter Burns-Hildy Johnson conflict by not resolving it at all—by leaving the conclusion an unanswered question. Does Hildy really want to get away? Will his life with Peggy be fuller or richer than that with Walter? No wonder that the 1930 Lewis Milestone film of *The Front Page* (which did cleverly sneak the "son-of-a-bitch" line onto the sound track) ends with an image of an immense (and rather silly) question mark between "The" and "End."* The evasive ending of *The Front Page* is consistent with its moral evasions throughout. The actors who play the two roles must find particular answers to these moral and motivational questions, but Hecht-MacArthur allow several alternative choices.

But in *His Girl Friday* when Walter-Grant tells Hildy-Russell that he wants to do something noble and wants her to go off with Bruce, we know he does not mean what he says. Like Hildy's talk in the film's beginning, his words are at odds with his feelings (although much more consciously so). The two have truly switched emotional places—in a typical piece of Hawksian symmetry. Everything he has done in the film reveals how much he wants to keep her with him—at home and at work. Why, then, does Walter say what he does not mean in this scene?

First, Walter must finally allow Hildy to make the decision, to verbalize the discovery, that he has tried to help her make. He cannot make that final decision for her; she must make it herself. If she still really wants to go to Bruce after what they have done and been through and lived through together in the past twelve hours, then Walter is ready to accept his defeat and ready to acknowledge his error: that she *really* wants to go to Bruce. He wants her to do what *she really* wants to do—because he really loves her.

Second, Hildy must come to a conscious and verbal realization that she is a newspaperman and a woman at the same time, and that she

---

* Although the conventional wisdom describes the superiority of *His Girl Friday* to Milestone's earlier film version of the Hecht-MacArthur play in terms of its speed, this description seems imprecise, a response to an effect not a cause. As opposed to the Milestone version, Hawks's film: (1) tosses the dialogue away in a casual manner rather than orates it; (2) converts the play's structure into a film narrative (indeed into a movie genre, a "screwball comedy") rather than retains the play's theatrical structure; (3) converts the play's decor, a mere backdrop, into cinema decor with meaning (the power of coats and doors and telephones); (4) knows where to locate the story's moral and psychological point-of-view; and (5) uses the camera and the frame to produce coherence, not to amuse with its own choreography (following Milestone's camera tricks becomes a dizzy game of "follow the bouncing ball"—quite literally in one absolutely dreadful sequence). All of these differences between the two films relate to the essential Hawks strengths.

cannot be a real and full "woman" if she denies being the newspaper-man she also *really* is. Walter's taking Hildy's previous argumentative position forces her to realize and to refute the spiritual, moral, emotional, and psychological errors of that position.

Third, Walter is also punishing her for those initial errors. Hildy's comic flaw (her self-deception about what makes a life meaningful and what makes her life meaningful) leads to a comic discovery of that comic flaw and (as is typical of many comedies with this structure) that discovery must be accompanied by a comic punishment that restores the moral and psychological balance (like the demise of David's dinosaur). Hildy must beg, plead, wheedle, and whine for Walter to take her back, whereas he now pretends to be sending her away. Only the final phone call from Bruce, announcing he has again been arrested for passing counterfeit money, reminds her that Walter *really* wants her (again, like Kid's two-headed coin), for she now remembers that all of Walter's strategies have been aimed at separating her from Bruce and keeping her with him.

Feminist critics and social moralists may again be upset by the film's "comic" resolution, for, as in *Twentieth Century,* the film celebrates a woman's accepting her slavery and her subservience to a man; she makes no linear progress but returns in a repetitive circle to exactly where she was before. Hildy-Russell's movement, gestures, posture, voice all reflect her reduction and belittlement.[15] She no longer walks strong, fast, and firm as she did at the film's beginning but cowers and cringes in Walter's presence. She no longer keeps up with Walter's verbal pace but says curiously little; indeed, she has said much less since Walter entered the pressroom to supervise the transportation of Earl Williams. She has surrendered her visual rights in the frame to Walter, who has dominated our visual as well as verbal attention since he entered the pressroom. Indeed, in the Pettibone scene Hildy has been almost cropped from the frame altogether—although one possible reason is that Rosalind Russell looks as if she is in perpetual danger of reacting to the improvisation by erupting into a laugh and spoiling the take. And the storyteller who is composing these visual frames, and who has sided with Walter's strategies throughout, unashamedly seems to stand with the triumphant Walter and against the submissive, whimpering Hildy in the film's final scenes.

Hildy's submission can only seem comically and morally satisfying

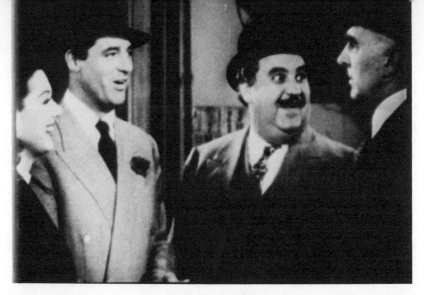

Hildy almost cropped from the frame with Walter, Pettibone, and the Mayor.

if we view it as comic punishment for her original comic sin. She is paying for her mistake of not knowing herself, not knowing life, not knowing the meaning of personal fulfillment, destroying her happiness (and, by the way, Walter's) by trying to divorce herself from both a person and from a vocation which she requires in order to survive. Like Lily Garland and Oscar Jaffe, Hildy Johnson and Walter Burns of *His Girl Friday* are a matched spiritual set who can only live fully as individuals by living fully as complements. There is no gulf between a personal need (home) and a professional need (work) because (for Hawks anyway) work is a personal need. By not working at what she loves to do and does well, Hildy can only betray herself, can only not be herself. Although Hildy returns full circle to where she was before—the same job and the same marriage—she returns with greater knowledge. Her human education, if not her human vocation, has progressed—the typical result of such comic structures (as opposed to the conclusion of *Twentieth Century,* which shares the same structural pattern but in which the characters, by definition, are not capable of such rational and conscious education).

The film's ending celebrates their reunion, their remarriage, and Hildy's rediscovery of values when Walter tells Duffy (over the telephone again) that Hildy will write the story of Earl Williams's reprieve. "Of course she's not quitting. She never intended to. We're gonna get married." Walter has known Hildy's real intentions from the beginning. As the two plan to honeymoon at Niagara Falls, Walter learns about a strike in Albany. Of course they can cover the strike on their way to Niagara Falls. As they set off toward another honeymoon that they may never take, in this synthesis of love as work as love, Hawks ends the film with another comic stage exit, accompanied by a dazzlingly comic exit line. As they leave the frame of the screen-stage in unison, the frame of the pressroom's doorway serves as their mock proscenium arch; Walter, who always walks ungentlemanly ahead, tosses the observation over his shoulder: "What a coincidence. We're going to Albany. I wonder if Bruce can put us up." And off they go, taking the energy of their private world with them, out the door, into the larger world itself.

The script planned to bring the couple back to the newspaper office for a shotgun wedding (the barrel trained on a still recalcitrant Hildy). A verbal-visual battle erupts after the "I Do's," a cacophonous battle of sound that duplicates the verbal war that closes *Twentieth Century.* As the fighting rages, Louie observes, "I think it's gonna turn out all right this time." And the script indicates a final fade-out on this unresolved resolution. Although the sexual shift of the shotgun's usual target is cleverly consistent with the film's sexual reversals, Hawks foregoes this kind of cleverness for the psychological solidity of an ending that evolved on the set—combining the pattern of the film's narrative structure, the definitions of its decor (that door), and the harmonious playing of its star performers. When Walter claims that Hildy "never

The pressroom door as mock proscenium arch.

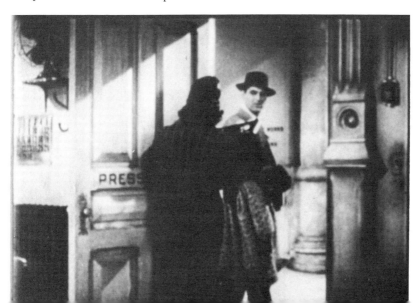

intended to" leave, he, like the psychiatrist in *Bringing Up Baby*, has analyzed a person's feelings far more knowingly than she herself has been able to do. Walter's smug pronouncement in the film's opening scene—that he would know Hildy's desires and intentions "anytime, anyplace, anywhere"—turns out to be quite true. The storyteller, in identifying from the beginning with Walter's perceptions, has consistently revealed Hildy's real intentions merely by her vocal patterns, her rhythms of movement, her posture, her handling of objects. Hildy's discovery of this underlying intention has made her whole again. She needs no shotgun to convince her. She has learned the lesson for herself (with Walter as her professor). When the two set off together—to Albany or Niagara Falls, for a honeymoon or to cover a strike—they are both going "home," for Hildy now knows that her home is wherever she is working with Walter.

8

Hemingway and Chandler into Bogart-Bacall and Hawks:
To Have and Have Not and *The Big Sleep*

I talked with Hemingway. I was trying to get him to do some writing for me. He said, "I don't want to go to Hollywood." We were sitting in his boat, fishing. I said, "We can meet here, Sun Valley, any place you want, or Africa, and write a story. You're always broke and can use the money." He thought a minute and said, "I don't want to do it." I said, "I can make a picture out of the worst book that you ever wrote." He said, "What's my worst book?" I said, "That bunch of junk called *To Have and Have Not*." "Well, you can['t] make a picture out of that," he said. So we sat around for two weeks and evolved the story that we did which was the meeting of the two people in his story and it had very much the same background.[1]

So I told Bogart, watch yourself because you're supposed to be the most insolent man on the screen and I'm going to make a girl a little more insolent than you. . . . In every scene in the picture she's going to walk out and leave you. You're going to be left standing with egg on your face. He said that isn't fair, and I said I know but I'm the director and I can do that.[2]

We were having an argument one time about who killed Owen, and no one ever knew who did it. After we had argued about it a lot I sent Chandler a wire and said, "Who killed him?" and he said, "So and so." He couldn't have, he was down at the beach at the time. So we didn't bother about it—we just tried to make good scenes.[3]

McBRIDE: It seems that you were more concerned with the relationship between Bogart and Bacall than anything else in the film.
HAWKS: Definitely.[4]

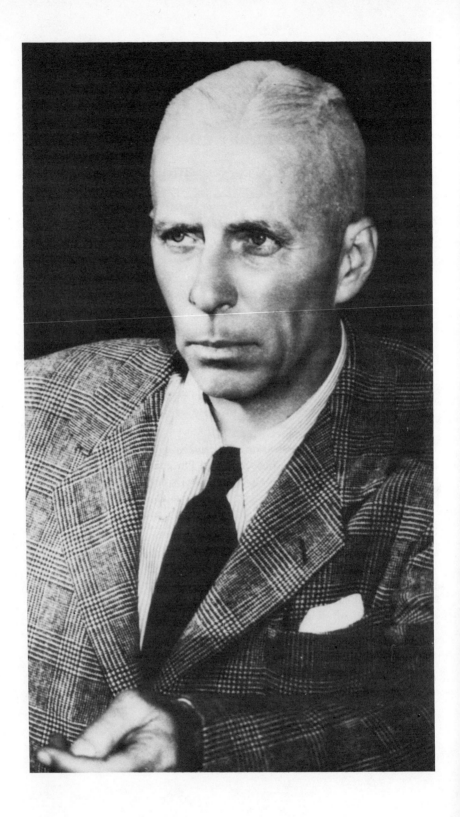

IT SEEMED INEVITABLE that Howard Hawks would film a Hemingway novel. Hemingway was one of Hawks's favorite writers: "I liked anything that Hemingway wrote."[5] For years he had planned to film one of Hemingway's greatest short stories, "The Short Happy Life of Francis Macomber." But after each announcement of the project in *Variety*, Hawks perpetually put it aside for another. John Wayne's confrontation with an angry elephant in *Hatari!* would be Hawks's closest approach to "Macomber." Although Hawks bought the rights to one of Hemingway's greatest novels, *The Sun Also Rises,* he never filmed that story and sold those rights to Twentieth Century-Fox; Henry King made that film in 1957. Instead, Hawks filmed "that bunch of junk," *To Have and Have Not,* in Hawks's opinion (without much argument from Hemingway) Hemingway's worst book: "Hemingway explained that he had written the story in one sitting when he needed money"[6] (another of those anecdotes that cast some doubt on the clear distinction between the debased commerciality of movies and the artistic purity of "literature"). In truth, the movie that Hawks made of this book bears little resemblance to it except the title, the name and a few traits of the leading character (Harry Morgan), the name of his woman (Marie), the name of his "rummy" companion (Eddie), and the name and character traits of the clumsy, dishonorable fisherman (Johnson), who not only fishes poorly but swindles Harry out of the money he owes him for chartering his boat. Johnson is the one figure from the Hemingway story who remains intact through the many versions of the film's scripts and the final film of *To Have and Have Not.* All those characters and incidents in the film that bear even the vaguest resemblance to Hemingway's come from his first four chapters, the first 50-odd pages of a 262-page book.[7]

Although Hawks's narrative bears little resemblance to Hemingway's, there is an unmistakable Hemingway aroma and flavor about the film. But the same could be said of any of the Hawks "adventure" films. Certainly no major American filmmaker and American writer, who were contemporaries chronologically, were also such close complementaries spiritually. Both told stories of men in action, and that action

Howard Hawks in the mid-1940s

245

was a personal assertion of existential meaning in a universe of potential cosmic meaninglessness. Both had a special fondness for stories of "Men Without Women" and of men who tried to find and make a place for those necessary women. Both preferred characters who did more than they said, felt more than they spoke. Both built their narratives upon moral systems based on personal definitions of honor and integrity, rather than the societally accepted and acceptable ones, which their works overtly or covertly attacked. Both developed a style—either verbal or visual—which was distinguished for its spare, bare understatement. Interestingly enough, while literary critics praised Hemingway's austerity for the idiosyncracies of its bareness, to many film critics Hawks's functional style seemed simply styleless—"uncinematic" or typically Hollywood. This discrepancy partially accounts for the immense difference between the cultural reputations of these two artists and friends who were so similar in their aims and abilities—the one a Nobel Prize winner and pillar of the American cultural pantheon of the twentieth century, the other a commercially successful director of genre pictures who was not listed in *Who's Who* until some two decades after he had done his major work.

In its initial stages the film of *To Have and Have Not* was to have been much closer to the Hemingway novel. The Hemingway story is a kind of experiment (modeled perhaps on both Faulkner's *As I Lay Dying* and *The Wild Palms*) in split narrative focus—its attention divided between two major characters, the tough owner of a fishing boat, Harry Morgan, and the vapid but successful political novelist, Richard Gordon (along with several other rich and useless sophisticates in his "set"); its setting divided between Havana and Key West (and the illegal commercial links between them); its point-of-view divided between third-person authorial omniscience and the first-person reports of two characters (Harry and his friend Albert). Harry Morgan's luck turns sour early in the book. Johnson runs off without paying him for chartering his boat, so Harry must accept a series of increasingly dangerous and illegal jobs, the kind which he avoided when he did not need the money to support his wife (Marie) and children. First, he must smuggle Chinamen from Cuba to Key West, but the machinations of Mr. Sing, the Chinese entrepreneur who arranges the deal, require Harry to murder the man and dump his body. Then Harry must smuggle liquor from Cuba to Key West, leading to a skirmish with the Coast Guard in which

Harry loses both an arm and his boat. Finally, he must smuggle four revolutionary bankrobbers from Key West to Cuba with the loot they have stolen to finance their revolution. After these four bandit-revolutionaries kill his friend Albert, Harry disposes of them but loses his life in the process. Lying in his boat, shot in the stomach, delirious, an inarticulate Harry manages to articulate the book's moral point: "No matter how a man alone ain't got no bloody fucking chance." Hemingway's narrative voice comments: "It had taken him a long time to get it out and it had taken him all of his life to learn it" (p. 225).

Juxtaposed with Harry's steady decline, which he defiantly, stubbornly resists, is Richard Gordon's drifting, aimless decline—the loss of his wife to another man, to boredom, to idleness, to a life of talk and booze. Although Gordon himself never meets Harry, some members of his social set bump into him in the bar where Gordon also goes to drink (Harry doesn't think much of them). Gordon twice crosses the path of Harry's wife, Marie, and Gordon instantly believes he perceives the meaning of her life and the depth of her degradation.

> Her husband when he came home at night hated her, hated the way she had coarsened and grown heavy, was repelled by her too big breasts, her lack of sympathy with his work as an organizer. . . . It was good. It could be easily, terrific, and it was true. He had seen, in a flash of perception, the whole inner life of that type of woman. (p. 177)

The irony of Gordon's perception is that it is absolutely false—that he himself has the wife whom he repels and who repulses him in return, a wife in whom both love and lust have died, while Marie, the woman he will make a functional character in a hack novel, dearly loves and longs for her husband Harry, who adores her in return. Gordon's failures at perception, as both a person and a writer, are underscored by the genuine political problems of several characters in Hemingway's novel as opposed to those in Gordon's facile political melodramas. A group of American World War I veterans has been unemployed for years, the Cuban revolutionaries have committed themselves to a violent reform of their society, while Albert, like Harry, must accept the dangerous job that kills him because he can find no other means to support his family. Gordon's emptiness is also mirrored by the empty and drunken boredom of several other members of his social set; one of the final chapters leaps from yacht to yacht in the harbor of Key West, briefly anatomizing their spoiled and comfortable occupants, all of them corrupt, callow, debauched, or suicidal, while Harry Morgan lies bleeding to death, alone, in his boat. There is something richer, truer, fuller, nobler, more valuable about the active, brutal life of a Harry Morgan than about the useless bored passivity of a Richard Gordon and his sort.

The reason that Howard Hawks found the book a "bunch of junk" was probably because of this artificial splitting of its narrative focus and the pointlessness of its wandering point-of-view. The story of Richard Gordon and his crowd merely pulls the reader away from the story of Harry Morgan to permit Hemingway's abstract commentary on rich, spoiled, useless people who should know and live better but don't. Hawks would solve these problems by concentrating on Harry Morgan exclusively and by making him a more humanly sensitive and sympathetic center of the narrative. Although Hemingway takes special care to remove Harry's moral responsibility for all his murders—each murder is a valid response to an unavoidable evil outside himself—this very moral exoneration would not exonerate him in Hawks's eyes. Hemingway's Harry passively suffers a lot of bad luck; he is precisely the kind of loser Hawks did not like. Hawks would convert this loser into a loner who finally rebels against his luck by taking action against it. He becomes the master, not the slave of his fate. In Hawks's film, Harry Morgan's discovery about the worthlessness of being "a man alone" would not manifest itself in a blatantly verbal statement that took him "all his life to learn," nor would it get lost in a sea of other characters and other story lines. That discovery, as is typical of Hawks films, would be the underlying, subtextual basis of the entire narrative's construction. Once Harry makes that discovery he takes action (as is typical in Hawks) on the basis of it.

In the first draft of the script (dated November 22, 1943), the story's setting is still Havana.[8] Harry Morgan, swindled by Johnson, takes on both the liquor smuggling job and the bank robbery job. The central location is a typical Hawks-Furthman hotel-restaurant-bar, run by a comical Cuban couple, Decimo and Benicia (this couple, which would be replaced by Frenchy in the film of *To Have and Have Not*, would return as Carlos and Consuela in the Hawks-Furthman hotel-restaurant-bar of *Rio Bravo*). There is a "new girl" in the bar, Corinne, who sings and plays the piano. And there is an old flame of Harry's, Sylvia, who comes to Havana with her new husband (a shift of *Only Angels Have Wings* from Barranca to Havana, from Geoff Carter to Harry Morgan, and from Judy to Sylvia). The script lacks any political dimension, its central government authority personified by the prefecture of police, Caesar, a good enough fellow for a cop who merely does his job. The second, revised version of the script expands this political dimension, setting the film more firmly within the Cuban political revolution against a corrupt Machado; Caesar becomes the head of the less sympathetic Cuban secret police. Corinne's name has been changed to Marie, the old flame now calls herself Helen, and there is a piano player named Chuck.

Several touches which find their way into the film have already been written into the script. Eddie, the "rummy," already asks his cryptic question, "Was you ever bit by a dead bee?", as a personal initiation rite, testing his respondent's imagination and friendship. Harry and Marie inexplicably call one another "Steve" and "Slim" for no reason established in the script. The Cuban revolutionaries use Eddie as a pawn in the game to hire Harry's boat for their bank job, knowing that Harry will not abandon his friend. Harry merely wants to go about his business, to run his boat, taking no interest at all in political quarrels ("Sorry, I'm not interested in politics"); he is eventually dragged into the political battle because he needs the money and he likes his friends.

Less than three months later, *To Have and Have Not* went into production, set in Frenchy's Hotel Marquis in Martinique, its political backdrop changed from the Machado revolution in Cuba to the European conflict between Free and Vichy France. Critics, then as now, assumed that *To Have and Have Not* was a deliberate attempt to remake *Casablanca.*

> Having once cornered Humphrey Bogart in a Casablanca café and beheld his tremendous potential in that sultry and colorful spot, it was logical that the Warners should have wanted to get him there again—or in some place of similar nature where the currents would flow much the same.[9]

The shift from Havana to Martinique, from Hemingway's story of smuggling and bank robberies to Hawks's film about taking a political-moral stand against a Nazi government, was obviously no deliberate, "logical" plan of "the Warners" but a sudden, spontaneous shift—an improvisational response to governmental pressure on Warner Bros., who were financing the Hawks production. An article in the *New York Times* of April 2, 1944, reported that the Office of Inter-American Affairs was so upset by the filming of Hemingway's *To Have and Have Not*—its depiction of corruption, smuggling, and brutality in the Cuban government and society—that it had pressured the Roosevelt administration to halt production of the film altogether. The Roosevelt administration, in turn, sensitive to the official "good neighbor policy" it promoted between the American nations, also pressured Warners to cancel the film, threatening to withhold the export license required for a film to be shown (and earn money) abroad. But studio research revealed that one Caribbean nation was outside the jurisdiction of the Inter-American office—the Vichy-dominated island of Martinique. "That immediately struck a happy chord," said Hawks. Hemingway's story would be told against a background of conflict between the Vichy and Gaullist French. "The script is being written, just ahead of production." Given the fact that Hawks's work always thrived on this kind of spontaneity, evolving a story from the characters, talk, and incidents that developed on the set, writing the script just ahead of production must have "struck a happy chord" indeed.[10]

The narrative "happy chord" which the shift to Martinique struck was to enable the film to set its action within a political context that was also, for the American audience of 1944, a moral context. The vagaries of Cuban politics made the political issues of the film's original script (and of the novel as well) almost apolitical; although the audience might feel some sympathy for the revolutionaries as romantic rebels (given Hollywood's romanticizing of such rebels) they would certainly feel little sympathy for bank robbers and brutal murderers. But in the film of *To Have and Have Not*, Harry Morgan's original decision to keep out of politics ("I don't care who runs France—or Martinique") seems, at least partially, a personal and moral evasion, while his ultimate decision to help the Free French ("Maybe because I like you and I don't like them") unifies his personal and moral commitments. It is this unity of personal, moral, and vocational commitments that very much makes *To Have and Have Not* a Howard Hawks film rather than a remake of Michael Curtiz's *Casablanca*. Whether deliberate or not, the Hawks film seems a rebuttal of *Casablanca*, in which the American loner portrayed by Bogart must choose between love and duty—either to consummate his personal love for a woman or to send her away with her heroic, freedom-fighting husband. Rick-Bogart eventually does the "right thing," preserving the traditional, classical dichotomy between personal need and moral obligation. But for Hawks, no moral obligation is greater than a personal obligation; only by synthesizing the two can a human being achieve a spiritual unity.

That spiritual unity, which increases our sympathy for Heming-way's original Harry Morgan, also serves as the film's narrative remedy for Hemingway's wandering narrative focus. Harry Morgan's percep-tions exclusively control the film's narrative point-of-view; there is not a single scene in which Harry is not physically present. Hawks takes Hemingway's first-person attachment to Harry in the first section of his novel and sustains it through the entire film—in the usual way that Hawks translates first-person narration into cinema. Rather than peer-ing directly through the character's eyes, Hawks makes the character an object in the frame while, at the same time, never constructing a frame in which the character is not or might not be present. This typical Hawksian balance of objective reportage and subjective perception would serve identically in the Bogart-Bacall companion piece, *The Big Sleep*, which also translates first-person narration into the Bogart character's presence in every shot or scene. With this new unity of the narrative's central character and its point-of-view, the film's narrative structure be-comes the evolution of not just Harry Morgan's discovery but, like Hildy Johnson's in *His Girl Friday*, his conscious and explicit expression of that discovery in action. Harry's personal system of morality, which underlies all his actions and values early in the film, must eventually manifest itself in physical—and political—action.

Into this familiar Hawks narrative pattern *To Have and Have Not* weaves two corollary Hawks themes. First, there is Harry Morgan's love for Marie, the woman who just got off the boat (like Bonnie Lee) in Fort-de-France and whose wit, cool, and toughness precisely match Harry's own. Hawks knew that he was going to use his "new girl," Lauren Bacall, whom he had signed to a personal contract after his wife, "Slim," showed him Betty Bacal's picture in *Harper's Bazaar*. Hawks changed her first name to Lauren (like Oscar Jaffe's changing Mildred Plotka's), added a second *l* to her last name (Bacall had herself changed her original last name, Persky, to Bacal) and sent her off to a vocal teacher to drop her voice into the sultry lower registers. Hawks also knew that he was going to team the "new girl's" sultry insolence with the established tough-egg insolence of Humphrey Bogart. (In the revised script, Marie even asks a bartender who the guy is that looks like Humphrey Bogart—a typical piece of Hawksian self-reference which Hawks this time chose to eliminate.) The basic problem confronting Hawks in making this narrative was to work this complex emotional relationship into the smuggling activities of Hemingway's novel. The political-moral shift to the struggle of the Free French allowed Hawks to work the love story into the adventure story in his familiar way. The two lovers demonstrate their love by working together.

The film's second narrative strand is Harry's friendship for the "rummy" Eddie, who, according to Harry, used to be a good man (and shows that he still is). Eddie, like Marie, becomes a victim and a pawn of the Vichy Gestapo, further strengthening Harry's sympathies in favor of their enemies. Walter Brennan's quirky, jumpy, jittery performance as Eddie—one of the very best of his very distinguished career—took its cue from a single descriptive sentence in the Hemingway novel: "He walked with his joints all slung wrong" (p. 9). Brennan accompanied his "slung-wrong" walk with a mind that also seemed to bounce off in odd directions and at odd angles, climbing aboard a train of thought, riding it a while verbally, then suddenly stopping to return to a crucial turning point, starting to run off on that train of thought again for a while, then stopping, returning, and so on. While Eddie's mind seems to work three paces slower than Harry's (hence the perpetual need to stop and turn back and jump forward), it works three paces ahead of his Gestapo interrogators (who can make no sense at all of his camouflaging babble of contradictory, "slung-wrong" talk). Eddie's spiritual extension in the film is Frenchy, the man who owns the "clean, well-lighted place," and who, like Harry and Marie, answered Eddie's cryptic but probing question of ritual initiation, "Was you ever bit by a dead bee?" correctly (*i.e.* playfully): "Was you?"

Like many of the greatest Hawks films, *To Have and Have Not* gets its depth, complexity, and vitality from its characters as performers and its performers as characters—Harry-Bogart, Marie-Bacall, Eddie-Brennan—none of which characters existed in precisely this rich and vibrant form in the original novel (and one of which did not exist at all). As in *Only Angels Have Wings,* the film of *To Have and Have Not* allows these characters, and particularly its central male character, to synthesize the demands of work, love, and friendship. His decision to work for the Free French allows his love and his friend to work with him and allows that work to become an expression of that love and friendship. This "conversion" from political neutrality to moral commitment may seem typical of the Bogart persona, whose conversion is never really a conversion but an evolution and external manifestation of a personal morality that has been evident beneath the surface throughout. That kind of evolution is as typical for the Hawks film as for the Bogart persona, making the pairing of the two in this film and in this political context particularly felicitous. The evolution of Harry-Bogart's sympathies is mirrored by "Slim" (Marie, according to her passport) who has the opportunity to protect herself, to "mind her own business," by leaving Martinique on the morning plane (like Johnson) and returning home. But like Bonnie Lee in *Only Angels,* Slim shows her sympathies by deciding to stay in a place that is stranger, more disturbing, and less safe than home: she feels more complete in the strange land with the strange man. It is difficult to imagine how Hawks would have been able to solve his narrative problem—to get Bogart and Bacall into this Hemingway story—without the shift from Havana to Martinique.

A corollary shift from the first Furthman script to the final film was a major change in the newcomer couple. As opposed to the script's uninitiated, youthful husband (starchily named Essex), who eventually proves his mettle and passes his initiation under fire by helping Harry Morgan exterminate the bank robbers, and to his wife, the former flame who once burned Harry's romantic fingers, the film's newcomer couple is the French freedom fighter, de Bursac (Walter Molnar) and the self-sacrificing wife (Dolores Moran) who accompanies him. Although the pretty young wife allows Slim some competitive cattiness, this new couple keeps the film's moral focus on the issues of heroism, integrity, and commitment rather than on romantic entanglements. More than any other element of the film (except for the presence and "conversion" of Humphrey Bogart), the freedom-fighting pair of de Bursac and sacrificing wife were probably responsible for the assumption that "the Warners" intended to remake *Casablanca.* Even if this motif were borrowed from the earlier film, it has been transformed in *To Have and*

Have Not into a Hawks (or Hawks-Furthman) motif, at least as similar to Bat and Judy, the newcomer couple of *Only Angels Have Wings,* as to the political couple of *Casablanca.* Like Bat and Judy, the de Bursacs enter the film to begin a new narrative section (the third), immediately after the section in which the new girl (Bonnie or Slim) has forged a strong bond with the tough man (Geoff or Harry). Mme de Bursac even looks like Rita Hayworth's Judy of Hawks's earlier film. The newcomer couple in both films then shifts the narrative toward its ultimate external action, allowing the other more central couple to demonstrate their unity and their feelings in taking or responding to that action.

As these structural parallels indicate, the four parts of *To Have and Have Not* mirror the narrative construction of *Only Angels Have Wings.* In the first section we are transported to an exotic foreign setting where we encounter a strong, tough man who is committed both to his work and to his strange but strong personal code of morality. We also encounter a strange set of cultural conditions that differs radically from our own (not the existential honor code of fliers but the battle between the Free and Vichy French) and a woman who, like ourselves, has just arrived there. While the conflict of *Only Angels* is the clash of values between those fliers who inhabit the world of Barranca and that female figure from the outside world who comes to Barranca with those outside values (hence she is our guide into that world, for her values are also ours), there is no conflict of values between Harry and Slim, who are spiritually one from their first meeting. Both honor their private, personal codes of morality, and both codes are identical. Their need to demonstrate that oneness to each other becomes the action of the film's second section. That demonstration takes the form of their similar reaction to the brutality of the Gestapo (and is confirmed by the distasteful Gestapo chief's similar distaste for both of them) and the sharing of cigarettes and drinks in the private, upstairs region of Frenchy's hotel, as they glide back and forth across the corridor to each other's rooms. In the third section, Harry and Eddie work together to carry the de Bursacs into Fort-de-France on Harry's boat, and after de Bursac's injury in the skirmish with the harbor boat (a transformation of the Coast Guard incident in the Hemingway novel) Harry and Slim work together to remove the bullet from his shoulder. In the fourth section, Harry and Slim directly confront the Gestapo together to save Harry's friend, Eddie, and at the end of the film this ideal Hawks community of man, woman, and friend rhumbas off to its next experience or adventure.

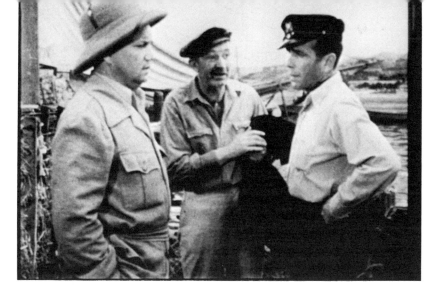

Johnson, Eddie, and Harry.

The film's first section is built around Hemingway's Johnson, beginning with his inept fishing trip and ending with his inept death. The contrast between Johnson's (Walter Sande) ineptness and Harry's competent strength establishes the essential traits of Harry Morgan which the remainder of the narrative will need. Harry's loose, casual clothing contrasts with Johnson's carefully selected, bindingly tight fishing "outfit." Johnson's haggling with Harry over the money he owes him contrasts with Harry's sense of money as a tangible sign of honor that does not bear haggling. "That's what you owe me and that's what I want." The relationship between honor and money is a major thematic ribbon that runs all the way through the film. Harry's trust in Slim can evolve only when he discovers that, despite her financial needs, money for her, too, is merely a tangible sign of personal integrity. Johnson's superficially hostile moral attitude toward a Vichy flag-raising ceremony—"That's Vichy for you"—contrasts with Harry's disinterested and pragmatic refusal to take a political side—"It's their flag." Johnson ignores Harry's orders to keep plenty of drag on his fishing line (just as de Bursac later ignores Harry's orders to stay down), so Johnson loses the line and takes a ridiculous pratfall as a result. Finally, Johnson feels a lordly contempt for the "rummy," Eddie—"What do you look after him for?"—while Harry responds to him as a comrade and equal: "He thinks he's looking after me."

Appropriately enough, Harry and Slim get to know one another after her theft of Johnson's wallet. Despite Johnson's ineptness (and, as

Harry later discovers, outright dishonesty), Harry treats Johnson's wallet as a token of honor that Slim must return. The two had briefly met before when she came to Harry's room to ask him for the inevitable Hawks-Furthman match. Then Harry goes to Slim's room to retrieve Johnson's wallet. This first pair of meetings between them sets the pattern that the later sections of the film will follow.

First, the film makes a major contrast between the downstairs and upstairs, the public and private regions of Frenchy's hotel-restaurant-bar. While *Only Angels Have Wings* took place primarily in the public downstairs world of Dutchy's hotel-restaurant-bar, punctuated by an occasional retreat to the private domain upstairs (the emphasis of downstairs over upstairs is about the same in *The Dawn Patrol* and *Barbary Coast*), *To Have and Have Not* is exactly the reverse. Much more of its action takes place upstairs (the scenes of sexual-emotional interaction between Harry and Slim, the secret meetings with the French freedom fighters, the final confrontation with the Gestapo), punctuated by occasional public scenes downstairs, where Frenchy (Marcel Dalio of Renoir's *Grand Illusion* and *Rules of the Game*) presides behind the bar and Cricket (Hoagy Carmichael—the well-known songwriter whose potential as a film persona Hawks discovered at a party—in his first film role) rules at the piano. Although Slim participates in this public downstairs world (like Bonnie, she joins in the music, becoming a spiritual extension of Cricket and his songs), she needs the private of the upstairs world to express her feelings for Harry, who is a much more private, "upstairs" character than Geoff Carter. This alternation of the

Slim with Cricket.

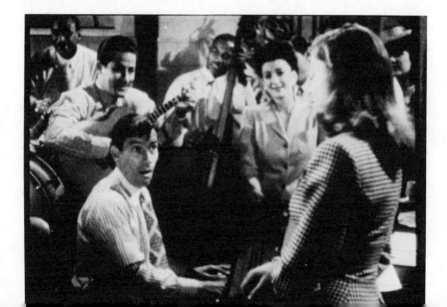

private and public regions of the film's setting is a metaphor for the film's conflict of personal and public expressions of morality, which Harry initially tries to juggle, like Hildy Johnson with two telephones, but he then discovers must be synthesized. Harry can preserve his honor and integrity only by taking it out of his room and going with it into the world.

This use of the upstairs is quite intentional in the film. In explaining the film's famous "whistle" line, Hawks relates,

> I was making a test of Bacall, so I wrote the scene just for the test and it went over so well we had an awful time trying to put it into the picture. Faulkner was the one who found a place to put it. He said, "If we put these people in a hotel corridor where nobody else is around, then I think we can make that scene work." [11]

The scene actually takes place in Harry's room, not in the corridor, but both Slim's and Harry's rooms are across from one another, off that hotel corridor, and both rooms allow them to play scenes where "nobody else is around." Hawks called in Faulkner for the film's final shooting script, the one that converted Hemingway-Furthman's Havana into Hawks's Martinique; the film's many upstairs sequences are Faulkner's primary contribution to the film's conception, since Furthman consistently prefered to write scenes for the downstairs regions of his hotel-restaurant-bars. Within that upstairs region the two characters move back and forth across the hall, from his room to her room to his room, in a kind of measured dance that mirrors the alternation of night and day in *Bringing Up Baby* and *Rio Bravo*.

Second, as is typical of the Furthman scripts for Hawks, the emotional dynamics of the film's narrative pirouette around the exchange of matches and cigarettes. Slim first comes to Harry's room to ask for a match; he tosses her the box of matches so she can light her own (like Walter Burns tossing matches to Hildy Johnson). In their second scene, the dispute about Johnson's wallet which takes place in Slim's room, Harry lights her cigarette for her for the first time. In the next scene, downstairs, when an angry Harry moves aggressively toward Johnson, Slim strikes a match in front of Harry's face to make him conscious of his action, bring him to his senses, cool him down (like Geoff striking

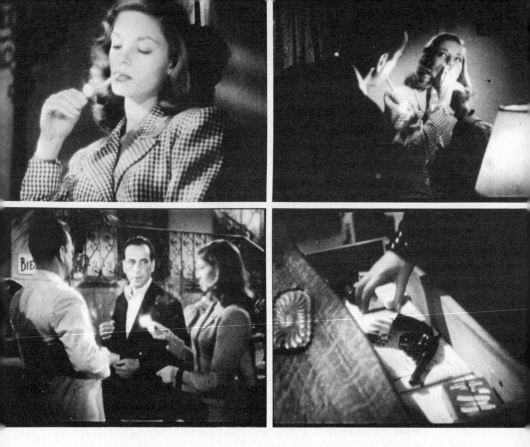

the match that brings Kid to his senses after Kid recognizes Kilgallen).
To emphasize each of these lightings, Hawks uses a tiny spotlight to
play on Bacall's or Bogart's face for a few seconds as the match approaches.* Later, Slim hustles money for drinks from a stranger by asking him to light the cigarette she just borrowed from Harry. Finally,
Harry collaborates with Slim in the assassination of the silent Gestapo
thug when he asks her to fetch him a cigarette and some matches from

* The play of this spotlight is so subtle and seems so naturally linked to the
illumination of the match that I didn't even notice it until I was making frame
blowups for this book. Bacall's face came out terribly overexposed in several
different frames when a match glowed nearby, although I had used the same
f-stop to shoot each frame. A match alone could never produce this effect on a
film frame (since films are shot in studios with hundreds of instruments required
to make even the darkest-seeming images). This extremely small and subtle touch
is another sign of Hawks's sensitivity to the operations of light.

the drawer that contains his revolver; she spontaneously understands that she should leave that drawer open so Harry can use that gun. The sharing of cigarettes became such a Bogart-Bacall trademark that *The Big Sleep* begins with a silhouetted Bogart lighting a shadowy Bacall's cigarette. The credits follow, superimposed over an image of two burning cigarettes lying together in a single ashtray, an image with no connection to that particular film at all except its evocation of two unseen people who, by implication, are smoking cigarettes very intimately (perhaps lying together, like the cigarettes), sharing the same ashtray.

Accompanying the cigarettes are the voices of Bogart and Bacall. Like *His Girl Friday, To Have and Have Not* is a film of verbal "singing" in which vocal harmonies imply spiritual harmonies. The dropping of Bacall's voice allowed her vocal purr to "sing" duets with Bogart's mellow growl, wrapping their low and lowing voices around the terse but measured cadences of the dialogue that Furthman-Faulkner-Hawks wrote for them. While the verbal "singing" of *His Girl Friday* was a breathlessly rapid, crackling, pattering scherzo (the parallel with the Lucky Strike auctioneer is an apt metaphor for that whole film's verbal music), the verbal "singing" of *To Have and Have Not* is a languid, liquid, stately largo. Both Bogart and Bacall "sing" in terse, simple phrases, dominated by monosyllables, their voices perpetually falling at the end of each phrase, then rising again at the start of the next and falling at its end. Their "songs" are dominated by rests and caesuras.

"You're sore aren't you?"
"Why should I be?"

"You were pretty good at it too."
"Would you rather I weren't?"

"This is about the time for it, isn't it?"
"The time for what?"
"The story of my life."

"Remind you of somebody, Steve?"
"It's brand new to me. I like it."

"What ya do that for?" (*after a kiss*)
"Been wondering if I'd like it."
"What's the decision?"

"I don't know yet. (*another kiss, a long one*) It's even better when
you help."

And even the famous "whistle" line is composed of a series of tersely
hypnotic, purring phrases, punctuated by brief musical rests:

> You don't have to say anything,
> And you don't have to do anything.
> Well, maybe just whistle.
> You know how to whistle, don't you?
> You just put your lips together
> And blow.

With these monosyllabic verbal arias and duets Hawks-Bogart-
Bacall succeed in transforming the style of Hemingway's terse prose
(surely the inspiration for this kind of dialogue) into a musical, mysterious free verse. That Hawks realizes the power of these arias becomes
clear in his camera strategy for shooting them, which is markedly different from that in other films. The tendency of the camera is to work
much closer to the two "singers" than it has in previous films, to frame
them in very tight two-shots falling somewhere between the standard
American shot (from the knees up) and the facial close-up. Hawks, for
example, frames Bogart and Bacall much more tightly than Grant and
Arthur in *Only Angels Have Wings,* the film with which *To Have and
Have Not* has so much in common. The Bogart-Bacall relationship is
both hotter and more mysterious than the earlier one. Rather parallel
to the shooting style of *Twentieth Century*—in which the fact of shooting inside a train necessarily confined Hawks's camera to the energetic
faces—Hawks deliberately confines himself to the faces of the "singers"
in *To Have and Have Not,* allowing their vocal energy to fill the frame
and allowing our eye to appreciate the irony and mystery of these cool
faces that reveal so little and warm voices that reveal so much.

The underlying energy of this camera strategy and verbal music
produces the undercurrents of sexual intensity and spiritual unity which
run between the two stars. The overt metaphor for these mysterious
undercurrents is the film's biggest (and resolutely unanswered) mystery—the names they invent for one another, "Slim" and (especially)
"Steve." It might be understandable for Harry to feel and see Marie-

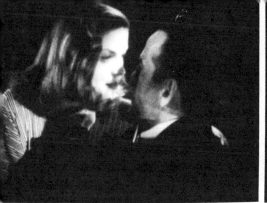
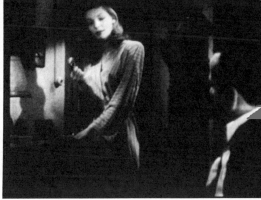

The "whistle" scene.

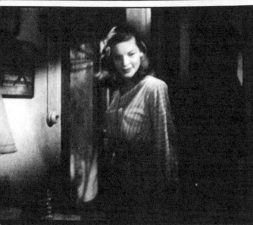

Bacall as "Slim" (although she is not so slender as Mme de Bursac), but why exactly does Slim call Harry "Steve"? And why does he never bother to correct her? And why does he accept the name of "Steve" without ever asking her why she calls him "Steve"? Both accept their nicknames (and, of course, the nickname is another familiar Hawks motif) without question; both assign the nicknames without explanation. And Hawks feels no narrative need to remove the two mysteries. Like Eddie's question about the dead bee, these nicknames clearly mean something to their coiners, and to accept the coiner as an intimate and an equal means participating in the nickname (like participating in the dead bee catechism) without question. The film's implication is that the explanations for these mysteries are far less interesting and vital than the willingness of the characters to live with one another's mysteries. The unexplained mystery (as *The Big Sleep* would develop at even greater length) becomes an essential element of the Bogart-Bacall relationship in their two Hawks films. The second section of *To Have and Have Not* devotes itself to showing the willingness of the central couple to play with each other's mysteries.

The third section complicates the narrative with the addition of the de Bursacs. Harry's agreement to carry de Bursac on his boat, initially because he needs the money, drags him inevitably into conflict with the Gestapo because he does not like them or the way they use people as pawns to achieve their ends. In response to the fat Gestapo chief's question, "What are your sympathies?", Harry initially answers Renard (Dan Seymour), "Minding my own business." Harry's "sympathies" for the people he likes, however, will require his political "sympathies" to evolve as well. The film builds this evolution of Harry's attitude around the deliberately recurring use of the slap across the face. The silent Gestapo assistant slaps Marie's face with her passport during the first interrogation session; he uses the legal document bearing her legal name for his illegal abuse. Then Harry slaps Eddie's face before leaving to fetch the de Bursacs; but Harry's slap, unlike that of the Gestapo, is a slap of affection, of human concern, his means to keep Eddie from going with him on a dangerous mission (there will be slaps of affection in *Red River* as well). Eddie, however, does not heed the slap (just as Chance's friends in *Rio Bravo* do not heed his orders to keep away from the final gun battle); only after Harry discovers him aboard his boat does Eddie, in one of those backward leaps, realize, "You was thinking of me." Slim gives Harry a similarly affectionate (but much more playful) slap across the face in his room when she tells him he needs to shave before she will kiss him again. But Mme de Bursac attempts to slap Harry angrily, even as he prepares to help her husband, reacting to his gruff speech, his words, rather than to his action, his deliberate descent into the hotel's basement to offer his aid. Finally, Harry slaps Renard's face with a pistol after using it to eliminate the silent Gestapo thug who initiated the cycle of slaps with Marie's passport. The Hawks circle of retaliation closes with the revolver that comes to Harry's hand as a result of Slim's partnership in the drawer-play improvisation.

The meeting with the de Bursacs also furthers the film's moral contrast of honor and money. Johnson initiated this narrative contrast with his lie to Harry: he needed to get money from the bank to pay Harry for chartering his boat, although he actually had $1400 in traveler's checks in his wallet and a ticket to leave Martinique on the morning plane before the bank opened. Johnson pays for this lie by earning the

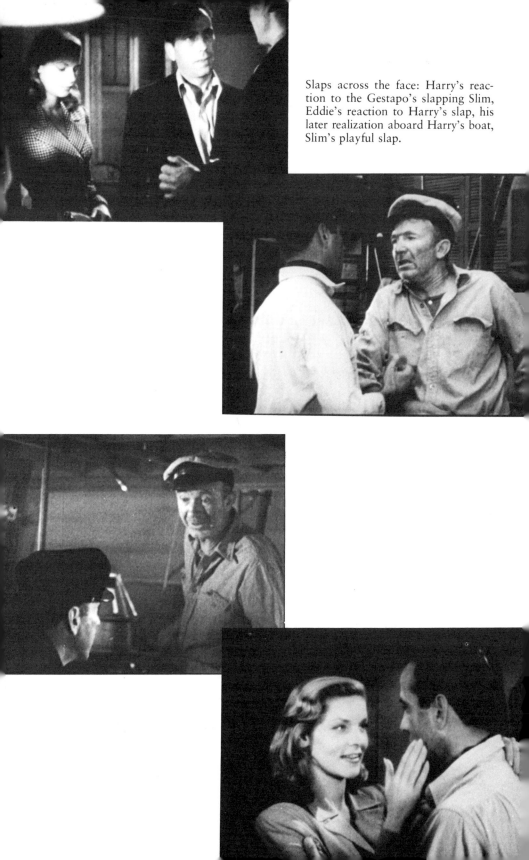

Slaps across the face: Harry's reaction to the Gestapo's slapping Slim, Eddie's reaction to Harry's slap, his later realization aboard Harry's boat, Slim's playful slap.

contempt of both Slim (who steals his wallet and repulses his physical advances) and Harry ("He couldn't write any faster than he could duck"). Ultimately, Johnson pays for his dishonor with his death. Renard reveals the same dishonorable attitude toward money when he himself keeps Johnson's wallet (which Harry refused to steal) as well as Harry's own money. And when Harry finally agrees to do the job that Frenchy and his Free French friends have begged him to do, to bring the de Bursacs into Fort-de-France on his boat, he claims he is helping them only for the money:

> "Why have you changed your mind?"
> "I need the money now. Last night I didn't."
>
> "I'm glad you're on our side."
> "I'm not. I'm getting paid."

But when Frenchy asks Harry to remove the bullet from de Bursac's shoulder (Harry's medical background is another of the film's deliberately unexplained mysteries), Harry refuses to accept Frenchy's monetary offer, to confuse these upstairs and downstairs responsibilities— performing the surgery without getting paid for it. After he has recovered, de Bursac observes, "There are many things a man will do. But betrayal for a price is not one of yours." De Bursac is quite right, for when Renard offers Harry a large sum of money ($500 plus the $825 Johnson owed him) to betray de Bursac, Harry toys with Renard and his offer (which would be the safest, most expedient, and most profitable for him to accept), but he cannot and does not accept it. After Harry has taken the irreversible step—killing the silent Gestapo agent and pistol-whipping Renard to release Eddie from jail and get safe-conduct passes for them and his boat—Frenchy asks him, "Why are you doing this, Harry?" He responds, "Maybe because I like you. Maybe because I don't like them." He follows this admission with the Bogart-esque joke to undercut his confession, "No kissin' Frenchy." Harry cannot maintain his personal integrity and honor, his friendship for the people he likes, without taking a political and public stand against those he does not. There is no conflict of love and duty; love *is* the duty.

Finally, the two de Bursacs contrast spiritually and pragmatically with both Harry and Slim, ennobling the more competent but superficially less noble couple. Despite Harry's apparent callousness ("Get down on the deck flat. You save France, I'm gonna save my boat."), his courage and competence contrast with de Bursac's panicky cowardice. De Bursac is ready to surrender to the Vichy patrol boat, and the enemy's bullets teach him his moral lesson—as they do Johnson—about cowardice and disobeying the wiser captain's orders. The storyteller implies that a man must save his boat before he can save his country, and only competence at the smaller task gives one a chance of succeeding at the larger one. Harry's competence, a typical Hawks virtue, is more valuable than de Bursac's abstract and patriotic ideals. So much for Rick-Bogart's noble, idealistic sacrifice in *Casablanca*.

Precisely the same contrast differentiates Mme de Bursac from Slim. Although de Bursac's wife sacrifices her own safety and comfort for an ideal, she is incapable of performing the small but necessary tasks. She faints when assigned the job of administering the chloroform to her wounded husband, so Slim takes over the wife's duties and performs them well (the first time she and Harry work together in the film). Slim does not allow these Florence Nightingale moments to pass without humor. As she fans away the fumes from the chloroform which Mme de Bursac spilled, Slim takes special care to fan them toward the fainted form of her rival lying on the floor. Hawks cleverly juxtaposes the visual motion of the fan in the lower right-foreground corner of the frame with Harry's doctoring midground center, a perfectly framed expression of their working together. When Harry picks up the lady to carry her to purer air, Slim asks, "What are you trying to do? Guess her weight?"

Working together: Slim's fan in the foreground, Harry doctoring in the midground, Frenchy and the inevitable Hawks lantern in the rearground.

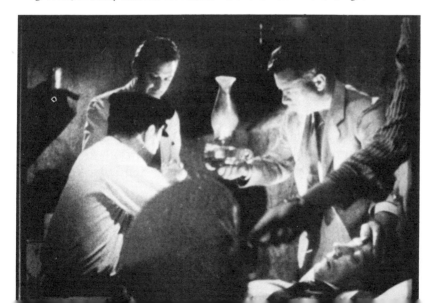

(A joke which Hawks and Furthman repeat, word for word, from Sternberg's *Morocco*.) And when Harry assigns Slim to watch her rival, Slim asks if she can give her a few more whiffs of the chloroform for good measure. Slim's jealousy of "Steve's" feelings for Mme de Bursac are more jocular than serious, as even "Steve" knows. When a scantily clad Slim tells Harry to give Mme de Bursac her love, he playfully responds, "I'd give her my own if she had that on." As in *Only Angels Have Wings,* people who "belong" together in the Hawks world must be able to joke together. Like Harry, Slim is tough and good enough, wise and clever enough, witty and sensible enough, to conquer the smaller tasks, which eventually will allow her to conquer the bigger ones.

The film's fourth section is surprisingly upbeat—and surprisingly musical—built around four Hoagy Carmichael musical numbers, played and/or sung by Cricket in the public bar downstairs. The first of the songs, which Cricket sings to begin the section, sets its theme. The song, an ironic blues, is about "a poor unfortunate colored man" who is arrested in Hong Kong: "I need someone to love me / need someone to carry me / Home to San Francisco." Its theme—of a foreigner far from his native land, in an alien culture, who longs to return home—echoes the plight of the Americans Harry, Eddie, and Slim in Martinique, who, at the end of the section and the film, leave the foreign place to go somewhere else—perhaps home. The second song, Slim-Bacall's number, "How Little We Know," also fits into the film's specific and Hawks's general themes—that experiences are transitory and surfaces deceptive, that appearances are merely apparent and constantly shifting, and that things often turn out differently than expected because of inconstant forces beneath the visible surface. How little Harry Morgan knew, for example, at the beginning of the film that he would take a moral and political stand against Vichy.

The third of the musical numbers is Carmichael's off-frame playing of the bluesy "Baltimore Oriole," which drifts upstairs from the public room below while Harry finally asserts his will and his anger against the Gestapo in his room. The ironic contrast of tones—the playful music off-frame as opposed to the serious action in the room—serves as a metaphoric reminder that personal, "upstairs" expression can never be divorced from the public, "downstairs" world, to which the upstairs is necessarily and architecturally attached. And the fourth musical number

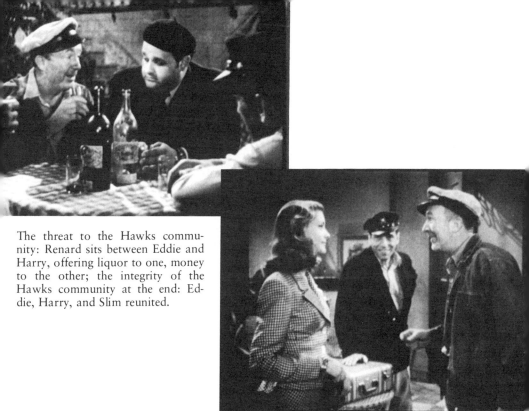

The threat to the Hawks community: Renard sits between Eddie and Harry, offering liquor to one, money to the other; the integrity of the Hawks community at the end: Eddie, Harry, and Slim reunited.

is an upbeat, instrumental reprise of "How Little We Know," played in a rhumba rhythm and tempo by Cricket to accompany the final stage-exit of Harry, Slim, and Eddie. As the three leave Frenchy's place, the door that leads to the street outside the hotel serves as the mock proscenium arch of their stage (like the door of the pressroom in *His Girl Friday*). Harry and Slim rhumba out that doorway, followed by the jerky Eddie, who holds a pair of suitcases, jerkily bouncing and shaking them in tempo like a pair of giant rectangular maracas. To emphasize that this is indeed a stage-exit, Eddie executes a very artificial, very sharp, 90-degree right turn, just outside the doorway, then disappears behind the doorway's arch as the music swells and the film cuts back to Cricket, the musical partner, before its final fade-out.

Like Hildy and Walter at the end of *His Girl Friday*, the three unified spirits go off, out a door, to new experiences and unknown adventures, either at home or "home," for wherever they are together doing what they do together is essentially and spiritually "home." Contrary to the schematic opposition in *Casablanca* of love and honor, of tough pragmatism and noble idealism, of selfishness and sacrifice, of private and public morality, *To Have and Have Not* synthesizes these oppositions, which Hawks finds facile and deceptive. Love (either romantic, friendly, or some synthesis of the two) is itself honorable; tough, selfish pragmatism gets the job done better than noble, idealistic sacrifice; and a public, political morality can only rest on the foundation of a private, personal morality. And as opposed to the analytic disjunctions of the Hemingway novel—between Harry Morgan and Richard Gordon, living life and writing about life, political necessity and political dilettantism, assertive action and passive observation—the Hawks film of *To Have and Have Not* achieves a synthesis of his personal concerns and commitments: the synthesis of work, love, and friendship, of personal honor and integrity with political sympathy and action, of inner feeling and its outward expression, of talk and action, of speech and music. The titles of the Hemingway and Hawks narratives, though using the identical words, mean opposite things. Hemingway's title emphasizes a disjunction—having *but* not having. Hawks's title emphasizes a conjunction—having *and* not having, like having one's cake and eating it too.

According to certain cultural values, *Casablanca* may seem more entertaining or more inspiring than *To Have and Have Not*. The film has always been more popular, perhaps because Rick-Bogart's climactic self-denial is more unabashedly romantic and hence more comforting than Harry-Bogart's refusal to betray his code and his self. And according to certain critical values Hemingway's accomplishment may seem more significant than Hawks's.

> And with *To Have and Have Not* Hollywood demonstrated that it could turn a conjunction of geniuses into a perfectly ordinary vehicle for Humphrey Bogart.[12]

> Faulkner proved the he . . . could hack away with the best (and the worst) of them, as witness . . . his efforts . . . on the hilariously pulpy version of Hemingway's *To Have and Have Not*. . . .[13]

Such opinions ignore the fact that *To Have and Have Not* may be Hemingway's worst novel, that "hilariously pulpy" and "hack" films (whatever these terms mean) may be superior to pretentiously chaotic novels, that Humphrey Bogart as Harry Morgan may be more interesting than

Harry Morgan as Hemingway wrote him (or as Hemingway didn't write him), and that this film was not presided over by an anonymous "Hollywood" at all but by an artist, craftsman, and storyteller named Howard Hawks, whom that "conjunction of geniuses" seemed willing to accept as one of its own.

The offbeat attractiveness of the Bogart-Bacall team in *To Have and Have Not* led Warners to ask Howard Hawks for another Bogart-Bacall vehicle. Hawks still owned half of Bacall's contract, having sold half to Warners in 1944 in exchange for their financing *To Have and Have Not.* Warners advanced Hawks $50,000 to buy the film rights to the Raymond Chandler novel, *The Big Sleep,* for which Hawks paid $5,000, keeping the remaining $45,000 for himself.[14] These kinds of favorable financial agreements were typical of Hawks, who used such strategies to maintain his independence from any single studio. For example, Hawks claimed that Hemingway made $10,000 from the film of *To Have and Have Not,* Furthman and Faulkner $75,000, and he himself $1,500,000.[15]

But *The Big Sleep,* in its original form, like *To Have and Have Not,* was a very unsuitable and unlikely basis for a love story, even the offbeat, sultry, witty, insolent kind of Bogart-Bacall love story. The male protagonist of Chandler's *Big Sleep* was a loner who took his knightly virginity seriously—at least when working on a case. And the novel's two women, the Sternwood sisters, as is common in the detective-mystery genre, were both morally poisonous.[16] Carmen, the younger sister, turned out to be the story's primary murderess; her other amusements included posing nude for pornographic photographs, imbibing exotic drugs, and crawling into men's beds without an invitation and without any clothes. Her older sister, Vivian, had been married and divorced three times; she also served as Carmen's accessory in the murder of her own third husband, Rusty Regan. How could Hawks make a Bogart-Bacall love story out of such unpromising material?* That was the narrative problem which confronted Hawks, Furthman, Faulkner, and Leigh Brackett in making a film of *The Big Sleep.*

---

*The 1976 film of *The Big Sleep,* with Robert Mitchum, is not so much a "remake" of Hawks's narrative as an original making of Chandler's, preserving most of the novel's incidents but inexplicably transporting them from 1930s Los Angeles to 1970s London.

First, Hawks's film made some necessary alterations in the moral clothing of Vivian Sternwood, the older sister, to draw a distinction between her values and those of her vicious sister, Carmen (Martha Vickers). In the film, Vivian has been divorced once, not three times. According to the Hollywood symbology, which mirrors the values of the culture as a whole—then as now—one divorce implies the kind of mistake that anyone can make, but three divorces indicates a three-time loser—a sign of moral instability and emotional superficiality. Vivian's former husband has become the anonymous "Rutledge" rather than the murdered man himself, Regan. And even the name "Rutledge," with its sturdy Anglo-Saxonness (like "Essex"), implies there may have been something cold and bloodless about the man; the marriage's failure may have been his fault, not hers. Indeed, the ambiguity surrounding Vivian's divorce is carefully related to the moral ambiguity surrounding Vivian's character and values in the film as a whole—until its final section—an ambiguity that is a deliberate and essential element in the new narrative's logic and construction.

Second, the film's moral alterations in Vivian's character accompany a corollary adjustment in Marlowe's. Chandler's Marlowe insists on keeping himself sexually pure, absolutely detached from the dangerously beautiful women who attempt to attach themselves to him. When Chandler's Marlowe orders the naked Carmen out of his bed, into her clothes, and out of his room, he tells us:

> I looked down at the chessboard. The move with the knight was wrong. I put it back where I had moved it from. Knights had no meaning in this game. It wasn't a game for knights. (p. 146) [17]

Hawks's Marlowe (or Marlowe-Bogart) is much more playful and much less knightly around these (and other) women. The delightful sexual intimacy and casual play which Marlowe exhibits with the eyeglassed woman who works in the bookstore (Dorothy Malone) and with whom Marlowe "takes shelter" from a rainy afternoon is the most obvious example of Marlowe-Bogart's sexual comfort, ease, and casualness with women. But Hawks deliberately adds several other women to Chandler's tale with whom Marlowe-Bogart can reveal this same playful and witty equality. The taxi driver who follows the book-filled station wagon

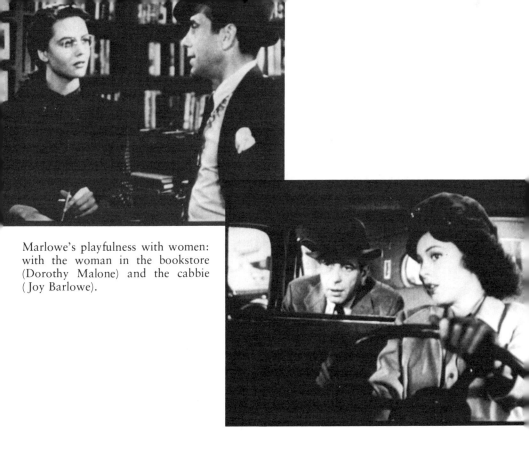

Marlowe's playfulness with women: with the woman in the bookstore (Dorothy Malone) and the cabbie (Joy Barlowe).

from Geiger's bookstore to Brody's apartment, a "fresh-faced kid" in the Chandler novel, becomes a witty woman in Hawks's film. She hands Marlowe-Bogart her card, asking him to call her if he has another "tail job" for her (that imagery once again). Marlowe pointedly asks, "Day and night?" She answers, "Night's better. I work days." This kind of sexual playfulness not only makes Marlowe-Bogart less self-righteous and less defensive in his treatment of women than Chandler's Marlowe but suits the breezy Humphrey Bogart persona much better than the sexual idealism of Chandler's knight—just as Vivian's moral ambiguity and mystery perfectly fit the Bacall persona.

Third, Vivian must simply play a more important role in the film than she does in the novel, where she plays second lead to her murderous younger sister. She must play a major role in several scenes from which she is absent in the novel, and her contribution must be expanded in several of those which Chandler originated. While the first meeting between Vivian and Marlowe in the film is identical to Chandler's—Vivian seductively tries to discover why her father has engaged a private detective—in their second film meeting, Marlowe deposits the drugged and dozing Carmen with Vivian when he retrieves her from the scene of Geiger's murder. In the novel (and in every version of the script as well) Marlowe leaves her with Norris, the butler, because Vivian is out playing. Hawks added this scene between Marlowe and Vivian during retakes, well after the rest of the film had been completed—at the same time that Hawks shot the famous "horse-racing interchange" between Marlowe and Vivian. Hawks added both scenes almost six months after the film had been released for viewing by the armed forces.[18] The third scene between Marlowe and Vivian, which takes place in his office, was greatly expanded from the novel, in particular Hawks's improvised addition of the comical telephone call to the police in which Marlowe and Vivian spontaneously play-work together, improvising nonsensical nonsequiturs as each other's father, daughter, mother, and son. The film adds Vivian to the scene in Joe Brody's apartment, where Marlowe goes to retrieve the lurid photographs which Brody plans to use to blackmail Carmen. In the film's narrative, adding Vivian to this Chandler scene both complicates the Vivian-Marlowe relationship and provides the basis for its eventual resolution. Marlowe wonders why Vivian has lied to him, why she has gone to Brody's without telling him: how deeply is she implicated in this nasty business? Vivian gets the opportunity to watch Marlowe at work, how well he does his job; eventually she will decide that Marlowe's competence and integrity will protect her better than buying protection with her own money. Finally, Hawks adds Vivian to the scene in the house next to Art Huck's garage, where, in the novel, only Mona Mars, Eddie Mars's missing wife, resided. This addition allows Vivian to aid Marlowe's escape from the killer, Canino, a part reserved in the Chandler novel for Mona Mars, who, for some reason or other, decides to aid this absolute stranger rather than her own husband's hired man.

Fourth, and the most complicated narrative change of all, Hawks must remake the story's ending completely, from the moment when Marlowe wakes up in Art Huck's house to his final clinch with Vivian. How can Hawks get this Bogart-Bacall film to that necessary final clinch? The many versions of the script indicate Hawks's difficulties in resolving this narrative problem. How can one conceive a climactic scene between Vivian-Bacall and Marlowe-Bogart if Carmen Sternwood is the story's ultimate murderess and the final piece of the puzzle Marlowe was hired to assemble? The novel's climactic scene appropriately takes place between Carmen and Marlowe, set in the metaphorically dank and drear oil fields out of which the Sternwood money flows. Carmen attempts to murder Marlowe, just as she murdered Rusty Regan, in revenge for his sexual rejection. Marlowe, however, cleverly filled Carmen's little pistol with blanks when he returned it to her (Chandler cutely fails to inform the reader of this little substitution). How can this Bogart-Bacall film effectively avoid or diminish this climactic scene between Marlowe and Carmen, which grows inevitably out of the narrative logic of Chandler's tale?

With great difficulty. In the first version of the script (dated September 11, 1944), Marlowe and Carmen play the attempted murder scene, as Chandler conceived it, in the oil fields. Then they return together to the Sternwood greenhouse (a familiar Hawks circle, the return to the physical setting of the beginning), where Marlowe explains Carmen's guilt to Vivian and General Sternwood; he intends to turn Carmen over to the police. Carmen, who refuses to be shut away "out of the sunlight," grabs her pistol and stages what she thinks is a fake suicide attempt (she assumes that her pistol still contains blanks). However, Norris, the butler, has substituted real bullets for the blanks, so goodbye Carmen. (Don't ask why Norris takes this action. After all, Marlowe is not supposed to tell the butler his duties.) With Carmen gone, Vivian and Marlowe can clinch.

In the revised script (dated September 29, 1944) Carmen does not go to the oil fields but returns to Geiger's house, where Marlowe has also returned to look over Geiger's things. (This version already moves closer to the film's final solution.) Carmen begs Marlowe to love her, to reform her, but he rejects her again. So she turns her pistol—as in the novel, filled with blanks—on Marlowe. As the defeated Carmen walks out the Geiger doorway, she is cut down by the machine-gun bullets of Eddie Mars's men, who wait for Marlowe outside the door. Then Mars comes into the house, alone and unarmed. (Don't ask why; he thought that Carmen's corpse was Marlowe's.) Marlowe shoots him without a word of warning or explanation. Marlowe then recounts all these doings to Vivian in a final scene at the Sternwood manse. Vivian asks, "Would you really have sent her to . . . to the . . . ?" Marlowe answers, "You don't kill people for free, you know." Vivian apologizes to Marlowe for her role in disposing of Regan's body but allays our moral qualms by telling Marlowe that she engaged a priest to say prayers for Regan's departed soul. Finally, Marlowe tells Vivian, "I've decided myself already to stay." And we get the final clinch. Both of these narrative solutions are far-fetched because they attempt to do the impossible—to resolve the Eddie Mars problem, the Carmen problem, and the Bogart-Bacall emotional problem as three separate actions. Such a narrative strategy could only diminish the ultimate Bogart-Bacall scene as an anticlimactic, parenthetic explanation of more interesting events. The final scene in the film, however, unites Bogart and Bacall against Mars, treating Carmen's murder and murderousness as the mere parenthesis: Mars will take the rap for killing Regan if Carmen goes somewhere to take some kind of cure.

The solution that Hawks forged, like the resolution of *His Girl Friday,* grows not out of the narrative logic of the original material but the alternative subtextual energy of his own character-performers, discovered and developed in the course of telling this particular film story. The underlying energy and evocations of Hawks's *Big Sleep* provide a new and higher narrative logic for the film, growing out of this alternative and subtextual logic, produced by the playing of Bogart-Marlowe and Vivian-Bacall. In Hawks's film, Marlowe never separates physically from Vivian from the time he awakes at Art Huck's. Their physical union represents and conveys their ultimate spiritual union, which has been felt—by one another and by the audience—throughout the film. As in *To Have and Have Not,* the Bogart character and the Bacall character, each of whom has a personal code of morality and integrity, must demonstrate that integrity to one another. Their evolutions of trust in each other's offbeat code of behavior eventually allow them to reveal their spiritual affinity, after which they demonstrate that spiritual union in action, by working together. The obstacle to the overt expression of their spiritual union is the very moral and legal darkness in which the two find themselves—the blackmails, the murders, the gambling, the corrupt physical world surrounding them.

Vivian must distrust Marlowe (because she has something to hide, because he is a hired detective, because perhaps he can be bought, because she does not know his "sympathies"—to use a term from *To Have and Have Not*). Marlowe must distrust Vivian (because she lies to him, because she is clearly implicated to some degree or other in the

274

nasty Sternwood business—whose depth he has yet to sound—because she is Carmen's sister). The conclusion of the film, the resolution of this new narrative, allows the undercurrents of trust and feeling between Marlowe and Vivian (whose potential trust and feeling have been sensed throughout the film, if only because they are also Bogart and Bacall) to express themselves in action (the typical Hawks motif). In this respect, the relationship of Hawks's *Big Sleep* to an earlier major work of this type, John Huston's *The Maltese Falcon,* is precisely the same as the relationship of his *To Have and Have Not* to *Casablanca* (all four of them Warner Bros. films of 1941–46 starring Humphrey Bogart). *The Big Sleep* is a kind of reply to *The Maltese Falcon,* just as *To Have and Have Not* provides a response to *Casablanca.* In *The Maltese Falcon,* Spade-Bogart must rise above his sexual and romantic attachment, his personal feelings for the worthless Brigid-Astor, to do the right, honorable thing—just as Rick-Bogart must rise above his personal feelings in *Casablanca.* To be true to his personal moral code, Spade-Bogart must abandon his love for a duty to his murdered partner—a man worthy neither of respect nor of Bogart's sacrifice—in order to preserve his own integrity and honor. But in *The Big Sleep,* as in *To Have and Have Not,* the Bogart character can synthesize the demands of love and honor because the woman he confronts becomes a woman with whom he can work—for she, too, has a personal code of integrity and honor.

Viewing Hawks's narrative of *The Big Sleep* in this way casts doubt on two of the critical clichés that pass for wisdom about the film. The first is that the film's narrative somehow mirrors or duplicates the narrative of Chandler's novel.

> *The Big Sleep* . . . is never once unfaithful to its source; it is relentlessly simple-minded and moral, smart-alecky and kinetic.[19]

There is no question that Hawks's film of *The Big Sleep* is much closer to Chandler than his film of *To Have and Have Not* is to Hemingway. Its aroma, flavor, and texture also resemble those of Chandler's seamy world more closely than the 1976 film version does, despite the later film's preserving more of the novel's characters and incidents. Like Hawks's film of *To Have and Have Not,* the film of *The Big Sleep* preserves the spirit of the original author's world without preserving

the specific details and incidents of that world. But Hawks had to re-
write far more than the ending of Chandler's novel to make his new
narrative work. To pull the final and unexpected twist (unexpected for
a representative of the detective-mystery genre) of the detective's getting
the girl, Hawks had to alter the size of the girl's role, her character, and
her moral sensitivity, the detective's character and moral sensitivity, and
our responses to these characters as embodied by Lauren Bacall and
Humphrey Bogart. Whoever else these "characters" were, they were also
Bogart and Bacall. The Bogart character can reject Brigid O'Shaugh-
nessy at the end of *The Maltese Falcon* at least partially because that
character is embodied by Mary Astor. Both Ms. Astor's sputtering on-
screen career as a succession of shady ladies and her scandalous off-
screen career as an amorous accomplice of many moneyed men make it
probable that the Bogart character will reject her—preserving his own
worth by detaching himself from the worthless mate. This is another
clear sense in which the film actor becomes the narrative's character,
making the whole course of the action probable. The Bogart character
could never reject a woman embodied by a Bacall—particularly since
public knowledge of their offscreen marriage must again influence audience expectations for their on-screen union.

This new narrative strategy (largely dependent on the subtextual
energy and vibrations of the two stars, on whom Hawks knew he could
depend) also casts doubt on the most common, and most challenging,
critical cliché about the film—that its plot is confusing, chaotic, sense-
less, illogical, indecipherable, and unfathomable. Something about the
film is indeed inexplicable and confusing—the simple and precise explanation for the chronological sequence of the film's external events: who
did what to whom, who killed whom, and why. Whodunwhat? But
before accusing the film's plot, its narrative, of incoherence one must
inquire if this confusing sequence of blackmails and murders—its diegesis—is really its narrative, its plot—its discourse—at all. Perhaps this
sequence of external events (to which the original novel is completely
devoted) is merely a context and pretext for the real narrative of Hawks's
film (as is the hanging of Earl Williams in *His Girl Friday*): Marlowe's
and Vivian's discovery of one another. Clearly this view of the narrative
not only makes it consistent with Hawks's other narratives but makes
it make sense. Let me explore this possibility at some length.

Hawks himself confesses he never figured out who killed the Sternwood chauffeur, Owen Taylor, in Chandler's novel. He has frequently told the story of sending Chandler a telegram with the question, only to receive the reply that Chandler didn't know either. Christan Nyby reports that the entire company stopped production for two days to sit around on the set and try to deduce some killer who might answer to this question.[20] Well, who might have killed Owen Taylor? It could have been Joe Brody (who admitted slugging him and taking the roll of film which Taylor ripped from Geiger's camera, both in the novel and the film). But Brody seems to small a "grifter" to kill anyone (although he does carry a gun). Much more likely, it could have been Canino, Eddie Mars's hired gun, who might have been keeping an eye on Carmen and Geiger for Mars (he would have had no motivation for killing Taylor, but then he had no real motivation for killing Jones, either). Or perhaps Taylor, who had just killed Geiger and awoke from Brody's slugging to discover the film of his nude beloved stolen, committed suicide. The police suspect Taylor was murdered only because he received the wound on the side of his head before his car flew off the Santa Monica pier. But if Brody "zapped" Taylor and then Taylor tied down his own throttle to commit suicide, all the facts of this death have been accounted for.

But who cares who killed Owen Taylor? Indeed, who *is* Owen Taylor? He merits one brief descriptive sentence in the novel (Marlowe observes him polishing the Sternwood car, in which he will meet his death), but no such shot exists in the film. It does exist in all the scripts, including the "Cutter's Script,"[21] which means that Hawks shot the polishing chauffeur but deliberately cut him out. (Ironically, Roman Polanski puts the polishing chauffeur back—in *Chinatown*—but that is because the cream-colored car will be important, not its polisher.) If Hawks had wanted to do so, he could not only have shown us Owen Taylor washing the car; he could have invented an answer to the question of who killed him. He knew the question had no clear, explicit, single answer in his narrative (or Chandler's). He chose not to supply one. This choice—the deliberate suppression of information and answers—generates the entire film of *The Big Sleep;* Hawks deliberately leaves mysteries mysterious rather than supplies explanations. This is the consistent way his narrative treats the details of Chandler's narrative, which does supply all the other answers.

What goes on in the back room of Geiger's bookstore? In the novel, it is a private lending library of pornographic books where only sub-scribers are permitted. The first version of the film's script explained it away as the place where Geiger's blackmailed clients came to pay their dues. Indeed, the film's evolving scripts are full of these sorts of expla-nations, many of which Hawks filmed. He deliberately cut them all out, leaving the detail (for example, Geiger's backroom) without its expla-nation. What was Carmen doing at Geiger's house? In the novel, Mar-lowe discovers her there wearing a pair of jade earrings—and nothing else. The implication was that she enjoys getting high (we never find out about that liquid in the bottle which Marlowe-Bogart sniffs) and posing in the nude. What is Geiger's relationship with Carol Lundgren, the leather-jacketed "kid" who shoots Brody? In the novel, Lundgren is obviously Geiger's lover who shoots Brody in revenge. In the film, the excessive exotica and Orientalia of Geiger's house may serve as Holly-wood iconography to imply that its inhabitant is gay. The film's first script made Lundgren's relationship with Geiger clearer. The woman in the bookstore answers Marlowe's question, "Who's the other guy?": "Damon—or Pythias, I don't know. Geiger's shadow anyway." Hawks leaves this curious "shadow" even more shadowy.[22]

True enough, many of these seamy details could never have been very fully or clearly explicated by the film. The Production Code Ad-ministration was extremely worried about the potential "depravity" of this film story from its inception.[23] But Hawks could certainly have either cleaned up these incidents so they might have been made clear to a movie audience or he could have found veiled ways to make Chan-dler's original, sordid incidents clear by implication. Hawks has no dif-ficulty, for example, implying that Marlowe-Bogart and the bookstore lady shared a lot more that rainy afternoon than his bottle of rye. Hawks's career reveals a willingness and an ability to remake narrative details entirely when it suits him and a willingness and an ability to convey even the most lurid details clearly but within the bounds of the Code's restrictions when it suits him. Neither of these options suited him for this film. Hawks deliberately chose to keep all of Chandler's lurid incidents but then to provide no explanations whatever of their lurid actuality. Each successive version of the script reveals fewer expla-nations of these sorts of details. The film itself bathes these details in an explanatory fog and darkness that metaphorically answers the fog and darkness of its visual imagery. The question, "Who killed Owen Taylor?," is only one of many unanswered mysteries in a narrative that is devoted to such mysteries.

Why does the film make these incidents so murky? One reason derives from Hawks's handling of point-of-view in the film. Hawks chooses to confine the audience's knowledge of events to Marlowe's own knowledge, mirroring the novel's first-person narration, which comes to the reader through Marlowe's eyes, words, and deductions. The fact that Marlowe himself transmits the novel's events to the reader makes one wonder if Chandler was playing fair when Marlowe failed to mention that he put blanks in Carmen's gun after he tells us he cleaned and *loaded* it. The film of *The Big Sleep* gives us both an objective account of events (for Marlowe is an object in the frame, and the camera observes his actions without commentary) and Marlowe's subjective experience of them (for Marlowe physically is—or might be—present in every single scene and shot in the film).

Hawks found this controlled experiment in confined point-of-view one of the most interesting elements of his story's construction: "The audience saw everything that the detective learned. You could make up your own mind about it."[24] Hawks's subjective-objective tension is opposed to the more idiosyncratically arty choice which Robert Montgomery made in his Marlowe movie of one year later, *The Lady in the Lake,* in which the camera's eye literally becomes Marlowe's eyes, his voice a voice-over on the sound track, and the physical form of the detective can only be glimpsed as reflections in mirrors and windows. Instead, Hawks's camera confined the audience to Marlowe's perceptions without literally burying the camera inside Marlowe's head, reminding the audience of the storyteller's tricky cleverness in doing so. Montgomery buries his camera inside Marlowe's head, as if Marlowe's face were the stone mask with the camera inside it that snaps Carmen's picture. Hawks's camera remains outside Marlowe's head, so that we see his head (just as we see the head of the stone mask), but we can see nothing that his head could not also see (just as the camera inside the stone mask can only see what sits in front of it). That stone mask becomes a visual metaphor for Hawks's attitude toward point-of-view (and the way that film cameras record and convey point-of-view in film stories)—a cold, analytic observer of what the world permits and arranges for it to see. The stone mask is Hawks's abstract (and subtle) disquisition on cinematic recording, just as the eye test in *Only Angels Have*

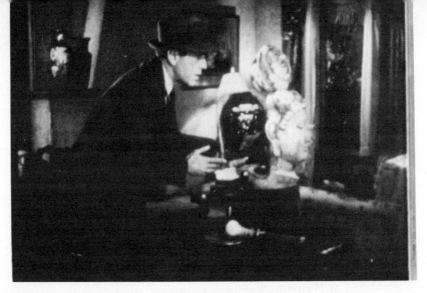

Marlowe examines the stone mask, another Hawks metaphor for the processes of cinema.

Wings is his parallel disquisition on the observer's perception of cinematic projection.

Hawks also refuses to use verbal voice-over, which would nullify the subtle and careful balance of his visual strategy. The Marlowe stories seem to demand telling in the first person, just as most Bogart stories do. A typical narrative device for tying an audience's sympathies to a potentially unlikable character is to tell the story through that character's perceptions (for example, Thackeray's Barry Lyndon, Camus's Meursault, Nabokov's Humbert Humbert, and Hawks's Harry Morgan). Such inside views convert the character-narrator into one of our friends, even if the friend is less than perfectly likable or admirable. When Hawks dispenses with Marlowe-Bogart's vocal commentary on what he sees and thinks, the audience receives the visual data without any ratiocination or explanation. Hawks's Marlowe-Bogart is no more talkative than that stone mask about what he sees. In the novel, however, Marlowe (using a familiar convention of first-person narration) comments to no one in particular about the data. As he walks up the steps of the Fulwilder Building, Marlowe describes what he sees and comments on it.

> The five stairs hadn't been swept in a month. Bums had slept on them, eaten on them, left crusts and fragments of greasy newspaper, matches, a gutted imitation-leather pocketbook. In

a shadowy angle against the scribbled wall a pouched ring of pale rubber had fallen and had not been disturbed. A very nice building. (pp. 159–60)

Robert Montgomery might have filmed this scene with a hand-held camera, ascending the stairway, moving from side to side to observe the crusts, fragments, matches (probably not the pouched ring—in 1946); a voice-over narration might have accompanied the visual observation of objects with the ironic verbal summary of their general impression: "A very nice building." If Hawks were to film this passage in his film of *The Big Sleep* (he does not) he would have shown us Marlowe-Bogart's climbing the stairs in a fairly distant shot, the litter juxtaposed parenthetically at his feet. But we would receive no verbal description of what Marlowe saw nor a verbal summation of what Marlowe thought of this "very nice building."

Hawks would have asked, to whom does Marlowe say "a very nice building" and why does he say it? If Marlowe thinks that the building is "very nice" how or why should he utter that thought aloud? Such generalizations never come to the audience verbally in this film (and rarely come to the audience directly or verbally in any Hawks film). Hawks requires both his characters and his viewers to make inferences on the basis of external signs—conversations, rhythms of speech, actions, movements, gestures, the handling of physical objects, compositional balances and imbalances within the frame—not on the basis of explicit verbal information. Throughout the film Marlowe may be making deductions—that the backroom of Geiger's bookstore is a lending library for pornographic books, that Geiger is a homosexual and Carol Lundgren his lover, that Vivian is paying off Eddie Mars and that the two are somehow in collusion. But he never states any of these general conclusions or deductions because he has no one to state them to and he certainly doesn't need to tell them to himself (this convention of talking to oneself in first-person narration would probably have struck Hawks as unacceptably explicit in a film). When Marlowe does say something aloud, for example the question he perpetually thrusts at Vivian, "What's Eddie Mars got on you?", he says much more than this (he in effect says that he knows, he has deduced, the two are in collusion) and he says it for a purpose (he cannot help Vivian or her father until he knows the answer to that question).

This synthesis of third- and first-person narration, objective and subjective points-of-view is deliberately designed to give us physical data without explicit explanation. Like Geiger's black book, apparently the names of his blackmail victims, we see the ciphers but, like Marlowe, we never succeed in decoding them. All we have are the visible ciphers. If nothing else, this strategy is a clever way to slip the seamy details of Chandler's sordid world through the restrictions of the Production Code. But it also plunges Marlowe (and the viewer) into a bewilderingly murky maze of almost faceless men (one of whom, Owen Taylor, is literally faceless; we only see his feet, Marlowe's subjective hearing of his running footsteps on the stairs), a proliferating series of blankly repetitive and undistinguished names: A. G. Geiger, Joe Brody, Owen Taylor, Carol Lundgren, Harry Jones, Eddie Mars, Art Huck. Many of these blank names/faces appear in only a single scene and then disappear from the film forever—making them seem more like way-stations on a journey than individuated human beings. Hawks increases this impression by giving General Sternwood only a single scene, making him the first of these way-stations (scenes with Sternwood run through Chandler's novel like a ribbon). Certainly Hawks could have allowed Marlowe to link these stations for the viewer on a clear, single, and logical track. The various scripts of the film (like the novel) include several scenes with the district attorney, which allow Marlowe to explain to an outsider exactly who has done what to whom and why. The cutter's script reveals that Hawks even shot one of these scenes.[25] But Hawks's eliminating this sole surviving scene from the film is consistent with his narrative strategy to explain nothing. He even fails to explain the film's metaphoric title (the explanation existed in that district attorney scene which Hawks shot and then cut) with which Chandler's novel ends.

> But the old man [Sternwood] . . . could lie quiet in his canopied bed, with his bloodless hands folded on the sheet, waiting. His heart was a brief, uncertain murmur. His thoughts were as gray as ashes. And in a little while he too, like Rusty Regan, would be sleeping the big sleep. (p. 216)

Consistent with so many titles of Hawks films—*Bringing Up Baby, Only Angels Have Wings, His Girl Friday, To Have and Have Not,* and (we shall see) *Red River*—the title of *The Big Sleep* remains a deliberately unexplicated metaphor.

Against the film's fog of faceless males, one thing emerges clearly. Most of the men in the film who go off to their "big sleeps" go because of some worthless woman (Carmen or Agnes). The question for Marlowe is what kind of woman is Vivian Rutledge. By making Marlowe's professional quest a partial blur, Hawks throws the Marlowe-Vivian personal relationship into sharp foreground focus. One of the two scenes that remains in the film between Marlowe and his outsider friend on the police force, Bernie Ohls, explains nothing about the maze of murdered men but instead draws a contrast between the two Sternwood sisters (this conversation exists in neither the Chandler novel nor the first two drafts of the film's script). Marlowe tells Ohls that one of the sisters (Vivian) is "wonderful" and the other one is "not so wonderful." What puzzles Marlowe is whether "wonderful" (and the ironic quotation marks can be heard in the gravel of Bogart's voice every time he uses the word) is as deeply stuck in the criminal maze as her "not so wonderful" sister, whether "wonderful" is in fact wonderful or not. Marlowe does not intend to be the same kind of sucker over a woman as those other men who went to their "big sleeps." The central issue of the narrative for Bogart-Marlowe (as well as for Hawks) is not his successfully piercing the blurry maze of murdered men but finding out what Eddie Mars "has" on "wonderful." Or rather, Bogart-Marlowe knows that this question will also extricate him and her from the maze.

What is "wonderful" doing while Marlowe-Bogart goes about his work in the maze? There is an invisible yet inferable counterplot in Hawks's *Big Sleep:* the machinations of Vivian Rutledge in alliance with Eddie Mars against Marlowe's journey through the maze to its center, ever closer to discovering the murderer of Sean Regan—Vivian's own sister Carmen. As opposed to Raymond Chandler's explicit chessboard in the novel, Hawks makes his chess game invisible—figuratively and literally. We do not see any chess game or chessboard, but Eddie Mars and Vivian Rutledge are surely playing chess with Marlowe, countering each of his moves with a strategy of their own.

Let us trace the film's narrative as it might be seen from Vivian's, rather than Marlowe's, point-of-view. She first encounters Marlowe when her father summons him to the Sternwood house for some investigative purpose. She invites him to her bedroom, shows him her legs, offers him a drink (but never gives it to him), and tries to find out if Marlowe wants to find Sean Regan, who has disappeared. Vivian is most fearful and most suspicious of this purpose since she knows that Carmen killed Sean and that she hired Eddie Mars to bury the evidence and cover the traces of this murder. Marlowe tells her to stop cross-examining him, and she tells him to stop playing poker with her. The two are both playing very dead-faced poker, probing each other, seeking to discover what the other knows or wants to know.

Then Marlowe brings Carmen back from Geiger's house, telling Vivian that Carmen has never been out and he has never been there. Vivian realizes that the circumstances must be "that bad, huh?" She affirms her loyalty to her sister ("You'd do anything for her, wouldn't you?" "Anything!") and her father in this exchange with Marlowe. Hence the importance of adding this scene after the film was shot: it provides Vivian with a genuinely honorable set of motivations for working with Eddie Mars against Marlowe.

Next Vivian appears in Marlowe's office with the photograph of Carmen (the film never explains that it is a photograph of a nude Carmen), which Joe Brody is using to blackmail Vivian into paying for more silence. Vivian conveys her nervousness in a typically physical and subtextual Hawksian fashion—scratching her knee (Marlowe playfully quips, "Go ahead and scratch"), playing with her glove (Marlowe playfully observes that every glove has five fingers). In his office, Marlowe and Vivian not only play chess against one another but with each other. They both participate spontaneously in the jocular double-talk on the telephone with the police sergeant when Vivian forces Marlowe's intervention by calling the police. And they both play spontaneously with the locked door that briefly imprisons her in Marlowe's office. He playfully apologizes, "It wasn't intentional," and she playfully counters, "Try it sometime." Neither the telephone call to Sergeant Reilly nor the locked office door can be found in any of the film's scripts; they are typical bits of Hawks's improvisation, which convey the spiritual similarity of those—like "Steve" and "Slim"—who can play together so spontaneously and complementarily. Although Marlowe and Vivian are both still playing poker, they are enjoying the competitive game, an enjoyment which will lead to their ultimate union.

Next Vivian telephones Marlowe with a lie—that she has not received any further instructions about making the blackmail payment for the photographs. But Marlowe drives to Brody's apartment to watch Vivian walk inside the building alone. Vivian clearly believes that she

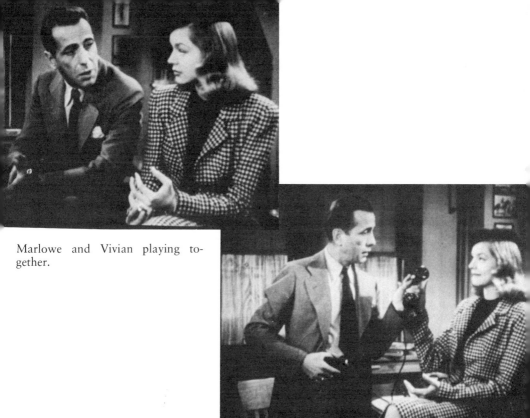

Marlowe and Vivian playing together.

can buy Brody (Louis Jean Heydt) off, quickly and easily, without Marlowe—just as she believes she can buy Eddie Mars, quickly and easily, to cover Carmen's murder of Sean Regan. Hawks gives her little to say in the scene, but her presence in the frame, like that of Hildy Johnson in the Mollie Molloy scene of *His Girl Friday,* makes her observations extremely important. Although Vivian first tells Marlowe, "You're spoiling everything" (this simple line implies her entire strategy—to juggle Eddie Mars and everyone else connected with the case by herself), she sees that Marlowe can get the photographs without recourse to her clumsy strategy (money) or her sister's (a gun). Like the villainous characters of Hawks's *To Have and Have Not,* Vivian believes that honor can be bought and sold; the Bogart character again knows that it cannot.

Vivian next meets Marlowe at a restaurant for lunch. Although Hawks's stated purpose of making this scene well after the film had been finished was to weave some sexual double entendres into their re-

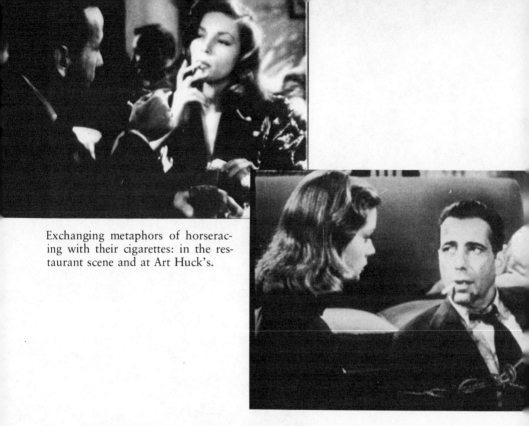

Exchanging metaphors of horseracing with their cigarettes: in the restaurant scene and at Art Huck's.

lationship,[26] their metaphoric conversation about horse racing (like the earlier added scene of Marlowe's bringing Carmen home to Vivian) relates closely to the invisible chess game that lies beneath the narrative of Hawks's *Big Sleep*. Most critics and audiences have paid attention to the clever sexual innuendoes of Bogart's observation, "You've got a touch of class, but I don't know how far you can go," and Bacall's response, "That depends on who's in the saddle." Perhaps the slyest sexual innuendo (especially given Hawks's fondness for "tail" jokes) is Marlowe's wondering whether Vivian is a front-runner or likes to "come from behind." But the other question that this conversation addresses is how much either of them can trust the other. "Speaking of horses, I like to play them myself. But I like to see them run. Find out what their hole-card is" (an interesting mixing of the horse-racing metaphor and the poker metaphor). In the Joe Brody scene, Agnes (Sonia Darrin) said of her blackmailer boyfriend, "Never once a man who's smart all the way around the course." Later at Art Huck's house, Vivian observes of the bound Marlowe, "You don't seem to be running in front today."

The point of these racing metaphors is simply that you don't bet on horses until you know how they run, you don't bet on poker games until you see all the cards and know how the players play them. Marlowe and Vivian are finding out about each other as "horses" and "card players." These pleasantries come to an abrupt end when Marlowe reveals he knows something about her hole card: "What's Eddie Mars got to do with this case?" He also knows that she wants to "sugar him" off it.

The next scene between Vivian and Marlowe appropriately picks up Marlowe's question and takes place at Eddie Mars's (John Ridgely). Although the previous restaurant scene was filmed some nine months after the rest of the film it fits seamlessly into the film's narrative fabric, which would be much weaker without it. Vivian wins a lot of money at Eddie's roulette wheel, and Marlowe foils an apparent robbery attempt in the parking lot to separate her from that money. But Marlowe believes that the whole scene has been faked and staged for his benefit—specifically to prove that there is no connection between Mars and Vivian. Ironically, it proves just the opposite, implying another unseen, unverified, and unverifiable strategy which Vivian and Mars have taken against Marlowe. As Marlowe drives her home, they share their first kiss ("I like that," she purrs, "I'd like even more") and their second ("That's even better"). But Marlowe again punctures the personal intimacy with his vocational question: "All right. Now that's settled. What's Eddie Mars got on you?" As is typical of so many Hawks films, the professional, vocational commitment (Marlowe's dedication to his job and his client, which is the basis of his honor) has come into conflict with the personal, emotional attachment. Marlowe told Vivian at the end of the restaurant scene, "We'll take up the question of you and I when the race is over." As is also typical of so many Hawks films, the conflict between the professional and the personal will be resolved when the two commitments become one, when the two lovers begin to work together.

Next Vivian tells Marlowe a second lie over the telephone—that Sean Regan has been found in Mexico and that she will drive off there to meet him. Instead, however, Vivian turns up at Art Huck's when Marlowe awakes from his beating by Canino. In a marvelous culmination of Hawks's physical business with coins, Canino (Bob Steele) slugs Marlowe with the whole roll of nickels he has been tossing (this roll of nickels can be found in both Chandler's novel and the filmscript), but the force of the blow breaks the roll, allowing Canino to jingle the individual coins in his hand after Marlowe has been knocked unconscious. These tinkling nickels exist in neither the novel nor the film's script; if the film were told purely within the first person, as the novel is, how could an unconscious man become conscious of the ironic tinkling sound of nickels? That Vivian waits for Marlowe at Art Huck's is the final and conclusive sign of the invisible chess game that Vivian and Mars have been playing with Marlowe throughout the narrative. Why and how did Vivian get there? Given all the puzzlement about Owen Taylor's murderer, it seems surprising that no one has been puzzled about Vivian's sudden and mysterious appearance at Art Huck's in Marlowe's hour of need (she is not there, of course, in the novel or original script).

We can again only speculate about this final move in the invisible chess game, for our understanding of Vivian's actions and motivation is dependent on our knowledge of what Vivian knows, but the narrative's construction and handling of point-of-view have made it impossible for us to know anything of what she knows. When Vivian told Marlowe she was going to Mexico to meet Sean, she used the same false destination, the same "cover story," that Mars used to explain the disappearance of Sean Regan and Mona Mars. Like Sean and Mona, Vivian is about to disappear; it would not be surprising for her to disappear to the same place where Mona Mars is hiding. Perhaps Eddie Mars and Vivian felt it would be safer for her to go where Marlowe could not find her. But Vivian might also have expected that Marlowe would indeed find her there. She now knows the way Marlowe "runs races"—that he does not stop until he gets to the finish line. Vivian knows that Mona Mars is hiding at Art Huck's in Realito, and she also knows that Mona is the final missing piece in the Sternwood puzzle. Once Marlowe finds Mona he will know that Sean did not run off with her—or anyone else; Marlowe will know that Sean is dead and will be able to narrow Regan's possible killers to three—Carmen, Mars, or Vivian herself. She certainly knows that when and if Marlowe does turn up at Art Huck's he will need her help because she knows that the brutal Canino stands guard there to protect that hiding place against intruders.

With their final reunion at Art Huck's she does help him, and they continue to work together (rather than apart and rather than on opposite sides of the chessboard) until the narrative conclusion. Vivian cuts the ropes that bind him; Marlowe-Bogart adds a delightful bit of spontaneous, almost motherly improvisation when he tells her to be careful of her fingers and not to cut toward her hand. Vivian screams to draw Canino's attention after Marlowe leaves the house; she then distracts Canino's attention with a second scream, pointing to the steering wheel of Canino's car, the place where Marlowe is not, exposing the hired killer to Marlowe's bullets (another "big sleep" caused by a woman). And at Geiger's house in the final confrontation with Eddie Mars, Vivian watches the back door while Marlowe watches the front (the backdoor-frontdoor strategy of two working partners returns in *Rio Bravo* and *El Dorado*). That Mars and Vivian have been partners in this invisible chess game against Marlowe is confirmed in the final scene at Geiger's house when Marlowe tells Mars, "She's all right, Eddie. She made a deal with you and she kept it." The comment reveals not only Vivian's personal standards of honor and integrity (which parallel Marlowe's own) but also Marlowe's awareness of the game that Vivian felt she needed to play with Eddie and against himself.

Vivian switches her allegiances when she realizes how well Marlowe runs and when she can overtly admit, "I guess I'm in love with you." As in *To Have and Have Not*, love is a much better source of loyalty and sympathy than money. Vivian has come to accept Marlowe's statement, in the restaurant scene, as a fact: "I don't want to hurt you. I'm trying to help you." Marlowe has also come to admit the realization that "I guess I'm in love with *you*." He has come to realize that "wonderful" has been playing with the not-wonderful Eddie Mars because she believes it is in her best interest—to protect her "not so wonderful" sister from a murder charge and, thereby, to protect her suffering father from even greater suffering. Her personal integrity also demands that she honor the agreement with Mars—just as Marlowe's agreement with General Sternwood links his personal honor and integrity with the demand that he do his job well. As opposed to *To Have and Have Not*, in which the Bogart character's trust in the Bacall figure must evolve until he accepts her as an ally and partner, in *The Big Sleep* the Bacall character's trust in the Bogart figure must evolve from enmity to partnership. In the conclusion of Hawks's *Big Sleep* Vivian and Marlowe achieve this synthesis of their personal and vocational "sympathies" by working together as partners. They simultaneously discover and reveal the strong feelings for one another that have run beneath their cool surfaces throughout the narrative by expressing those feelings overtly—in both words and actions. This synthesis, this discovery, and this expression provide the typical conclusion and resolution of a Howard Hawks narrative.

In trying to deduce what Vivian is doing off-frame, on the other side of the looking-glass of this narrative, the audience re-creates the deductive process which Marlowe himself experiences. It is precisely because this process requires such a high degree of inference with no explicit confirmation—by the characters or storyteller—of the validity of these inferences that the film of *The Big Sleep* seems incoherent, illogical, or unfathomable. One might simply agree with Hawks that the story itself makes no sense in or difference to the film, that all he wanted to do was to "have fun" by making "good scenes." But this temptation is too easy; it denies that there is some kind of spiritual, subtextual unity that links these "good scenes." Hawks claimed that in many films, particularly his later ones, he became more interested in characters than in stories.

> I'm using less and less plot and more characters constantly. I'm learning more about characters and how to let them handle the plot, rather than let the plot move them.[27]

His film of *The Big Sleep* is an example of the way that characters (or character-performers) not only "handle the plot" but become the plot. The events of Chandler's crime story are a mere pretext for that central human relationship in Hawks's human story, the background against which it is played and the narrative obstacle to its successful culmination.

Several other characteristics of the film's narrative construction confirm both the care of its making and its link to Hawks's other work. The perpetual return to Geiger's house, the location around which the narrative revolves, reveals that the deliberate elegance of Hawks's symmetries (particularly the symmetries of *Only Angels Have Wings*) have been carefully and consciously employed to build a solid pattern of structural probability for a potentially wandering and formless tale. When Hawks brings the narrative back to Geiger's house for its conclusion (as opposed to the return to the greenhouse in Chandler's novel and the film's original script), Hawks is returning his narrative to its true spiritual origin rather than to the literal, visual origin of Chandler's narrative. The return to Geiger's allows Vivian spiritually to undo what her sister Carmen had done to initiate the maze of men and murders, just as Marlowe's bullet shatters the stone mask which contained the camera that started the string of murders (the subtly symbolic closing of another Hawks circle).

As in *Bringing Up Baby* and *Only Angels Have Wings,* everything in *The Big Sleep* comes in twos. There are two scenes between Marlowe and Vivian in his automobile; two scenes in which a woman waits for Marlowe to arrive (Vivian at his office, Carmen at his apartment); two lying telephone calls from Vivian to Marlowe; two witty women outsiders who aid Marlowe's search (the bookstore lady with the glasses and the cabbie); two beatings that Marlowe receives from Mars's men (one from the two goons, the other from Canino and Huck); two male goons who work for Mars (they are a very comical team, The Two Stooges)

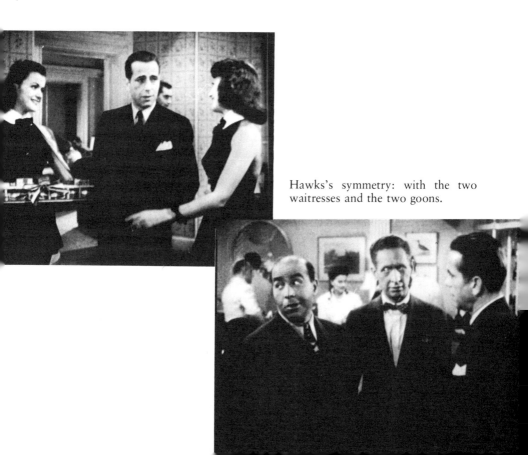

Hawks's symmetry: with the two waitresses and the two goons.

and two cocktail waitresses who work at Mars's casino (a symmetry underscored when both the two goons and the two girls deliver the identical message to Marlowe); two bluff telephone calls to the police (one in a scene between Marlowe and Mars, the other in a scene between Marlowe and Vivian—subtly linking Mars and Vivian against Marlowe); two real telephone calls to the police (Marlowe's summoning Ohls after the capture of Lundgren and the death of Mars); two telephone calls from Marlowe to arrange a meeting with Mars (the first at his casino, the last at Geiger's house); two scenes in which one character watches another take a beating while Mars's men "play out their hand" (first Jones watches the two goons work Marlowe over, then Marlowe watches while Canino poisons Jones); and two scenes in which a character threatens to count to three, "like they do in the movies" (in another ironic piece of Hawksian self-reference). Only one of these symmetries exists in the Chandler novel (the parallel of Vivian's waiting for Marlowe in his office and Carmen's waiting for him in his bed), and Chandler makes the parallel to equate the two women, not to differentiate between them, as Hawks does. Many of these symmetries do not exist in either draft of the screenplay, obviously built into the narrative structure (as so much is in a Hawks film) during shooting.

These structural symmetries accompany consistent visual motifs that reinforce the narrative's underlying unity by bathing it in a consistent (and consistently bleak) tone. Most of the film takes place either indoors and/or at night. The indoor shots are claustrophobic (especially the uncomfortably hot meeting between Marlowe and Sternwood in the greenhouse), heavily shadowed (typical of Hawks—especially the scene in which Marlowe watches a blurred two-dimensional reflection on rippled glass of Canino murdering Harry Jones, accompanied by the clarity of their off-frame voices), and atmospherically uncomfortable (the stifling ornateness of Geiger's house or the tacky gentility of Brody's apartment). The outdoor shots are cast in darkness, saturated with fog (the first scene outside Geiger's house when Marlowe sees the photographic flash and hears the three shots; the vision of Owen Taylor's heavy, black death car hoisted from the surf; the skirmish between Marlowe and Vivian's assailant in Mars's parking lot; the misty alley where Mars's two goons teach Marlowe a painful lesson; Marlowe's final confrontations with both Canino and Mars). There is very little daylight in the film at all. The few exceptions are the comical bookstore

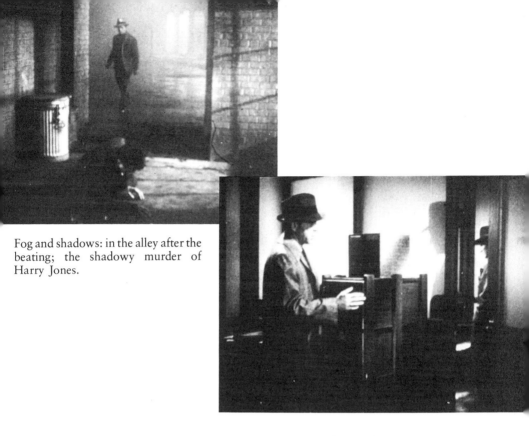

Fog and shadows: in the alley after the beating; the shadowy murder of Harry Jones.

scenes, Marlowe's first almost comical encounter with Mars at Geiger's house (where they will face each other less comically for the final time—at night), and the light which streams in the windows when Vivian enters the restaurant for her meeting with Marlowe (a decidedly bright scene). Hawks's camera tracks with her to reinforce the impression of her forceful and energetic walk as she moves from the light to Marlowe's table. This vigorous walk on this bright day in this added scene probably reveals the underlying strength and solidity of Vivian's moral character more forcefully than any other piece of data in the film. Although the foggy, shadowy, imprisoning darkness of most of the film seems prototypical for a post-war *film noir, The Big Sleep*'s imagery is also prototypical for Hawks, who had always known how night and shadows can suffuse and dampen a film's atmosphere—in *Scarface, Barbary Coast, Bringing Up Baby, Only Angels Have Wings.*

The Big Sleep is also built around two instruments of human communication—the telephone (like *His Girl Friday*) and the automobile (this film's replacement for *His Girl Friday*'s typewriter). The telephone

293

is the perpetual means for telling lies and spinning strategies in the film—Vivian lies twice to Marlowe, Marlowe plays telephonic games with both the police and Eddie Mars. Just when Marlowe fears that his quest has ended, after Harry Jones's death, the telephone rings; the call from Agnes allows Marlowe's race to continue. Marlowe uses the telephone to discover that Jones gave Canino a false address to Agnes's apartment. And he uses the telephone in his final strategy with Eddie Mars—telling him that he will meet him at Geiger's house, when his automobile has already carried him there.

The automobile is the film's extension of the telephone—Marlowe's car, Geiger's, the station wagon that transports Geiger's books to Brody's, the Sternwood car that contains Owen Taylor's body, Harry Jones's gray coupe, Marlowe's letting the air out of his car's tires in Realito, Vivian's false information to Canino that Marlowe sits behind the wheel of Canino's car, Marlowe's taking that car for his final appointment with Eddie Mars. The automobile becomes Marlowe's sanctuary and refuge—the place where he expresses his feelings for Vivian, the place where he hides the guns that permit him to perform the most difficult jobs. As opposed to Chandler's metaphoric symbols (Marlowe's chessboard, which has no function in the novel other than to comment on Marlowe's knightliness and the chess-like action in which he has become engaged), Hawks's symbols must *do* something—must be able to move or be handled or be used—in the literal, surface narrative as well.[28]

The result of these structural symmetries, the consistent atmosphere and lighting, the consistent reliance of the narrative upon the telephone and automobile, both functionally and metaphorically, is to reinforce our sense of underlying unity about a narrative whose real sense is also underlying and underneath—not a detective's search for clues to crimes but a human search for meaning and value, the synthesis of personal integrity, vocational honor, and emotional fulfillment. This *Big Sleep* is not Chandler's story of Philip Marlowe, Knight, but Hawks's story of the kind of insolent, intelligent, sexual love a Bogart-Marlowe and a Vivian-Bacall can discover and express, a love that, along with a human vocation, is a personal assertion of meaning and value in a dark, murky maze of a potentially chaotic universe. One of the essential assumptions of the detective genre—from Huston's *Maltese Falcon* to Polanski's *Chinatown*—is that the goal of the detective's quest, which seems so clear to him at the beginning, becomes steadily more distant and elusive as he pursues it, constantly changing, constantly drawing him forward down strange paths and around strange corners. As he weaves his way through the labyrinth, the detective ultimately discovers something quite different from what he started out to find. In Hawks's *Big Sleep,* the detective ultimately and unexpectedly discovers both himself and his fulfillment by another. That is the sense that this narrative makes for those who sense that it makes sense—as much sense as any Hawks film does, in the way that Hawks films make sense, and about the matters about which they wish to make sense.

9

The Genre Epic:
Red River

Red River made Wayne a good actor, because he does *not* try too hard, to do things he's not capable of doing. He's a hell of a lot better than most people think he is.[1]

Wayne . . . has more power than any other man on the screen. The only problem with Wayne is who do you get to play with him? If you get somebody who's not pretty strong, why he blows them right off the screen. He doesn't do it purposely—that's just what happens. In *Red River* he had Monty Clift, who was a pretty fair hand.[2]

There are about thirty plots in all dramatic literature which have been done by very good people and if you can think of a new way to do it, you're pretty good. But if you can put characters in there, you can forget about the plot. Let them tell your story for you and don't worry about the plot.[3]

When I made *Red River,* with thousands of cows, I had enough of them. I no longer wanted to work with anything but human beings.[4]

R*ED* R*IVER* OCCUPIES a unique place in the work of Howard Hawks. The film is one of Hawks's biggest, most ambitious, and most expensive undertakings—for which the director-producer paid dearly in time, money, and trouble. Budgeted at $2,000,000, a significant sum for an independent production in 1946, the film's actual costs ran $800,000 higher than that. Injunctions were threatened against the film's release: by the Teamsters, who represented the cowhands in Arizona, owed over $20,000 for their services when the production company ran out of money; by the Pathé film laboratory, which had not been paid for processing the film;[5] by Howard Hughes for Hawks's supposed "theft" of the ending of Hughes's *The Outlaw* (which Hawks had devised himself).[6] The film's financial problems led to the bankruptcy of Hawks's Monterrey Productions, his first independent producing company (he would later found Winchester and Malabar Productions). Finally released some two years after it had been shot, the film eventually was successful—both in the opinion of viewers at the box office and in the critical responses of reviewers. *Red River*, like *Sergeant York*, won Hawks wider and more enthusiastic attention in the nation's press than any of his more modest productions.

But this very attention in the "majority" press has led many of Hawks's admirers to dismiss *Red River* as one of the director's less remarkable accomplishments—like *Sergeant York*. Many committed Hawksophiles, like Robin Wood, prefer both *Rio Bravo* and *El Dorado*, two more modest westerns, to *Red River*. The French dismiss *Red River* for what seems its lack of humor,[7] while some American critics find its score bombastic,[8] its plot meandering, and its historical context atypical of Hawks. More than anything else, some seem disturbed by Hawks's denying his own more modest concerns, his attempting to make a "Ford western" rather than a "Hawks western." *Red River* is an awesomely outdoor film, shot on location, unlike his later and more modest westerns, which are primarily indoor, studio-interior films. As the cattle trader, Melville, tells Matthew Garth at the end of the film's cattle drive, "There are three times in a man's life when he has the right to yell at the moon: when he marries, when his children come, and when he finishes a job he had to be crazy to start in the first place." Like the cattle drive in the film, the very making of *Red River* may have been something that Hawks had to have been crazy to start in the first place.

But like the cattle drive, Hawks started it and finished it, and the result was as impressive as the attempt. Hawks himself felt *Red River* was the best of his westerns:

> The one I like best is *Red River*. . . . When you have to shift 3,000 head of cattle every time you shoot a new scene, that's hard work.[9]

Like so many of the vocations in Hawks's films, the task of making the movie parallels the task within the movie. Christian Nyby reports that Hawks wanted to save money on the film (an idea rejected by the film's financial backers) by buying the cattle rather than renting them, then selling them back at a profit (since each cow would have gained fifty to a hundred pounds over the months of filming).[10] No clearer parallel between making movies and raising cattle could ever be found.

Hawks's shaping of his narrative, his adapting Borden Chase's serialized story, "The Chisholm Trail," into his film, *Red River,* reveals his usual perceptions and procedures. For anyone who has read the Chase story, it is simply amazing that Hawks could make such a good movie out of such terrible material. Hawks had purchased the film rights to the story even before it appeared in the *Saturday Evening Post,* between December 7, 1946, and January 11, 1947. He even tried to convince the *Post* to use his title, "Red River," rather than Chase's.[11] There must have been something Hawks saw in that story, for he never bought any property unless he liked the story.[12] But Chase's narrative, as is typical of many serialized stories, is remarkable for the plethora and proliferation of its incidents rather than the care and depth of rendering any one of them. In Chase's story, Tess Millay manages romantic attachments with Thomas Dunson, Matthew Garth, Cherry Valance, and several other gents; Chase gives us not one but three stampedes; during the cattle drive north the herd is attacked by border gangs, by Indians, and even by Cherry Valance and the gamblers, who try to steal the herd from Matthew; there are gun duels between Cherry and the Donegal (a gambler who is Tess Millay's "protector"), between Dunson and Cherry, and, finally, between Matthew and Dunson. At the climax of the serialized story, Dunson shoots directly at Matthew but shoots wildly (because he has been injured in the duel with Cherry), while Matthew draws his gun but does not shoot at Dunson (because his hand suddenly becomes paralysed and his finger will not squeeze the trigger). At the end of Chase's story, Dunson, Matthew, and Tess return toward Texas and, just after Dunson crosses the Red River on this southward journey, he collapses and dies on Texas soil. In the *Post* story, Nadine Groot (named Groot Nadine, as he is in the original filmscript), is an unimportant cook on the cattle drive (no more important than a dozen other cowpunchers), there is no woman (Fen) whom Dunson initially deserts, and there is no snake bracelet.

As is typical of Hawks's method of telling stories, he pares down the quantity of Chase's incidents to develop their quality, their texture, their underlying resonances. For a very long film (originally 127 minutes),* it is remarkable how little actually happens in *Red River*. Most of the incidents which the film promises never take place (they all take place in Chase's story—and more); many of those promised incidents also take place in the film's first screenplay, the only version of the script on which Borden Chase worked, and most of them Hawks deleted or altered. (Despite his credit for the screenplay, dictated by the Screen Writers' Guild, very little of Chase survives in *Red River*.) We hear there are border gangs in Missouri; we never meet them because the men go to Kansas instead. We hear there are Indians; they are dispersed with less than two minutes of shooting and whooping. We are told that one day Cherry Valance and Matthew Garth will surely shoot it out; they become close friends and fight alongside, not one another. Finally, we are promised a climactic gun battle between Dunson and Matthew, and it never takes place either. Even Groot observes that this battle seemed inevitable for fourteen years. Apparently not. If Hawks's narrative strategy in *The Big Sleep* was to build a bewildering series of many incidents and then refuse to explain them, the narrative strategy of *Red River* is to promise many incidents and then refuse to depict them.

Despite the differences in these two narrative methods, their general strategy is identical—to shift the emphasis away from the external incidents and toward the underlying psychological and emotional interactions beneath the incidental surfaces. The blurring of external incidents in *The Big Sleep* throws the entire film into the hearts and minds of the central couple—Marlowe-Bogart and Vivian-Bacall. The stripping away of incident in *Red River* throws the entire film into the hearts and minds of its central couple—Thomas Dunson and Matthew Garth. Hawks dispenses with all those incidents that do not relate directly to this "story of friendship, which is really a love story between two men" (as Hawks described the Wayne-Mitchum relationship in *El Dorado*).[13] The link between Hawks's three major westerns is that he is "much

---

* There is a serious textual problem with *Red River*, which I explicate in the note appended to this chapter. One extant version of the film is some seven-and-a-half minutes longer than the other. There are several other significant differences. My discussion of *Red River* assumes that the longer version of the film is the authoritative text, a point I will argue in detail in the appendix to this chapter. As the reader will discover in that appendix, there are those who could argue otherwise.

more interested in the story of friendship with the two men than . . . about a range war, or something like that."[14] Each of the successive scripts of *Red River* pared down the scenes and incidents that did not relate directly to the love-friendship conflict between Dunson and Matthew, including several very lengthy scenes between Tess Millay, Cherry Valance, and Matthew.[15] Although one explanation for the vestigial shards of Tess's and Cherry's roles in the final film is that Hawks did not much care for Joanne Dru or John Ireland (according to Borden Chase because the two were having the affair that would lead to their marriage and about which Hawks was jealous, but according to Christian Nyby because John Ireland was lazy and refused to work very hard at his role[16]), this is the sort of gossip that seems to delight a certain kind of cinephile who believes that such explanations really explain things. Another possible explanation is that Hawks's narrative sense convinced him that anything in his story that did not relate directly to its Dunson-Matthew love-friendship center was indeed peripheral and inessential, and ought to remain vestigial.

At the center of Hawks's narrative is the contrast and complementarity of Dunson-Wayne and Matthew-Clift. Just as Hawks had previously teamed a "new girl" with an "established man"—Lombard with Barrymore, Bacall with Bogart—Montgomery Clift (not Joanne Dru) is the real "new girl" of *Red River* who has been teamed with the established John Wayne. Clift, a trained Actor's Studio newcomer from New York, had been discovered and tested for his first appearance by Hawks. Many of Hawks's "new girls" (or old girls in new roles) took advantage of a reversal of sexual stereotypes and cinema expectations (the "maleness," toughness, and shrewdness of Dvorak, Lombard, Russell, Bacall). Montgomery Clift allowed Hawks to manipulate the opposite sexual expectation—the male who seemed gentle, sweet, sensitive, and "soft"— in contrast to Wayne's indomitable hardness. This softness-hardness duality becomes the center not only of the film's contrasting acting performances but of its narrative issues as well.

Dunson is firm and Matthew is flexible; Dunson is the man who repeats that "nothing you can say or do" can change his opinion, while Matthew is the man who changes the drive's destination from Missouri to Abilene. Dunson is committed to the fulfillment of a goal by means that have been previously determined (like his absolute demand to fulfill an obligation after "signing on"); Matthew is committed above all to the fulfillment of the goal and is willing to modify the means to accomplish that end (he can only hope that there is a railroad in Abilene, but he knows that the drive has no hope at all if it continues toward Missouri). Dunson has a ferocious sense of justice and honor, while Matthew is mercifully sensitive to human weakness and insufficiency. Dunson believes that a man must be hard by seeming hard, while Matthew believes that a man can be hard by seeming soft; when Cherry tells Matthew that his softness will hurt him one day, Matthew answers, "Could be. But I wouldn't count on it." While Dunson is consistently called by his last name (only Fen and Groot call him "Tom," and Groot reverts to "Dunson" or "Mr. Dunson" whenever Groot believes him wrong), Matthew is always called by his first. The herd itself has been produced by Dunson's bull and Matthew's cow—Matthew supplying the female principle that Dunson has lost with the death of Fen and both his cows. Even in his love scene with Tess Millay, Matthew-Clift seems to play the more passive, feminine role—her face and body in the upper half of the frame, hovering above his face and body, which recline in its lower half.

This contrast between Dunson-Wayne's stereotypic "maleness" and Matthew-Clift's soft and beautiful "femaleness" (certainly Montgomery Clift has never been more clearly and healthily beautiful in any other film, nor has any other figure in any other Hawks film been quite so purely beautiful as Clift in *Red River*) is not meant to imply any kind of overt or covert homosexual longings between them.[17] Hawks uses the two men as a metaphoric paradigm of the meaning of "maleness"; in one of his typical reversals of sexual stereotyping, Hawks reveals that the more superficially male of the two men is not the man who can get the job done. The "soft" "womanly" man turns out to be the better man for this particular difficult task (and the accomplishing of difficult tasks has always been a virtue in Hawks's moral system). But the power of Clift's soft beauty could never have played this metaphoric role, giving a shape and a focus to this Hawks narrative, without a shift and a more precise definition of the established persona of John Wayne. Just as the established Katharine Hepburn, Cary Grant, or Rosalind Russell first played a kind of role for Hawks that afterwards became an essential characteristic of their screen personas, the inflexible indomitability of John Wayne became one of the dominant traits of his screen being after Hawks developed it. Wayne had never played quite this kind of role before *Red River;* he was far more often the romantic, beautiful young outlaw—for example, the Ringo Kid in John Ford's *Stagecoach,* made just seven years earlier—more like Clift himself. Once Wayne had played this unbendingly hard (yet vulnerably insecure) male for Hawks he would play variations on it forever (and would seem as if he had played it forever).

All of Hawks's changes in the Borden Chase story can be traced to his making the Dunson-Wayne/Matthew-Clift contrast the center of his new narrative. In Chase's story, Dunson and Matthew are two of a kind. Chase described Matthew as a "male creature, loaded with threat in every movement" (Part I, December 7, 1946, p. 152) [18]—not exactly the Matthew Garth embodied by Montgomery Clift. After Matthew takes command of the herd away from Dunson, Chase turns Matthew into the same kind of tyrant as Dunson. Cherry observes, "Grow a little gray in your hair and I'd swear Thomas Dunson rode beside me" (Part IV, December 28, 1946, p. 54). The initial script of the film (the one on which Chase worked most closely and the one which most resembles his own story) similarly depicted Matthew as driving the men as hard as Dunson. In Hawks's film, however, Matthew is a much more supple and likable commander than Dunson, earning his men's admiration and compassion, not their fear. Matthew's ability to convert Cherry Valance from menacing foe to comradely friend in the film is a sure sign of his ability as a leader of men, who appeals to the best in men (this important conversion is Cherry's only function in Hawks's narrative—and the film needs no more from him).

With the Dunson-Matthew contrast as the pole around which everything else in the narrative revolves, Hawks shapes the originally sprawling, serialized tale which wanders from incident to incident into the elegant symmetry of his familiar four-part construction. The most important section of this structure—preparing for the events to follow and shaping their pattern—is, as usual, the first. The three-part prologue of *Red River* (like the three-part prologue of *Twentieth Century*) plants every narrative seed that Howard Hawks will need for his narrative at its climax; almost none of these seeds come from the original package. Thomas Dunson has made up his mind to leave a wagon train on its journey west—and nothing anybody can say or do will change that mind (just as almost nothing anyone says or does changes it during the rest of the narrative). Dunson owes no debt of honor (that essential

Hawks trait) to the wagon train of settlers because he never signed an oath to finish the journey; he joined the train after it had left St. Louis.

His friend and traveling companion, Nadine Groot, the outsider on the wagon rather than the cowboy on a horse, leaves the train with Dunson. Groot, played by that familiar Hawks comrade, Walter Brennan, becomes, like Kid, Eddie, and Stumpy, the moral interpreter of and commentator on his friend's deeds and values. Groot-Brennan explains his friendship with Dunson without explaining it: "Me and Dunson . . . well, it's me and Dunson." This kind of verbal incompleteness, in which subtextual inference must replace explicit information, is typical of the sympathetic pattern of communication throughout the film between Groot and Dunson, who do not need words to talk. This choice, typical of the verbal ellipses of Howard Hawks, was emphasized during shooting by Hawks's extensive pencilled deletions and rewrites in the shooting script, replacing large chunks of explicit dialogue with terse, understated, incomplete verbal phrases, which implied far more than they said.[19]

Dunson's woman, Fen, also begs to accompany him. She asks him to listen with his heart as well as his head. These two metonymies for the conflicting psychological and emotional bases of human action will later be embodied in the narrative by Dunson's progressive retreat into his own head and Matthew's ability to balance the claims of head and heart. Fen also reminds Dunson that the sun shines only half the time— the other half is night. And this separation of the male and female, public and private worlds is reminiscent of Hawks's visual alternation of night and day in so many films (including this one) as well as the downstairs and upstairs regions of his hotel-restaurant-bars. Dunson refuses to bend to her insistent and powerful pleas. By giving her a dominant position in the frame—we see Fen's face and Dunson's back, as their two complementary and harmonious bodies stand straight and firm in a full shot against the sky, plains, and wagons—Hawks lets us know that Dunson is making a serious mistake. Instead, Dunson promises to send for her after he has settled and started his spread, giving her, as a token of his sincerity, a curious, coiled snake bracelet that belonged to his mother. In the film's original script, the bracelet belonged to Groot, not Dunson's mother, eliminating its essential link to Dunson's female, domestic side.

After their separation from the wagon train, as they reach the

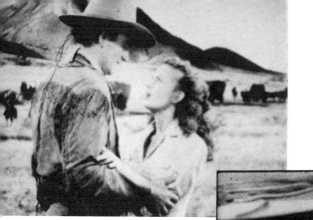

The power of Fen's appeal.

northern bank of the Red River, Groot and Dunson see smoke on the horizon—accompanied by Indian-like, tom-tomish music on the sound track—clear signs of a deadly Indian attack against the settlers. Groot's immediate verbal reaction, with no grammatical antecedent, makes no logical sense but clearly reveals the way he has sympathetically, almost telepathically realized what Dunson is thinking without his saying it aloud: "Shoulda took her with us." That night, along the northern bank of the Red River, Groot and Dunson fight together for the first time against the small war party of Indians (they will fight together again a second time) who have come to make sure there are no survivors. As Dunson battles an Indian brave in the river, the first baptism in the Red River (there will be a second), Groot tosses Dunson a weapon (a knife—in a later battle Groot will toss Dunson another weapon, a rifle) that allows the friend to conquer the enemy. Already in this early sequence, with the fight, the weapon, and the river, Hawks has begun to build the symmetries that will lock the narrative into its shape, none of which exist in the Chase story. According to Christian Nyby, both Jules Furthman and Leigh Brackett worked with Hawks on the screenplay of *Red River,* uncredited; such symmetries are much more typical of their collaborations with Hawks.[20]

Dunson finds his snake bracelet on the slain warrior's wrist, implying, subtly yet clearly, in the physical way that Hawks establishes narrative information, the fate of Dunson's Fen. Groot, seeing that bracelet, makes another sympathetic yet elliptical leap that never quite concludes. "Oh, Tom, that's too bad, we shoulda took her with. . . ." Womanless, Dunson slips the bracelet back on his own wrist. The mistake has been his first, the death has been his fault. He will not make this mistake again. The prologue's first part seals Thomas Dunson off from the world of women, mildness, and flexibility.

In its second part, which begins the next day, Dunson meets the boy who will replace the woman in his heart and his life. The alternation of day-night-day in the prologue is a familiar Hawks piece of metaphoric intensification and structural precision. As opposed to *The Big Sleep, Red River* is predominantly an outdoor, daytime film; its beneficial, positive events occur in the daylight, its most troublesome and disturbing events at night. The appearance of the boy who replaces the woman (Dunson will even give him the snake bracelet) the very next morning is the first of the film's indications that it is absolutely impossible and improbable that Dunson will really kill this boy in the daylight duel of the film's climax. He has already killed the woman; he will not kill her replacement. The narrative game that Hawks will play in *Red River,* however, will be to build one set of genuine probabilities into the film (that Dunson will not and cannot kill Matthew) that will later be obscured by an apparent set of probabilities (that Dunson means what he says rather than what he feels, that gunfights are inevitable at the end of westerns) only to emerge as the real set of probabilities after all. There are those who find the narrative of *Red River,* like that of *The Big Sleep,* confusing: somebody ought to kill somebody at the film's end.[21] The prologue of *Red River* works as hard as possible to substitute a different series of expectations for the film—or, at the least, to establish one set of expectations which can play off against another.

The second major section of the prologue develops these expectations—constructed as a series of lessons for Matthew (and us) about Dunson. The boy, leading his cow behind him, has been stunned by the visions of murder and burning he has witnessed; his brain and his mouth wander as aimlessly as his body, muttering the words "Burning, it was all burning" to no one in particular. The aimless stream of sound is again more meaningful for Hawks than any specific words in the stream. Dunson slaps the boy twice to stop the stream and bring him to his senses (as in *To Have and Have Not*, a friendly, beneficial slap); the boy does not feel the slap that way. He draws his child-sized gun very quickly and warns Dunson, "I wouldn't do that again." At the film's climax Dunson *will* do that again, and Matthew will not act upon his childish threat. Dunson then turns away from the boy, tricking him into lowering his guard, then lunges quickly toward him, slaps him a second time, and takes that gun away.

Dunson now gives the boy his own warning in return: "Don't ever trust anyone 'til you know him." The boy answers, "I won't." And he won't either, for at the film's climax Matthew knows that Dunson's code of honor will not permit him to shoot a man who does not intend to shoot him. Then Dunson gives the little gun back to the boy—a sign of Dunson's confidence in the boy, that he now "knows" the boy. It will be the first of two guns that Dunson will give him. Dunson taunts him comically, "Well, are you gonna use it?" "No. But don't ever try to take it away from me again." In the film's climax, Dunson will take a gun away from him, and he will taunt Matthew again by reminding him of this child's warning. But the child who has become a man will no longer attach any importance to these childish words. Dunson observes to Groot—in one of those familiar, terse Hawks statements of one character's respect for the strength and competence of another— "He'll do."

Matthew's education continues in the next sequence—Dunson's first gun battle with another to defend his land and his rights. After crossing the Red River together for the first time, Dunson devises a brand for the bull and the cow—two wavy lines, representing the banks of the Red River, with a large block *D* beside it—the Red River D brand. Matthew observes, "My name is Matthew. I don't see an *M* on that brand." Dunson replies, "I'll put an *M* on it when you've earned it." "Fair enough. I'll earn it." And Matthew will. The adding of that *M* to the brand will be the final incident of the film. In the original script, a small *m* was to accompany Dunson's large *D;* Hawks sharpens the issue by omitting any initial at all until the boy demonstrates he has become a man.

Another man has a quarrel with Dunson's claim to the land and his brand. The Mexicanish music on the sound track (the film's use of unmotivated music for this kind of information is a sign of evolving musical styles in Hollywood films) accompanies the fast approach of a rider, who informs Dunson that the land belongs to Don Diego, who lives 400 miles to the south. For Groot, "That's too much land for one man. That ain't decent." And Dunson tells Don Diego's man that the Mexican's spread ought to end at the Rio Grande—warning Matthew with a gesture to back away because trouble is about to begin. Here Groot and Dunson are moral allies in their casual formulation of the proper national boundaries between the United States and Mexico. Hawks already developed his view of the illegitimate rule of these Mexican Dons in *Viva Villa!*.

The Mexican goes for his gun, but Dunson outdraws him. Matthew asks how Dunson was able to outdraw his opponent, since the Mexican went for his gun first. "How'd you know when he was gonna draw?" "By watchin' his eyes," Dunson answers. "Remember that." "I will," says Matthew. And he will. At the film's climax he will demonstrate in his eyes that he will not draw his gun (and Hawks will give the viewer several powerful close-ups of those eyes for Matthew's demonstration). Dunson has given the young Matthew two pieces of information which he has told the boy not to forget—not to trust a man until he knows him and that he reads a man's eyes to know when to draw. Despite the clarity and explicitness of this information (added by Hawks in pencil to the original typescript), some two hours of film will separate this clear expository information from that gun battle, and Hawks will later pass the viewer a conflicting kind of information that will, ironically, lead us to forget what Hawks has made very sure we know.

Even the beautiful, luminous shots of the vast western spaces in the prologue serve an essential narrative function, for this will be a story of men in those spaces and in that light. The action will chronicle the conquest of these vast spaces, of human beings asserting their power and determination over those spaces. The journey that the three men make southward in the prologue will be retraced by the journey that the men and cattle make northward in the main body of the narrative (just as the camera retraces its steps in *Scarface* and *His Girl Friday*). The visual metaphor for this assertion of human beings against the spaces of the earth and the vastness of the sky can be found in the prologue's

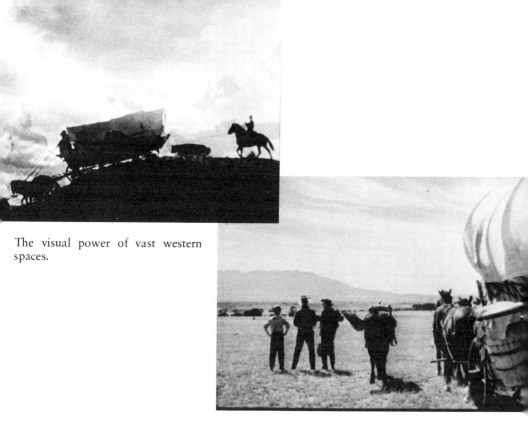

The visual power of vast western spaces.

awesome, low-angle shot (no eye-level here, unless it is a toad's eye) of Dunson, Groot, and Matthew, standing tall and firm against the heavens. This shot not only declares their human assertion against the vastness which surrounds them (such an assertion parallels that of the men against gravity and the sky in *Only Angels Have Wings*); it also links them as another ideal Hawks community—old teacher and commentator, man, and boy (the boy who has become both son and "wife" to the man).

Another of the prologue's functional visual images can be glimpsed during Dunson's first reading of the Bible over the body of the slain Mexican. These "readings" become one of the film's dominant running motifs; the first one immediately precedes the first branding of cattle. Juxtaposed with the branding iron in the foreground of Hawks's frame is the cross on the Mexican's grave in the rearground. The allegorical link of these two actions and objects ("reading" and branding, cross and branding iron) reveals that for Dunson his vocational sense is one with his spiritual sense, his commitment to vocational action related to

309

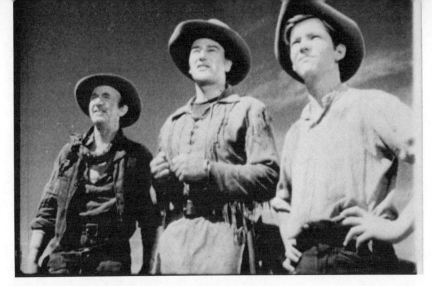

The power of the film's community, emphasized by the low angle (Brennan, Wayne, and Mickey Kuhn).

a belief in the cosmic significance and value of his efforts. The branding iron is an extension of the cross; the settling and crossing of these vast spaces is a partnership between God and human beings, the cosmos and the earth. Allegorically, the two parallel objects imply that American history itself—the settling of the West by the ownership of land and cattle—is an embodiment of the Divine Plan.

The third (and final) section of the prologue establishes the precise social and economic conditions that make the film's cattle drive necessary. Hawks begins this sequence in "the present" (*i.e.* 1865) with a dissolve and a very clever juxtaposition of verbal narration and visual demonstration. Dunson describes the plan of his ranch for Groot and the boy Matthew, and, as he verbally sketches its buildings, dimensions, and locations, the film's visual imagery shows the ranch to be not an idea but a physical fact. Hawks effortlessly leaps fourteen years, his camera coming to rest on the same ideal community—Groot, Dunson, and Matthew—all older but still united. It is this unity that the film's action will test. At the end of Dunson's transitional speech, he observes that they now have the land, and the spread, and the beef, but their entire effort has been for naught. There is no money in the South after the Civil War to pay for that beef. They must drive the cattle north.

The potential tension between Matthew and Dunson begins almost immediately. When Matthew suggests one route for the drive, Dunson tells him, "That's the long way around." And when Matthew continues

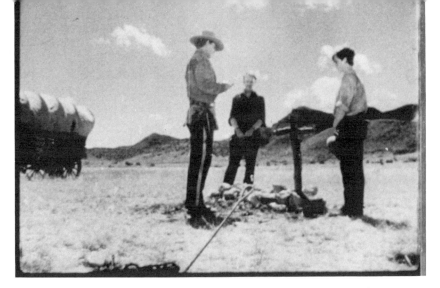

Juxtaposition of the cross in the rearground, branding iron in the foreground.

to outline this plan, Dunson interrupts him again, "I said, that's the long way around." The issue is settled; they will go Dunson's way. In his haste Dunson resolves to brand every steer on his land, regardless of its actual owner. Matthew, however, respects the cattle's brand and the principle of ownership; he frees those belonging to Meeker (a neighbor) or Don Diego (the Americans and Mexicans now live peacefully). When Dunson explains to Matthew that he hasn't the time to separate the cattle so particularly, Matthew accepts the pragmatic sense of Dunson's argument: "Brand him." But there has been a comical (or is it comical?) skirmish between them. Matthew observes, "You'll wind up branding every rump in Texas except mine." Dunson answers, "Hand me that iron, Teeler. (*Pause*) You don't think I'd do it?" Then Dunson backs away from this challenge to reveal he was only joking. In the original script, however, he is not joking at all. Dunson tells Matthew, "Afraid, Matthew boy? Afraid of what an old man can do?" The line, typical of Borden Chase's rhetoric, both demeans Matthew and conveys no sincere affection of the man for the boy at all. Hawks understandably got rid of it.

Groot plays a pivotal role in this early tension. Groot, the film's moral barometer, participates in the Dunson-Matthew skirmishing. He surprisingly yells, "Draw!" provoking both men to wheel around, their guns drawn. This comic duel will be answered by the film's conclusion

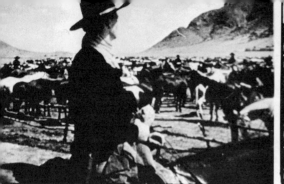
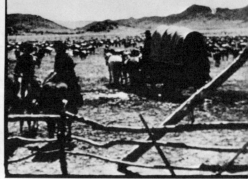

The counter-clockwise pan (read from right to left),

when the boy refuses to draw on command. Groot observes that he is not sure which of the two would win such a duel, but he teasingly tells Dunson that Matthew seems just a bit faster. Groot also shows his fondness for Matthew, his acceptance of Matthew as an extension of Dunson, by his verbal welcoming him home from the war. As is typical of Groot (and Hawks) it says more than it says, ends without concluding, and leaves both the listener and the audience to fill in the three dots: "I'm glad you come home cause . . . well, I'm glad you come home." It is Groot who tells Bunk Kennelly (Ivan Parry) that Matthew and Cherry Valance, a gunslinger hired by Meeker who decides to work for Dunson instead, will tangle in the future for sure. (They won't.) It is Groot who playfully lashes Bunk with a whip for stealing sugar from the chuck wagon. Dunson will attempt to whip Bunk severely when his later sugar theft causes that chuck wagon's collapse and the resulting deadly stampede. Already Hawks has planted this narrative seed. It is Groot who provides the film's consistent comic echo, losing a half-share of his false teeth, the comic symbolic counterpart of the snake bracelet, to his Indian companion, Quo, in a poker game. Like Dunson and Matthew, Groot and Quo (Chief Yowlachie) make an unlikely "marriage"—a very odd couple who are spiritually one, though physically opposite. (In the original script, the tooth gags built around their shared teeth run relentlessly through the entire story, until Quo dies in a river stampede, and Groot buries the teeth as an amulet with his friend.) And it is Groot who first signs the oath which pledges to finish the drive, giving his word as a pledge of his honor to Dunson. As Groot implants his large X on the agreement with a comical flourish, the scene fades out, and the film's lengthy prologue—the three narrative subsections which precede the cattle drive itself—concludes.

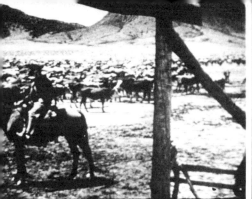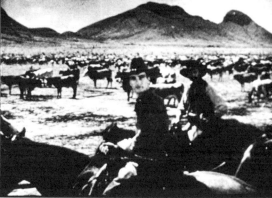

beginning with Matthew and ending with Dunson.

The film's second major section chronicles Dunson's leading the drive, which provokes the growing tension between Dunson, the rest of the men, and Matthew, until Matthew takes possession of the herd himself. The section begins with a series of shots that are as visually dazzling and psychologically perceptive as anything in the work of Howard Hawks. It is an early morning scene, and the earth is strangely quiet. Neither the men nor the cattle make any noise. The light is strangely dim. And even the shot's depth-of-field, ordinarily very crisp and deep throughout the film, seems softer, flatter, narrower. The moment seems almost otherworldly, almost silent slow-motion, and yet obviously not precisely either. It is a moment of departure, of leave-taking, of drawing a final physical and spiritual breath before jumping off the edge of the world.

For the shots do enclose a world—Dunson's world (or rather, Dunson's and Matthew's world). Dunson surveys his world from his horse's saddle, with Matthew sitting on the horse alongside him. At this point, Hawks's camera executes what is probably the most idiosyncratic camera maneuver in the entire work of Howard Hawks. What is striking about the maneuver, however, is not merely its visual idiosyncrasy but its complex manipulation of narrative point-of-view—no other Hawks shot attempts in a single shot to show simultaneously that there are two physical points-of-view which are really a single spiritual point-of-view. Here is what Hawks does and how he does it.

The camera makes a circular pan, a full 180-degree half-circle, in a counterclockwise direction, surveying the entire visible world in the direction the drive is headed—as far as the eye can see. The shot surveys the plains, the cattle, the mountains, the men on their mounts. It clearly circumscribes the world with which these men are familiar, which these men know, and to leave this world is to embark upon the dangerously unknown. But whereas the shot begins by surveying the world from Dunson's point-of-view, from the position established to be occupied by Dunson and his mount, it ends by looking *at* Dunson from Matthew's point-of-view, from the position established to be occupied by Matthew and his mount. In other words, the shot begins as Dunson's point-of-view, looking at Matthew, and ends as Matthew's point-of-view, looking at Dunson. The 180-degree arc circumscribes not Dunson's world but Dunson's *and* Matthew's world—the world in which the two are linked as the two inseparable poles of a complete spiritual and physical circle:

The parallel physical figure which this shot describes is the film's central Hawksian object and token of love—the snake bracelet. Like the bracelet, this is a shot with two heads, two rounded poles, bound by a circularly continuous band. Like the bracelet, the shot conveys a two that is one and a one that is two. The shot not only imparts the difficulty and the danger of leaving "home," of leaving one's world; by linking the hearts and minds of the two contrasting men, whose vision is so spiritually one that they see the world together and they see it as one, the shot makes the film's ending, the gun battle that does not take place, completely probable. The 180-degree circle implies that, although Dunson and Matthew may leave their physical world, their physical home, they cannot leave the emotional circle that constitutes their spiritual "home" wherever they may go. Their real "home" is their feeling, their affection, their love for one another (making the film consistent with the definitions of "home" in *His Girl Friday* and *To Have and Have Not*). Matthew's supplanting Dunson as leader of the drive does not break that circle but sustains it. Dunson's fear is that Matthew's specific usurpation has broken the emotional "bracelet" that links them. The final gun battle is Dunson's test—in action not in words—of whether that circle has been broken or not. Matthew has, in reality, sustained the circle that binds him to Dunson by offering a more applicable form of leadership to the particular task that faces them, a task in a strange land where Dunson's particular qualities of leadership no longer suit. By getting the cattle to market, by receiving the check made out in

Dunson's name (as in the Bogart-Hawks films, money is a token of honor in *Red River*), by refusing to draw his gun even when provoked, Matthew proves that the circle still binds the two men and that the two of them have come "home."

Hawks then punctures the mood and mystery of this lyrical shot and moment with a very opposite cinematic device. At the end of the 180-degree pan Dunson gives the order—and Dunson is always giving the orders—"Take 'em to Missouri, Matt." Hawks then executes a montage series of cowboy whoops, yells, and "yahoos," a visual-vocal symphony of energetic faces and determined yowls. This picture-sound montage, which parallels the two montage sequences of reporters' tense faces and terse comments in *His Girl Friday*, emphasizes the men's need for courage, stamina, and commitment in the face of the task and the danger that lie before them. The whirling faces, widening mouths, hooting voices convey the men's attempt to summon the determination and

The montage of "yahooing" faces.

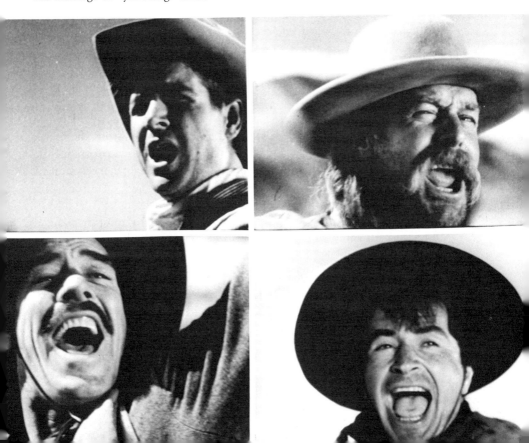

the strength that the drive will demand of them. But Hawks does not allow this heroic moment to pass without its comic echo. Groot, the outsider, the old man on the wagon, tries to summon up his own exuberance with a "yahoo" as well. Unfortunately, his wheezing "yahoo" degenerates into a cackling cough. After this sputtering cough, the drive gets underway, underscored by the vibrant male singing of the song Dimitri Tiomkin composed specifically to "establish the mood" of this heroic journey.[22]

The remainder of the second section, chronicling the degeneration of both Dunson's mind and the men's spirit under the older and harder man's command, is built around three incidents: Bunk Kennelly's theft of the sugar, which produces the stampede of the herd and the death of one of the men, Dan Lattimer; the open rebellion of three cowhands, whom Dunson, Matthew, and Cherry cut down in open combat; and the sneaking away of three more cowhands, whom Dunson sentences to hang when Cherry brings two of them back. This final pronouncement of Dunson justice affronts Matthew's moral sense so violently that the younger man, in preventing the hanging also seizes command of the herd. The strategy of such a section, then, must be to show each of these three incidents as signs of Dunson's progressive spiritual and moral decline, each of the three incidents as furthering Matthew's own sense of his values and their differences from Dunson's.

Hawks does as much as he can to balance our moral sympathies between Bunk Kennelly and Thomas Dunson. In Chase's story, the stampede (the first of three) begins accidentally; Kennelly's saddle strap breaks, his rifle slides out, and the rifle goes off (Part I, December 7, 1946, p. 160). In *Red River,* Hawks converts this pure accident into a moral action. Kennelly has been caught stealing sugar from the chuck wagon twice and punished twice—with a playful whiplash and knife toss—by Groot, once in the prologue and once in a lighter moment near the beginning of the cattle drive. The way that Hawks carefully prepares for the climactic sugar theft which causes the noisy collapse of the wagon's pots and pans, then the stampede (even the script planned for Groot to catch Bunk only once, not twice), reveals Hawks's sense of constructing probabilities. When a man's death—not to mention the loss of several hundred head of cattle—occurs because of another man's childish and selfish action, that other man is indeed morally responsible, guilty of a crime.

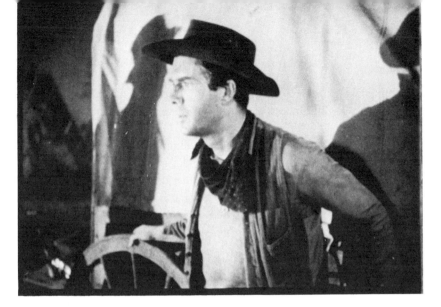

Bunk Kennelly alone with the shadows.

But what is to be gained by the justice, the punishment which Dunson intends to exact upon this guilty man for his childish theft? No punishment could be worse than Bunk's own sense of his guilt and his responsibility for the death of a friend. The shot that Hawks devised, which leaves Bunk standing alone in front of the very wagon from which he stole the taste of sugar, while the shadows of the men troop past him, without speaking, gives Bunk his ultimate moment of shame, penance, and sorrow. He has been banished from the group and stands in a world by himself—quite literally, since shadows are two-dimensional and he is a three-dimensional body.

Dunson lacks the human understanding to realize that Bunk has been punished enough. When Bunk resists Dunson's whipping and goes for his gun, Matthew usurps Dunson's power for the first time, drawing his gun faster than Dunson, shooting Bunk in the shoulder (Dunson would have shot him "right between the eyes"). As Bunk lies on the ground, the other men surround him, sympathizing with his pain and his plight, somehow realizing that he has paid mightily for a crime that was thoughtless, not intended. With this shot of the men surrounding Bunk, Hawks subtly conveys that Bunk has been reunited with the group, accepted back into it, no longer an outsider to a group of trooping shadows. It is Dunson who has become the outsider. Although correct in his abstract moral judgment that Kennelly deserves punishment, Dunson-Wayne's error is the human one of not realizing that Kennelly has punished himself already, that any further physical punishment would serve no human, social, or moral purpose. For the first time, Groot tells Dunson, "You was wrong, Mr. Dunson."

The second of the section's three rebellious incidents lacks the moral complexities of the Bunk Kennelly episode. It is a simple and open rebellion by three cowhands who do not intend to continue the drive any further. The food is bad, the coffee undrinkable, Dunson inflexible, and failure inevitable. Despite the justness of many of these complaints, the men's decision to leave violates their oath of honor which they gave to Dunson by signing on for the drive in the first place. To allow these men to leave would threaten the entire society of men who have joined to perform this action essential to their own survival and that of the land on which they live. If Bunk Kennelly's crime was personal, moral, the rebellion of the three cowhands (three deliberately anonymous figures on this cattle drive) is a social crime, a violation of the film's "social compact." Dunson reminds the men of their obligation openly. When they openly support their rebellion by preparing to draw against an unarmed Dunson, Groot, Matthew, and Cherry all side with the social leader. Groot tosses Dunson a rifle, while Matthew and Cherry each cut down one of the other rebels.

Despite the social rightness and necessity of this killing, Dunson pays for his responsibility both physically and morally. His foot has been struck by one of the rebel's bullets. When Groot comes to take a look at the wound, and to cleanse it with some whiskey, he takes special (and comic) delight in pouring even more whiskey than necessary into the wound, to make Dunson wince with even greater pain. Matthew is also disgusted—with himself and with Dunson—at the necessity of the murder. He tells Dunson, "I'll take your orders, but don't tell me what to think." Soon, what he thinks will make it impossible for Matthew to take his orders. Dunson starts to sleep with a pistol in his hand after this open rebellion, and, like Shakespeare's Lady Macbeth, he finds it impossible to sleep at all.

Hawks interrupts this steady degeneration for a moment of triumph and assertion—the epic crossing of the Red River. While in Chase's story the crossing of the Red is another scene of violent chaos and destruction (the river has become swollen with rain, both men and cattle drown), in Hawks's *Red River* the crossing is a monument to human exertion and accomplishment, to the potential harmony of men, horses,

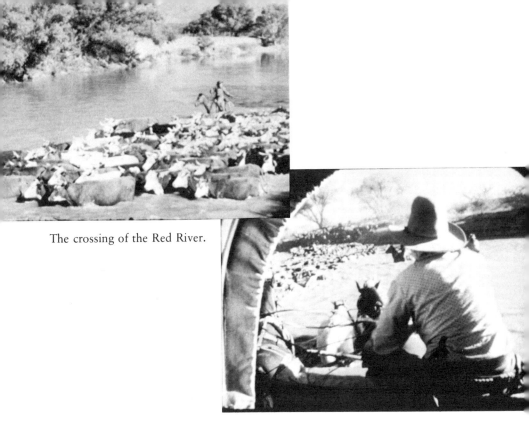

The crossing of the Red River.

cattle, sky, and water. There was no other way to shoot this scene of men driving cows across a river, of course, except to show these men driving these cows across this river. The act of shooting this event becomes as strenuous, as demanding, indeed the same as the event itself. The same will and spirit required to take such an arduous action were necessary to make such a film of this action almost a century later. The parallel accomplishment of both film plot and film production is underscored by a recurring shot in this sequence of crossing the Red River; the camera sets itself up inside Groot's wagon and rides with him, looking over his shoulder, using the curved cover of the wagon as a frame within a frame. Groot, the choric outsider, merely observes the deeds of the cowhands, just as the camera is an outside observer of those deeds. The unity of a real camera, living actors, and fictional characters, all crossing that river, has been established, linked by the simple fact that in both 1865 and 1946 the central task was getting "thousands of cows" across a body of water.

The moment of triumph is succeeded by Dunson's ultimate moment

319

of degradation. Cherry brings the two surviving rebels back to Dunson's camp for judgment. Their crime is a synthesis of the two crimes that preceded it; they are guilty of theft (like Bunk's stealing sugar) and of desertion (like the three overt rebels). Teeler and Laredo—unlike the previous rebels, they are familiar, established members of the film's community—counter Dunson's moral accusations with their own. Their defense is not concern for their own personal safety (like that of the previous rebels) but their being morally justified in deserting Dunson and his now corrupted social purpose. Teeler accuses Dunson of not being the same man who started the drive (the storyteller has provided evidence—Dunson's maniacal sleeplessness—to support this claim) and of forgetting that the herd is not really his own but belongs to the whole region (another moral position with which the storyteller is in sympathy; the drive began with this devotion to a regional and national purpose). Dunson is now the one who is acting selfishly, concerned more with expressing his own will and his own power than with accomplishing the task that needs doing. Dunson's response is merely a naked expression of that will and power: "I'm gonna hang 'em."

With the storyteller's detachment of moral sympathy from Dunson's actions and principles, Matthew detaches himself from them as well: "No, you're not." "Who'll stop me?" "I will." Matthew has heard Teeler's words; he realizes the strength of Teeler's moral argument; Matthew is still committed above all to getting the job done. But Matthew need not face Dunson alone. The community of men joins him, shooting Dunson's gun out of his hand, then continuing to fire so Dunson cannot retrieve it. They too have decided to follow Matthew.

Matthew, however, refuses to allow Teeler to take personal revenge on Dunson, to murder him. He slaps Teeler's gun away from him (another of those slaps in the film), goes for his own gun, and then catches himself. "You're a lucky man, Teeler. That's how close you came." This "coming close" line is identical to a line and situation in *To Have and Have Not*, Humphrey Bogart's warning to Renard after slapping him. It is remarkable that the same line could be uttered by two actors and characters as different as Harry-Bogart and Matthew-Clift (Hawks penciled the line into the script of *Red River*). In both films, the line suggests the character's careful balancing of unchecked emotion with conscious self-control, of head ruling heart. While in *To Have and Have Not*, Harry-Bogart's expressing the line reveals that his anger and emotion have finally risen to the surface to guide his actions, that he can keep control over his feelings only with great difficulty, in *Red River* the line suggests precisely the opposite. Matthew-Clift is telling Teeler (and us) that despite his strong feelings he remains the master of his emotions, conscious of his duties, his obligation to the men, and his debt to Dunson. At the film's climax both Dunson and Matthew will reveal themselves as masters of their emotions, of thinking with both their heads and their hearts.

For a second time Groot tells Dunson, "You was wrong, Mr. Dunson." Although Groot offers to stay with Dunson (out of habit), Dunson sends Groot along with Matthew. Without ever explaining why he does so, Dunson may well be sending Groot to look after Matthew, as his surrogate "father," now that the genuine "father" has been left behind. Matthew's farewell to Dunson is remarkable for its quiet, its lack of movement, the spareness of its speech. Matthew walks over to the isolated Dunson (now it is Dunson, not Bunk Kennelly, who stands alone and apart) and tells him simply, "I'll get your cattle to Abilene." Without moving, without looking at him, without raising his voice, Dunson tells Matthew that he is "soft," that he should have let Teeler kill him because "I'm gonna kill you, Matt." According to Hawks, Montgomery Clift

> thought he had a great scene, but Wayne never looked at him or anything—he just looked off and said, "I'm gonna kill you." Monty didn't know what to do. Finally, he came out of the scene and came around to me and said, "My good scene certainly went to the devil, didn't it?" I said, "Anytime you think you're gonna make Wayne look bad, you've got another thing coming." [23]

Hawks's camera, of course, sympathizes with Dunson's sorrow and loss in this scene; despite the man's moral error, the camera sympathizes with the loss of his authority, control, and ability to lead men. It remains as motionless as Dunson and works toward his back, emphasizing the man's stooped figure, his separateness, particularly when the men ride off together, leaving him alone, a solitary figure in a vast framed space.

Dunson's telling Matthew that he will kill him initiates the film's

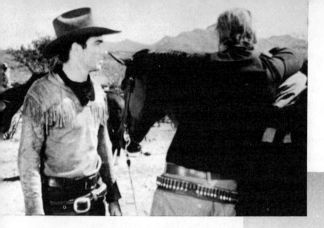

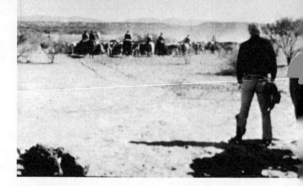

Dunson losing his herd—and the power of John Wayne's back.

conflicting series of probabilities that make the death of one of them seem inevitable. Does Dunson mean what he says? According to Christian Nyby, Leigh Brackett asked Hawks precisely this question at a story conference, after Hawks had decided upon the simple, direct, "I'm gonna kill you, Matt." Hawks's answer: Sure he does. At the time.[24] Times, of course, change. Dunson's verbal threat parallels the threats that the boy Matthew made to the man Dunson in the film's prologue—they are spoken by a person who means what he says when he is not in complete control of his real thoughts and feelings. Both express the warped feelings and intentions of that moment rather than what the characters really and more deeply mean and feel (hence the contrasting importance of Matthew's control over his feelings by coming "that close" but no closer to killing Teeler). When both the crazed boy and the crazed man fail to control their feelings, they are both, significantly, leading cows. At this midpoint of the narrative, Matthew and Dunson have not only reversed their positions of leadership and dominance in the cattle drive; they have also reversed the relative positions of rational control and mature competence, which marked their initial meeting in the film's

322

prologue. It is now Matthew who speaks as a man and Dunson who speaks as a "boy." Just as Matthew has grown up since the prologue, has come to know what a man knows and feels, Dunson will grow up again before the climax.

The film's third major section, Matthew's leadership of the cattle drive, revolves around a newcomer to the narrative (a typical structural shift for a Hawks film), a woman—Tess Millay. The return of a woman to the narrative contributes to two of its established motifs. First, she recalls the film's first woman, Fen, and even refers to her directly—particularly in her identical appeal to Dunson to take her with him (this time to Abilene). As opposed to his refusal the previous time a woman asked to accompany him, Dunson consents this time (revealing his growth and awareness—and again casting doubt on the sincerity of his threat to kill Matthew). Second, the woman furthers the film's fertility and historical themes—the passing of Dunson's spread to a future generation. This link, connecting Dunson to Matthew and Matthew to Tess, takes physical form with the snake bracelet which Matthew has passed to his woman (as Dunson previously did to Fen) after the night they spend "in the rain" (as in *The Big Sleep*, Hawks's subtle, understated use of wet weather implies sexual consummation). Cherry Valance's sexual ease, familiarity, and "hardness" has contrasted with Matthew's apparent distance from women throughout the narrative (another major shift from the Chase story in which Matthew is as experienced and promiscuous with women as Cherry). Among the scenes Hawks deleted from the original script was one that depicted Matthew's sexual ease with the prostitutes in the wagon train. Cherry's provocative observation that "there are only two things more beautiful than a gun: a good Swiss watch and a woman from anywhere," is followed by a provocative question: "Ever had a good Swiss watch?" It is possible that Matthew's answer to Cherry's real question—about ever having the other beautiful thing—is "no." His night in the rain with Tess would then signify his passing of another initiation rite.

Other than these two essential functions, Tess Millay's role, like that of Cherry, remains vestigial in the film. Joanne Dru was not Hawks's original choice for the role.

I had a great girl for *Red River*. She got pregnant two days before we left. Maggie Sheridan had more promise than almost anybody I ever knew. But she married a very nice, dull man, and after five years she wasn't the same girl.[25]

It sounds as if she might have married Bruce Baldwin!

My theory was that she was so good with cards that she didn't have to be a whore. Maggie worked for, oh, two months, beforehand. She could deal anything, flip cards all around and do anything with them.[26]

The woman who could deal cards would return with Feathers in *Rio Bravo*. At least thirty digressive pages of the script—scenes for Tess and Matthew, Tess and Cherry—were deleted from the film's third section.

What remains (and for many the shards of Tess's character, like Cherry's, are so vestigial that they seem incongruous) serves to keep the focus of the section on Matthew and Dunson, despite the addition of a new character. Matthew's love scene with Tess (or is it her love scene with him?) is so brief and understated as to be almost absent— we never see her receive the snake bracelet; we only note, like Dunson, that she wears it. Tess spends most of the section finding out about and talking to Dunson. She becomes the link between the two men, asking Dunson if he still intends to kill Matthew, to which his verbal response is the familiar "Nothing you can say or do. . . ." Dunson even asks her if she will consent to be his wife (the fertility-historical issue again) and bear him the son who will inherit the spread; Tess would agree only if he renounces his pursuit of Matthew. And these are words he will not say.

Matthew first meets Tess during an Indian attack on a wagon train of gamblers and prostitutes (the film blurs Tess's resemblance to her fellow travelers). The Indian attack links Tess to Fen, who lost her life in such an attack on a wagon train in the film's prologue. Like Dunson, Tess slaps Matthew the first time she meets him. And like so many Hawks women, Tess works alongside Matthew during the attack, proving her strength and her courage. This proof, by implication, speaks to Dunson's initial error in abandoning Fen—not giving her credit, because she is a woman, for having strength and courage. Tess also defines a function of speech and talk that differs radically from the tight-lipped ellipses of Matthew, Dunson, and Groot. Whenever she feels scared, frightened, excited, she talks, says anything that comes into her head, just to make noise, to release her feelings. "That's why I'm talking. Just talk and keep on talking." Like the crazed Matthew we first meet in the film's prologue, Tess's aimless stream of chatter is a sign of uncontrolled and uncontrollable emotion. Unlike the boy Matthew, Tess is conscious of her verbal streams—and conscious of their healthy, purgative effect. Hawks will use her babbling chatter at two crucial moments in the film's final section.

That section takes place in Abilene, where the weary cattle drivers experience both the relief and the joy of discovering that there really is a railroad in Abilene after all. As happens so often in Hawks, this discovery first comes to the men as an off-frame sound—the shrill hoot of the locomotive's whistle. As the men drive the cattle across the railroad tracks, we understand that, as with the crossing of the Red River, the men have crossed another boundary—this time the one that signifies they are "home" and safe. The film's final section is a mirror image of its opening prologue, built on an alternation of day (first encounter with the railroad; driving the herd into Abilene), night (an honorable settling of the financial details for the cattle; the reunion of Tess and Matthew in his hotel room), day (the final duel that does not take place).

That night scene in his hotel room reveals a familiar Hawks motif—sexual refreshment on the night before to give the man additional strength and courage for the task on the morrow. Hawks builds this indoor scene around Tess Millay's talk, talk, talk—accompanied by a subtle and ingenious visual device: the hanging kerosene lamp (a familiar enough Hawks object), which this largely outdoor film has had to do without (except for the lamp's privileged position during Groot's poker game with Quo before the cattle drive). The lamp hangs down into the upper-right corner of the frame as we observe Matthew alone, then in the upper-left corner in the parallel shot of Tess; the lamp has seemingly become the physical and spiritual force that separates the two of them, keeping them apart. But as Matthew overcomes his surprise and assertively moves toward her to conquer the gulf between them, he accidentally bumps into the lamp, brushing the obstacle away and walking right through it, as if it either didn't matter or weren't there. The lamp, however, continues to assert its troublesome presence in the room by projecting its shadow onto the wall behind the two lovers, swaying back and forth, back and forth, to accompany Tess's chatter.

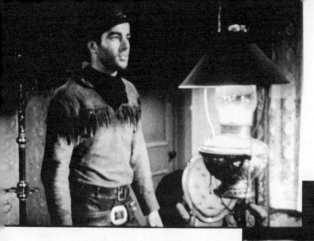

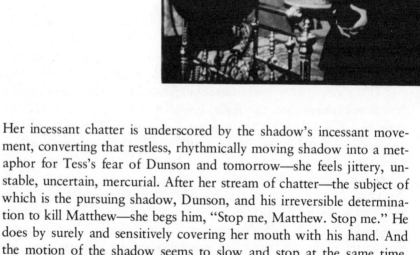

The lamp that hangs between Matthew and Tess (note that given the camera's chest-level position, the lamp had to be deliberately lowered into the frame).

Her incessant chatter is underscored by the shadow's incessant movement, converting that restless, rhythmically moving shadow into a metaphor for Tess's fear of Dunson and tomorrow—she feels jittery, unstable, uncertain, mercurial. After her stream of chatter—the subject of which is the pursuing shadow, Dunson, and his irreversible determination to kill Matthew—she begs him, "Stop me, Matthew. Stop me." He does by surely and sensitively covering her mouth with his hand. And the motion of the shadow seems to slow and stop at the same time. Matthew can take control of this scene (as he took control of the herd and will take control of the morning gunfight) because he knows Dunson as a man, not a shadow.

All the pieces are now in place for the climactic battle. Matthew emerges from the hotel into the sunlight—loose, casual, relaxed. This coolness and looseness will dominate Clift's playing throughout the final scene—implying Matthew's absolute confidence in what he alone knows about Dunson. He knows Dunson, and he knows he can trust

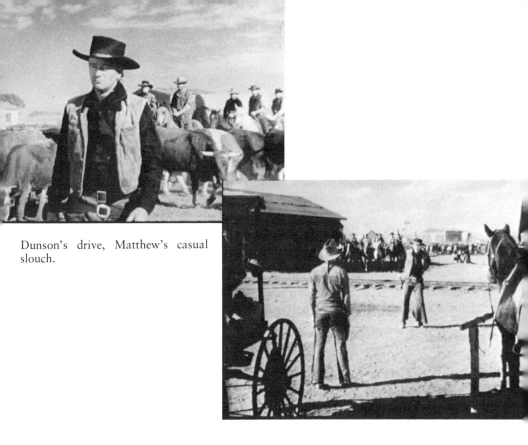

Dunson's drive, Matthew's casual slouch.

him. One of the cowhands passes Matthew a cigarette (the familiar Hawks gesture of affection that linked Matthew and Dunson earlier in the film). Matthew slouches casually, leaning on the horse railing outside the hotel, surrounded by the group of men who have come to love and respect him.

As opposed to Matthew's slouching stillness in a group is Dunson's driving, irresistible motion as a man alone. Dunson strides toward Matthew for this promised final meeting, the power of his walk undescored (as is typical of Hawks) by the striding of Hawks's camera with him. The film's score accompanies Dunson's ferocious walk with an insistent, rhythmic pulse. The film seems to be developing the collision of an irresistible force and an immovable object. On the one hand, there are the fourteen years of love and work that link the two men. As Dunson strides toward Matthew he must walk through the tangible, physical signs of that love and work—the immense herd of cattle that has sprung from the mating of Dunson's bull and Matthew's cow. The cattle which fill the frame during Dunson's final walk serve as reminders of the initial meeting of man and boy and of that circular survey of this very herd which linked the men's minds at the beginning of the cattle drive. The cattle also serve as reminders of the biological continuity and unity of life that link sky and earth, men and women, people, horses, and cattle, fathers and sons—the very biological unity which Dunson's walk threatens. On the other hand, there is Dunson's verbal oath, to which he has always been unswervingly true—"I'm gonna kill you, Matt." And there are the conventional expectations of the western genre, which lead us to anticipate a climactic gun battle, expectations which Dunson's walk, Hawks's tracking camera, and the rhythmic Tiomkin score all support.

At the center of what might seem an unresolvable narrative dilemma is John Wayne. The persona of Wayne, the moral and emotional characteristics of the star as a character, will provide the resolution of the film's narrative dilemma—just as the characteristics of the star persona have provided the "logical" solutions to so many Hawks stories. One of the stories about the film (for which I can find no support) is that Hawks originally wanted Matthew to kill Dunson at the end of the film but changed his mind because "you can't kill John Wayne." (I don't see why not; they kill him at the end of *The Sands of Iwo Jima*.) Hawks says otherwise:

> I certainly would have hated to kill one of them. It frustrates me to start killing people off for no reason at all.[27]

It would have frustrated his audience as well; our sympathies are too firmly attached to both of the men—and to their fertile union—to want to see either of them "killed off." There are no indications in either the Chase story or the film's original script that Matthew was ever going to kill Dunson. Hawks's film works hard and well to make what he must have considered the fuzzy probability of Chase's ending (the paralysis of Matthew's trigger finger, frozen by the inability to kill his surrogate father) absolutely necessary for his. Hawks knew that controlling the audience's moral and emotional sympathies at this climax would be both very tricky and the foundation on which his narrative absolutely depended:

We were walking a tightrope in telling a story like that. Are
you still going to like Wayne or not? [28]

We still like Wayne because the quality of the Wayne persona which
Hawks discovered, defined, and developed was that, regardless of what
Wayne *says*, he will always *do* right at the end of a film (as he would
then do in film after succeeding film—most memorably for John Ford
in *The Searchers*).

It may seem a hyperbolic claim, but no star in the history of film
other than John Wayne could play this role in *Red River* and make it
mean what it does and make the story mean what it does. But then the
same would be true of Cary Grant in *Bringing Up Baby, His Girl Friday,* and *Monkey Business* or of Humphrey Bogart in *To Have and
Have Not* and *The Big Sleep*. The complexity of Hawks's narrative puzzles requires the solid sense that these archetypal stars make of their
roles. Think of Gary Cooper marching toward Montgomery Clift at this
climactic moment (too soft and loose; Cooper doesn't march, he saun-
ters—hence Cooper's appropriateness in *High Noon* or Hawks's *Sergeant York*).[29] Or James Stewart (too calmly reasonable). Or Henry
Fonda (too sweetly mysterious). None of these stars can even walk the
way Wayne does, devouring space with his stride. And for Hawks, to
walk is to be.

The perpetual flaw of the Wayne persona is that he is stubborn—
intractable, unmovable, self-willed. This flaw, however, is balanced by
a more powerful virtue: his absolute honor and his ultimate affection
for others, particularly deserving others. Dunson-Wayne's march toward Matthew-Clift is the culmination of his stubbornness in the film,
but that stubbornness will be overcome by Matthew's appeal to Wayne-
Dunson's honor and affection (hence the importance of Clift's soft, loose
beauty). Matthew must demonstrate in action (not in talk) that he is
still "deserving." He will not draw his gun, as Bunk Kennelly started to
do (and Dunson-Wayne would never kill a man in cold blood). And he
will show in his eyes (and his totally relaxed, controlled body) that he
will never draw his gun. Dunson tries to provoke Matthew—grazing his
face with a bullet, taking his gun away (and reminding him of Matthew's boyhood threat), slapping his face. But Matthew's head is now
the master and ally of his heart; that mastery is what his growing up
has taught him. Matthew is demonstrating in action the love that he

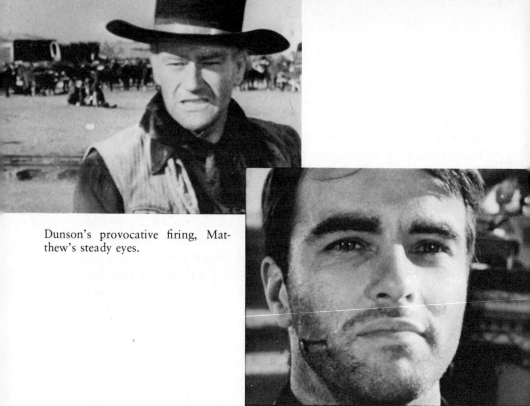

Dunson's provocative firing, Matthew's steady eyes.

still feels for Dunson; necessity may have required him to seize command of the herd but his heart and his mind have not altered in their regard for his father-lover-friend.

The expression of love between the two men consummates a bit raucously. Matthew answers one of Dunson's "affectionate slaps" with a slap of his own, socking Dunson in the jaw, which leads to a marvelously comic expression of puzzlement on Wayne's face as he licks the dust out of his teeth. This sock leads to another of Groot's elliptical observations, "It's gonna be all right. For fourteen years I've been scared, but it's gonna be all right." Groot reveals (for the first time in the film) that his real fear about these two men to whom he is so close has been their tangling with one another, not with outsiders. The affectionate brawl in Hawks's work, not so common as it is in Ford's, can be traced back to his silent film, *A Girl in Every Port*. This brawl ends when Dunson and Matthew ram into a supply wagon, sending its contents clattering to the earth. With the collapse of the wagon, the film closes another symbolic circle. The tension between Matthew and Dunson began with Bunk Kennelly's theft of the sugar, when the clattering pots and pans from Groot's supply wagon started the stampede. Now their tension ends with the clattering of a second wagon's pots and pans. In the original script, a symbolic wheel of fortune hung above Matthew's head, which Dunson's bullets set a-spinning. In the typical Hawks manner, he removes this obvious and fancy symbol for the much subtler, more functional, and more organic one of the supply wagon. Like the swaying lamp in the hotel room, the supply wagon is a richly suggestive symbol because it doesn't seem to be a symbol at all—merely an ordinary, unsurprising object that "just happens" to be there so the actors can "accidentally" bump into it.

Tess steps into the brawl to stop it, puncturing their combat with the firing of an off-frame shot (the third time she has handled a gun in the film). She begins once again her incessant chatter, the uncontrolled flow of emotion as sound, babbling that the two men got everyone worried when all the while they knew they would never really shoot it out because "everyone can see you two love each other." Hawks ends this

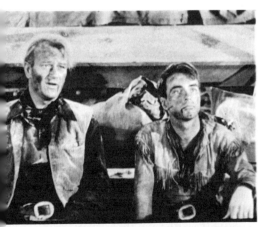

The harmony of the film's three final shots.

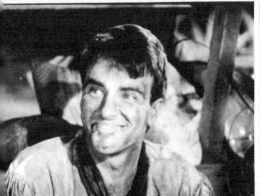

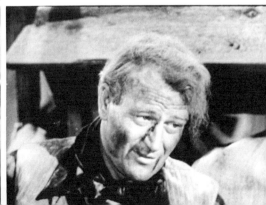

chattering outburst with a comic kicker that deliberately undercuts her hysterical babble—she thrusts the pistol into a cowhand's stomach, leading to his expulsion of a comic "oof." Her departure leaves Dunson-Wayne and Matthew-Clift alone for the film's final interchange (the fact that this pair gets the film's equivalent of the final "clinch" is a sure sign of Hawks's awareness of its centrality). Dunson quietly orders Matthew, "You'd better marry that girl, Matthew." And Matthew asks, "When are you gonna stop giving people orders?" "Right now." But then Dunson gives his final order, which completes the film's narrative circle: He'll add an *M* to the Red River D brand. The broadly smiling faces of Dunson-Wayne and Matthew-Clift confirm the affection and warmth of the two men as Dunson offers his final judgment of Matthew's growth to manhood, "You've earned it."

Despite the film's western, generic surfaces, like all Hawks's best films *Red River* is essentially an internal, psychological story of evolving thoughts and feelings. But the film transcends these usual Hawks strengths—the rich depiction of the spiritual inner life, the elegant symmetries of narrative construction—with its deliberate addition of a larger cultural issue. Hawks uses the film to examine the history and the values of American culture itself. The action of *Red River* takes place at the intersection of history and myth. The film begins with a shot of the cover of a book, titled "Early Tales of Texas." The volume is bound in cowhide, tied with leather thongs; its text is written in longhand, not set in type. This is very much a living history, a history that is still by the people and of the people. While one of the two versions of the film uses these handwritten pages for all its narrative transitions, the other uses a voice-over narration by Nadine Groot. In either form, as freshly handwritten description or as folksy oral history, the film's historical events are offered as a human story that still lives freshly in the memory and the imagination.

The historical pageant the film depicts—the first cattle drive on the Chisholm Trail, from Texas to Abilene, Kansas—is an important chapter in the history of the American nation. That trail represents the crossing of a vast space, in effect the conquest of the nation's vast spaces themselves. Hawks mentioned that the reason for the film's vast visual spaces is that its historical subject is the conquest of those spaces.[30] That conquest allowed a vast land to become one nation (under God), indivisible. The cattle drive, like the wagon train in the film's opening section, always moves across the frame from our right to our left, Western culture's familiar vectoral translation of westward movement.[31] Hawks's frame itself becomes an historical road map. Hawks might well have called his film *The Birth of a Nation*—if he were not given to metaphoric understatement rather than to Griffithesque hyperbole. *The Big Sky* is a glimpse at an earlier chapter in that same historical chronicle, the conquest of a river rather than of the land (unfortunately, that river allowed Hawks fewer visual and narrative opportunities). In *Red River*'s conquest of space, which occurs from 1851 to 1865, bracketing the years of the Civil War (like Griffith's *Birth of a Nation*), Hawks also shows the transition from one kind of cultural leader to another, from one kind of historical need to another. Dunson's virtue of single-minded determination is a lonely virtue. It is the kind of virtue that builds civilizations out of wildernesses, but it is not the kind of virtue that keeps civilizations together once they have been built. That second, more comradely virtue is Matthew's, who wins the gunfight by not drawing his pistol, because the ultimate weapon—and strength, and human bond—is love. Dunson's determination is that of the builder; Matthew's softness is that of the binder. While America required the builder in the period when the narrative begins (in 1851), it required the binder in the period when the narrative ends (after 1865). The events that the narrative chronicles are those of binding—binding men on a cattle drive, binding the vast spaces into a single nation, binding Texas with Kansas, binding Texas beef with the hungry needs of a whole nation.

Like John Ford's *The Man Who Shot Liberty Valance* (which uses the more familiar American symbol for the forging of national unity—the railroad), Howard Hawks's *Red River* is an allegory of historical transition from one kind of law, one kind of virtue, to another. It is typical of Hawks that, unlike Ford, he could handle allegory so casually that the film seemed a mere "action-packed western" (even if this western is actually packed with little action). Also unlike Ford, Hawks could develop an allegory without creating purely allegorical characters and events: like a black man's learning to read by stumbling over the words of "The Declaration of Independence." The differences between Hawks's and Ford's uses of the western as allegory give a clear indication of the two men's differing view of the connection between individual human beings, historical evolution, and moral purpose. For Ford, human beings—whether Abe Lincoln, Wyatt Earp, George Custer, or Ransom

Stoddard—were extensions and expressions of Divine Will, or perversions of that Will, human manifestations of divine purpose; the cosmic master plan required precisely these historical personages to enact precisely these historical-cultural-moral events at precisely this time. For Hawks, history itself is a product of human character and human will, a social manifestation of individual human purpose. History doesn't demand the coming of a Tom Dunson and a Matthew Garth; Dunson and Garth, who have come—and come in succeeding generations—demand that history serve them. In *The Man Who Shot Liberty Valance* the ideal, cosmic power of "the Law" itself demands the evolution from Tom Doniphon's gun law to Ransom Stoddard's book law, even if the gain for civilized society means a loss in natural spontaneity. But in *Red River* the evolution from builder of civilization to binder of civilization arises from the will of Tom Dunson, succeeded and conquered by the will of Matthew Garth.

To construct an historical allegory is to impose a fictional pattern upon historical events. It is to make myth out of history. The perfectly schematic opposition of the hard Dunson and soft Matthew is the stuff of fiction, not of life, the paradigmatic perfection of characters rather than the many internal contradictions of actual human beings. It is common for cultures to affirm their values and their purpose by converting history into myth. Homer's *Iliad* and *Odyssey,* as well as the Old Testament's five books of Moses, are among the most familiar examples of history as myth, myth as history. As Robert Scholes and Robert Kellogg argue in *The Nature of Narrative,* the Homeric epic was accepted as both historical and fictional by its listeners.[32] The two separate urges—to tell stories and to recount facts—did not exist then. The split between empirical narrative and patterned (or fictive) narrative developed many centuries after Homer, primarily with the histories of Herodotus and Thucydides.

Like Homer and the Old Testament, *Red River* is a juxtaposition of legend and history, myth and fact, oral tradition and written record. Like Homer and the Old Testament, *Red River* is an attempt to tell (or retell) to the culture a story of how that culture developed, what and where it had been, so its members could know what it was and, therefore, what it is. Just as these earlier historical myths came to and spread through the culture by the primary means of popular dissemination— the Greek singer and the Hebrew cantor (note the importance of singing in both)—Hawks used the most common form in his day for "singing" his culture's historical myths—the moving picture. Once one begins to think of *Red River* as the kind of historical myth which we call today "epic," it is amazing how many parallels one can find in the film to those epics.

The journey, of course, provides the structure for both *The Odyssey* and the Old Testament's Exodus. As in Homer, *Red River* develops the tension between the commander and his men, and the fact that, although the enemy appears to be natural, geographical, or external, the real enemy is psychological—in the hearts and minds of the travelers themselves (hence, Hawks's paring down the proliferation of Chase's external incidents). As in Exodus, the travelers cross a body of water called the "Red," and the magnificent crossing of Hawks's men and beasts through the real waters of the Red River seems far more miraculous than the crossing of Cecil B. DeMille's Hebrews through the process-shot waters of the Red Sea in *The Ten Commandments.* Once the travelers in both *Red River* and Exodus reach the wilderness on the other side of the Red, their troubles increase. Like Moses's reaction to the prostrate Israelites at the feet of the Golden Calf, Dunson's inflexible commitment to duty, honor, and the written law keeps him from understanding the weaknesses that have driven his weaker but equally mortal followers to the false idol. Like Moses, Dunson condemns his erring followers justly but harshly and, like Moses, he is repaid for his hubris, his harsh and inhuman sense of justice, by being deprived of his command. Joshua, not Moses, takes the children of Israel to the Promised Land, and Matthew, not Dunson, takes the men and the herd to Abilene.

And there are still other parallels. The union of calf and bull in the film's prologue, a marriage which also implies a kind of marriage between Matthew and Dunson (an implication supported by the gift of the bracelet as well as the male-female oppositions in their characters), evokes the mythic couplings of gods, humans, and animals in the Homeric world. Dunson's commitment to "read over" the men he kills reveals the same kind of doing honor to the remains of one's fallen adversary as the warriors perform for the corpses of Hector and Patroclus in *The Iliad.* Dunson's "signing on" the men to make the drive parallels the commitment of honor that the Achaian princes pledged to Menelaus before the journey to Troy. Nadine Groot is the film's choric

Nestor or Mentor, its old, wise man whose age and wisdom give him the privilege to console, criticize, and advise. As the men leave Texas for Missouri, their exuberant "yahoos" are an American western's translation of a warrior's vaunting on the Homeric field of battle. Finally, if *The Iliad* sings of the unbending, single-minded anger of Achilles, *Red River* sings of the unbending, angry single-mindedness of Dunson—quite literally sings of it since song is very much a part of the film's soundtrack, its folkloric evocations, and its heroic spirit.

How conscious was Hawks of these parallels? Christian Nyby, the film's editor, never heard any references to such epic works, although he believed the parallel to *Mutiny on the Bounty* was conscious.[33] And that sea story, with a screenplay by Jules Furthman, who also worked on *Red River,* is a much more obvious direct descendant of *The Odyssey.* Hawks's background and classical education, as well as his fondness for reading and for stories, probably led him to read these epic stories at some point in his life, perhaps at Phillips Exeter. That he knows something of the classic world becomes clear in one of Hawks's interviews where he refers to the original property of *El Dorado* as "a story that was sort of a Greek tragedy."[34] Perhaps the one concrete indication that Hawks might have been conscious of his story's epic parallels was his title, *Red River,* which no one else seemed to like or even find relevant to the narrative. The film's associate producer urged Hawks to change the title, either to something more specifically geographical (such as *In Old Texas*) or more specifically related to the film's heroic task (such as *The Great Cattle Drive*).[35] Hawks's title is a deliberate (and unexplicated) metaphor—like *Only Angels Have Wings* or *The Big Sleep.* Its most specific connection is not to a geographical body of water but to that Biblical body of water in Exodus. It is difficult to explain Hawks's insistence on keeping the title *Red River* except as a deliberate play upon the parallel between a Red River and a Red Sea. Once this single Biblical parallel falls into place, the others fall in line behind it.

What is significant, however, is not Hawks's consciousness of these epic parallels but the way that the particular narrative task he set himself called them forth. He might not have known he was going to make a classical epic, but he knew he was going to make a very big film. Its narrative would be a synthesis of historical fact and fictional story, of a culture's geographical history and its guiding moral myth, of social purpose and personal psychology, of external dangers and internal tensions. Hawks may well have realized, as did his friend John Ford, that the western was America's guiding historical myth, our cultural equivalent of the Trojan War or the exodus from Egypt. Significantly, these allegorical westerns which affirm the virtue and value of the American enterprise were made in the years that bracket the Second World War, when the strength and future of that enterprise was severely tested. Hawks certainly realized that the making of his film was as immense, as epic a task as the action which the narrative depicted, so that the making of the film in the present was not just a retelling of the past but a reenactment of it, bringing the cultural myth of the past into the cultural reality of the present.

It may just be that in telling immense stories of this type, stories which develop the unity of humans, animals, and nature, of past and present, of external and internal dangers, these mythic, epic parallels might necessarily arise. Whatever their source, the *Red River* that results from them is one of the major translations of classical epic and myth into native American terms. Like Twain's *Huckleberry Finn,* Melville's *Moby Dick,* Keaton's *The General,* and Faulkner's *As I Lay Dying, Red River* finds its closest epic affinity with *The Odyssey,* the comic rather than the tragic epic model: the long and arduous journey that tests the strength of the leader and the travelers from outside and inside. At the end of many of these American odysseys, the leader and the travelers pass those severe tests, learn a great deal about the dangers both outside and inside, and, like Odysseus, finally arrive "home."

A NOTE ON THE TEXT OF *RED RIVER*

Before making any critical or interpretive surmises about what an artist may intend in a text, it is obviously necessary to know precisely what the text is. The problem of determining the authoritative text precedes the problem of explicating any text's meaning. This determining of authoritative texts is a common enough problem in literary study—particularly with those early texts which were not personally and carefully prepared by the author for the printer (for example, Shakespeare's plays). It may seem strange that film, a uniquely contemporary art, should produce as many textual problems as these older literary texts, but indeed there is probably not a single major film whose textual authenticity might not be questioned or at least examined. As this study has shown, several different evolving scripts precede the filming itself. Many changes in that script occur during shooting. After the film has been shot, many filmed scenes never become part of the finished film. Even after the film has been "finished" (like *The Big Sleep*), the maker may desire to add or delete material. Many films are trimmed for television—particularly to expurgate "unwholesome" scenes or shots, or to fit into scheduled time slots. It has also become common practice for films today to go into initial release with a particular audience rating (say, an "R") and then for its producers to return to the Rating Board after its initial release to ask which scenes need be eliminated for the film to earn a more popular rating (say, a "PG"). There are enormous differences in the existing prints of even classic films like *The Birth of a Nation, Intolerance,* and *Potemkin.* To put the question into an historical perspective, when an audience one hundred years from now sees *The Big Sleep* or *Red River* or any other film by any other director, what film will they see? This kind of question bodes well for the cinema scholars of the future.

This general problem can be illustrated by attempting to determine an authoritative text of *Red River,* for two radically different versions of the film survive today, and both have some claim to authority and authenticity. One of the existing negatives, which I will call the "Book Version," uses the consistent visual imagery of handwriting on paper, clearly the pages of the book "Early Tales of Texas," for its essential narrative transitions. The second existing negative, which I will call the "Voice Version," uses the voice-over narration of Nadine Groot to provide those same transitions. The Book Version is about seven and a half minutes longer than the Voice Version. Some of that additional length can be accounted for by the slow transitional process that the history book as visual image necessitates. Reading the pages of this book requires three shots—a visual image which precedes the written page, a slow lap-dissolve to the handwriting on the page, the reading of that information, and then a slow lap-dissolve to the visual image that the written page describes or implies. The Voice Version, however, needs only two shots—the visual images preceding and following the written page—which are connected by the simultaneous verbal information from Walter Brennan. This transitional method not only eliminates one of

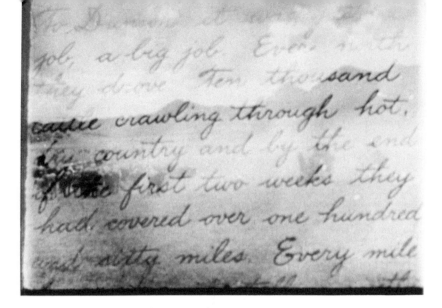

The Book Version's use of dissolves for narrative transitions.

the three shots entirely from the process (and it is a rather lengthy shot—long enough for an audience to read the important written words on the page) but it eliminates the languid dissolves both to and from that page.

There are several other differences between the Book and Voice Versions. A few scenes in the Book Version have been trimmed or eliminated altogether in the Voice Version. Although none of these is very important, the most significant one is Cherry's more detailed description of the particularly beautiful woman who told him about the railroad in Abilene, although he never saw it himself. Also omitted from the Voice Version is a scene conveying Matthew's nervous jumpiness at night, with the pursuing Dunson at his heels. Matthew's nerves parallel Dunson's previous nocturnal sleeplessness, revealing the weighty responsibility of being the group's commander. There is a tendency for the musical score of the Book Version to be more vocal, the score of the Voice Version more instrumental. There is also a bit more music in the Book Version, and that music tends to sound bigger, grander, louder than that in the Voice Version—but the differences are slight, subtle, and inconsistent (for example, at some moments the Voice Version will use grandiose singing where the Book Version uses muted orchestral playing).

These differences between the two versions are clearly matters of emphasis, tone, and color. They are slight and subtle variations and, as the discussion below will reveal, the arguments in favor of authorizing the one or the other will also be subtle. There is one major difference between the two versions, however, that is more pronounced and more important. The final gun battle between Dunson and Matthew differs markedly in the two versions. It is not that the two battles have difference emphases; quite simply, one of the two battles is longer and more complete than the other. At the beginning of the gun battle in the Book Version, Dunson issues Matthew the explicit verbal command, "Draw." His pistol rests in his holster. Dunson next says, "Then I'll make you draw," and he begins to fire. When Matthew refuses to draw after all this shooting, Dunson explicitly tells Matthew that he is "soft." In the Voice Version, however, Dunson starts firing at Matthew—and continues to fire—without saying a word. In the Book Version, there are recurrent shots of Matthew's steadfast eyes, each moving progressively closer to those eyes than the previous reaction shot. The Voice Version eliminates all but the last of these eye shots. Clearly, the problem of sorting out these variant endings is altogether different from that of settling the differences between a visual and a vocal principle of narrative transition.

Let me begin with the subtler issue—the preferability of the visual history book or the vocal narration as a general method for making narrative transitions in this film. The second question, the preferable ending, will require the telling of a story that is almost as interesting as the film itself. As I stated in a footnote to the text, I accept the Book Version as the preferable (i.e. authoritative) text of the film. First, the Book Version is longer; it contains everything that the shorter version does, and more. It had to have been made first (the history book could not have been added; it could only have been deleted). And it was indeed made first.[36] When the film first previewed, this is the version that patrons saw. But just because the version came first does not mean that it seemed preferable to Hawks or anyone else. The first released version of *The Big Sleep* lacked two scenes which certainly enrich the film and reflect Hawks's artistic intentions.

In its previews, audiences (and the film's financial backers) felt *Red River* was too long. United Artists, who were to distribute the film, also wanted it shorter. Further, reading the lengthy handwritten pages took too long—especially for slow readers. Although the clever use of illumination takes the viewer's eye directly to the important narrative passage on the page, there was still concern about losing a viewer who did not have time to read the entire page.[37] The shift to a voice-over narration allowed Hawks to impart the identical narrative information but in much less time, cutting what might seem like five dead minutes from the film's running time, satisfying both the audience and United Artists simultaneously. The fact that the Voice Version resulted from "extra-artistic" pressures in no way guarantees that the resulting version is artistically inferior to the original. Hawks had no objections to the voice-over version, may even have preferred it (he used voice-over transitions for his companion historical film, *The Big Sky*), and never expressed any feelings at all about the preferability of either of the versions (as opposed to his violent reactions to the bowdlerization of *Scarface*).[38]

There are a few minor inconsistencies in the Voice Version from which the Book Version does not suffer. First, the Voice Version begins, like the Book Version, with a shot of the same book, "Early Tales of Texas," and, after that book opens, a shot of the written history's same first page. The voice-over begins with the sight of that book page. For Hawks to establish a convention (the book and its page) and then to drop it is not particularly typical of his careful construction. This is yet another indication that the Book Version was indeed prior, and that priority gives rise to the question of whether Hawks would have used an initial shot of a book at all if he had planned the whole film from the beginning for a vocal narration.

A second inconsistency is that one of the scenes which a Groot vocal passage introduces—Dunson's meeting with Tess Millay—could not possibly have been witnessed by Groot himself. The advantage of establishing the presence of an authorial book to chronicle the film's events is that such a book, unlike any character in the story, stands outside the action and can report, therefore, on all actions. Another quibble about the Groot narration is that Hawks apparently felt he had to use the voice-over narrator more frequently than the history book, to keep that voice in the audience's memory as our guide and traveling companion. As a result, several of the vocal passages are narratively unnecessary, providing information that the visual images themselves supply without any additional aid. Groot's voice, for example, tells us that "Cherry come back, just like I knowed he would," but Hawks's shot makes it obvious that we are watching Cherry's return with the two runaways. This narrative redundancy is not typical of Hawks either.

Nor is it typical of Hawks to use voice-overs. He frequently uses printed visual material to supply transitional narrative information—the calendar whose pages are machine-gunned away in *Scarface,* a newspaper column in *Twentieth Century,* Carmen Sternwood's IOUs to A. G. Geiger or the page of code headed "STERNWOOD" in *The Big Sleep,* Professor Potts's handwritten notes on slang in *Ball of Fire.* Only in *The Big Sky* does Hawks use voice-over—although this film is clearly a sequel to *Red River.* I also wonder if the explicitness and directness of verbal address required for a voice-over narration is completely consistent with Hawks's usual dependence on verbal obliqueness and implication. Further, I wonder if Groot's explicit, direct, and articulate address is consistent with that character's usual evasiveness and ellipticality in his putting thoughts and feelings into words.

Those who favor the Voice Version prefer the folksy, human tone of our relationship with such a speaking companion, the "colorful, idiosyncratic quality of Brennan's voice."[39] Given Groot's role as chorus and commentator within the film's action, it is appropriate enough for him to serve as our narrative guide outside it; certainly no other character in the narrative is important enough and has enough objectivity to tell the tale. Groot's values and perceptions are as close to the storyteller's as those of any character in the tale (or any other in any Hawks tale). By speaking the story to us, Groot converts the film into a piece of oral folk-history, as if we were his listeners, sitting around the campfire, attending to a story that was close to us in spirit if somewhat removed in time. Such a folksy historian would be consistent with the Book Version's implication that this history is still alive and of the people, since the book is both handmade and handwritten. It would, of course, push the book's silent, stately detachment in a more folksy, more familiar, more conversational direction.

Unfortunately, Walter Brennan's narration also pushes *Red River* closer to the smaller, more domestic, more chamberlike, conversational western that *Rio Bravo* is. I prefer the Book Version precisely because it is more epic—not just in the Hollywood sense that big is better but in the classic sense of the term that underlies the film's conception. The languid dissolves from visual image to book page and back to natural imagery allow the eye and ear to luxuriate in the beautiful images and stirring songs without the punctuating crackle of Brennan's voice. The Book Version is lyrical and the Voice Version conversational. The slow, languid pace of the Book Version's visual transitions seems the appropriate poetic rhythm for this tale of heroic human action in awesome visual spaces. The film's epic mood and tone benefit from the leisureliness of these Book Version transitions. Without that mood, that tone, and that languid rhythm, *Red River* does not feel like quite the same film.

To prefer one of the two versions of *Red River* in its method of making these essential narrative transitions is clearly the result of very subtle and complex issues of argument and taste. The same, however, is not true of the specific problem of those two variant endings. The ending in the Book Version is quite simply superior to that in the Voice Version since the shorter duel omits essential narrative details—Dunson's sense of honor (the verbal challenge to draw, foreshadowed by Groot's comic verbal command in the prologue), his determined testing of Matthew ("Then I'll make you draw"), his reference to the film's central opposition (Matthew's "softness"), and the progressively closer shots of Matthew's eyes (which refer to the essential information Dunson imparted to Matthew in the prologue). It is possible that those who find the ending of *Red River* a narrative evasion have never actually seen the film's ending. If Dunson approaches Matthew shooting like a wild man (which he does in the Voice Version), the audience has no sense that the man's action is deliberate, rational, and controlled. It is essential that we understand Dunson at the film's climax as the mature, controlled man we met at its beginning, not as the crazed "boy" who loses his herd to the younger man in the middle of the film.

Not only does the truncated ending of the Voice Version fail to fulfill the narrative pattern which Hawks carefully establishes in the film's prologue but, in point of fact, Hawks had absolutely nothing to do with the continuity of this version of the sequence. The final showdown between Matthew and Dunson was shredded into artistic hash in the Voice Version for "extra-artistic" reasons. *Red River* was scheduled to open simultaneously in Texas, New Mexico, and Arizona the first week of October 1948. Four hundred fifty prints of the film had been struck. One week before the scheduled opening, Howard Hughes cabled Howard Hawks, telling him he was seeking an injunction against the film's opening: Hawks had "stolen" the ending of Hughes's *The Outlaw*, in which Doc Holliday commands Billy to draw, shoots at him to make him draw, and even nicks his ears with those shots. Of course,

Hawks himself had written that scene for *The Outlaw* (the friendly rivalry of Doc and Billy clearly prefigures that of Dunson and Matthew) and was simply using a variation on it again—as was typical of Hawks, who was always willing to use identical lines, business, and situations that had worked before (like "that's how close you came" of both *To Have and Have Not* and *Red River*). Hawks might even have deliberately done the similar scene to show Howard Hughes how to do it right.[40] So Hughes retaliated when he just happened to send this cable on the very day Hawks was leaving for Germany to shoot *I Was a Male War Bride*. Despite his wealth, his power, and his many other interests, that's the way Hughes played pool with Hawks for playing games with *The Outlaw*.

Red River had been shot two years earlier. The production ran $800,000 over budget. The film had been held up by unpaid bills and labor troubles. Hawks's Monterrey Productions was broke. United Artists needed the film's release—and so did Hawks. When Hawks left for Europe, he entrusted the film's release to his editor, Christian Nyby, asking him to speak to Hughes, to try to placate him with some judicious pruning of the final sequence, so the film could be released on schedule. Hawks had relied heavily on Nyby's abilities in the two years of assembling the film. When Hawks returned from shooting it in Arizona, two other editors had initially assembled the footage. Hawks found the result so appalling he telephoned Nyby, still under contract to Warners, at 10:30 one night to come over and salvage the project. Nyby pulled the entire film apart, putting it back into its pieces of individual dailies, then putting the pieces back together anew. Hawks's allowing Nyby to direct *The Thing* was probably his way of saying thanks for saving *Red River*.

Nyby met with Hughes in a screening room, made a few cuts in the gun battle sequence, showed it to Hughes—Hughes still said no. He made a few more cuts. Still no. A few more. Still no. After showing the sequence to Hughes "sixteen times," Nyby said enough. He walked out of the screening room to his car, followed by Eddie Small, "one of the guys who had money in the picture." A nervous Small asked Nyby if he could do anything else. Nyby told him that he couldn't but "I'll tell you what you could do. Howard Hughes *loves* to fool around with film. See what he can do with it." At midnight that night, Hughes phoned Nyby to come view his version of the sequence. Nyby looked at the

Hughes version a dozen times, "to pull a Howard Hughes," then ventured that the sequence would satisfy him if he could add two reaction shots, one of Joanne Dru, the other of the observing cowhands, to cover the fact that the action was "jumping around so badly." Hughes asked where those pieces of film were. Nyby answered, "In my pocket."

Nyby redubbed the sound of the Hughes-cut sequence the next morning, then sent the piece of film to the lab to make 450 copies. The next day he hired "24 or 25 assistant editors and editors" and sent them to all those film exchanges in Texas, New Mexico, and Arizona which were handling the release of *Red River*—to substitute the footage of the Hughes version of the final sequence for the film's original version in each of the prints. *Red River* opened as scheduled.

Several years later, when United Artists needed to strike new prints of the film, they sent their original negative—the Book Version—to the lab. Because of the last minute recutting of the release prints, they had never received a negative with the voice-over narration and with Hughes's cutting of the final gun battle. After the mistake had been discovered United Artists asked Hawks to clear up the confusion. For legal reasons (if not aesthetic ones), Hawks told them to "follow the original release," the authorized Hughes version of the film.[41] All prints that exist today of the complete Book Version descend from this United Artists confusion. Interestingly, none of those complete prints legally circulates. The only version of the film the public can see on television or in theatres is the tonally questionable and climactically shredded Voice Version. That the Book Version still survives can be attributed to United Artists' preservation of both negatives, one of which somehow arrived in the hands of private film collectors, who have continued to preserve the negative and prints of the film which Hawks originally intended. These collectors have performed the same service of preservation for any number of films (Hawks's *Scarface*, for another example).

The Book Version of *Red River* seems to me not only the version of the film Hawks initially intended but the version he really intended. Although he found the switch to Walter Brennan's voice-over acceptable and congenial, my view is that Hawks's original sense of the epic story he was telling, his sense of the film's mood and rhythm (always one of Hawks's strengths), his sense of the particular visual and musical underscoring this particular epic story required was right to begin with. When you add this tonal rightness to the fact that the final showdown between Matthew and Dunson is (understandably) incoherent in the Voice Version, failing not only to make narrative sense but to fulfill the careful pattern of Hawks's narrative plan, there is no question which of the two versions audiences should be able to see. Now that the combatants are all dead, perhaps the real *Red River* (like *Scarface*) might be rereleased. If you haven't seen the Book Version of *Red River,* you have probably not seen *Red River.* [42]

10

The Value of the Stories

Goldwyn said, "There has to be some way you would remake *Ball of Fire*." I said, "Probably could. For $25,000 a week I probably could." He said, "You made a deal." Oh, what the hell! Then he wouldn't let me do anything. . . . One of the things that I said was, "I don't have to use that—what's her name?—Mayo." Not only did I have to use Virginia Mayo . . . but he had her work and run all the scenes that Stanwyck did. Well, she wasn't Stanwyck. . . . It was completely awful. It [*A Song Is Born*] was the most unpleasant picture you'd ever known.[1]

We made a lousy picture that had a lot of great stuff in it called *Land of the Pharaohs*. Everybody in that was a jerk—you didn't have anybody to root for. . . . I didn't know what he [a Pharaoh] talked like either, and I did a lousy job. It was awful.[2]

I knew that he [Rock Hudson] had been in some successful comedies but I didn't know he couldn't be funny. On the first day [of *Man's Favorite Sport?*] I knew I was stuck.[3]

I made *Red Line 7000* and it doesn't work. Because you just get interested in one story and you drop it and go to another story. . . . over in England, they think it's a classic, they think it's one of the best pictures . . . I think it's lousy.[4]

As for *Rio Lobo,* I didn't like it. I didn't think it was any good. I only made it because I had a damn good story and the studio couldn't afford to put a[nother] man as good as Wayne in it, so we ended up with the cast we had.[5]

I<small>T IS NOT POSSIBLE</small> for a Hawks film to be more or less of a Hawks film, more or less "Hawksian." They all chronicle the same kinds of actions about the same kinds of people, told by the same storyteller, with the same attitude toward human psychology, human society, and human morality; they collapse facile, abstract cultural oppositions, by means of the same control of cinema style and narrative structure; they emphasize the communicative importance of concrete, physical data. But just because a Hawks film cannot be more or less a Hawks work does not mean it cannot be more or less good. Hawks himself was quite candid about which of his films he thought "lousy," and an implication of my detailed discussions of nine illustrative Hawks stories is that these films are good examples not only of Hawks's work but of his very best work.

The earliest of these nine major films was made in 1930, the latest (and it, I will admit, is the one film of the group about which there is the least consensus) in 1952. By implication, the nine films suggest that Hawks's richest creative period was his first two decades rather than his last two decades. These first two decades coincide with that period of American film history known as the "Studio Era" rather than the later two decades of increasingly independent production. By implication, this chronology suggests that Hawks, an independent producer, worked better within the commercial assumptions of the studio system than within a commercial system in which most film production had gone independent. By implication, the nine films suggest that Hawks's visual medium was black and white—which is most dependent on the contrast of light and darkness, Hawks's great visual strength—not color (or the wide screen).

Hawks's own assessment of his work suggests an identical pattern. The films that he called his worst—*A Song Is Born, Land of the Pharaohs, Man's Favorite Sport?, Red Line 7000,* and *Rio Lobo*—were all color films made between 1947 and 1970. Hawks has also been critical of all his silent films as well as three films—*The Big Sky, Monkey Business,* and *Hatari!*—released between 1952 and 1962.[6] Of the color films he directed since 1950, Hawks has been enthusiastic in his opinion of only three—*Gentlemen Prefer Blondes, Rio Bravo,* and *El Dorado.* I see no reason to quarrel with any of Hawks's assessments (although I might shade a few of them differently).

When Hawks finds fault with one of his films, where does he find the fault? First, and most frequently, with the stars who embody the characters. He dislikes (to put it mildly) Virginia Mayo in *A Song Is Born* (he seems to have forgotten Danny Kaye, who strikes me as even worse), Ginger Rogers in *Monkey Business,* Kirk Douglas and Dewey Martin in *The Big Sky,* all the "jerks" in *Land of the Pharaohs,* everyone but John Wayne in *Hatari!* and *Rio Lobo,* and Rock Hudson in *Man's Favorite Sport?.* Second, Hawks finds fault with the narrative structures of the films—no one "to root for" in *Land of the Pharaohs,* to concentrate on in *Red Line 7000,* and "not much story" at all in *Hatari!*[7] Hawks's self-criticism reflects an awareness of one of the most striking qualities of his best films—the stars are the characters and the characters are the story. The evocations and resonances of the stars create the nuances and depth of his characters, and those nuances and that depth provide the logic for the action in which the characters exist and which the characters propel. Without the subtlety and richness of Hawks's stars as characters and his characters as stars, we get the bare skeleton of Hawks's narrative patterns and symmetries without the flesh and sinews that make them live. The shape without the vitality produces a narrative that seems not only dead, but also overpatterned, overcontrolled, and therefore contrived, incredible, and false.

When a Hawks film fulfills its narrative conception and fills its narrative shape with the vitality of its characters-stars, it inevitably provokes the same kind of hyperbolic observation I made of John Wayne in *Red River*—no one else in the history of film could have embodied these characters and made both them and the film mean precisely what they mean. Of all the great Hawks films, *Scarface* (also the most mangled of the great Hawks films) seems least dependent on its equation of stars and characters—except that Hawks himself found Muni, Raft, and Dvorak specifically for their roles in the film. Barrymore-Lombard, Grant-Hepburn, Grant-Russell, Grant-Arthur, Bogart-Bacall, Wayne-Clift—these pairs simultaneously give life to the carefully patterned narrative structures and to the psychological and moral issues that lie beneath the structures. Imagine, for example, Rosalind Russell as Susan Vance (much sharper, more calculating, more acidic than Hepburn-Susan) or Katharine Hepburn as Hildy Johnson (more brittle, less cunning, more airy than Russell-Hildy). If Hawks was dissatisfied with Ginger Rogers in *Monkey Business* it was probably because any number of other stars might have played that role as meaningfully as she did. She played "Edwina" without becoming the role and without the role becoming her. So too, if Hawks and other critics have been dissatisfied with Joanne Dru in *Red River,* it is probably because any competent actress could have played Tess Millay and made Tess mean as much as Dru did. (For example, Dru and Coleen Gray, who played Fen, could have switched roles without affecting the film's meaning and resonances at all—except perhaps a slight diminution of the opening woman's power.) Hawks reveals his awareness of this fact by making Tess vestigial to the narrative's central love affair, making her the fourth-most-important figure in that narrative structure, not its essential, central partner.

Hawks's narratives lose much of their power when the star fails to fill the character and the character fails to become indistinguishable from the star. Hawks's perception of the physicality, the concrete physical data, of film sound and film imagery led to his awareness that the story lived or died on the face, voice, body, gestures, and walk of his stars—and on the explosive chemistry of mixing at least two of these faces, voices, bodies, gesturings, and walks together, letting them stimulate and release each other's energies. Hawks's personal theory of cinema required the vitality and the inextricability of stars as characters in order for his stories to seem warm, vital, electric, alive, credible, "fun." For Hawks, a narrative—whatever the beauties of its elegant shape and complex pattern—had to be credible to be "fun" and "fun" to be credible. The stars-characters were the source of both the credibility and the "fun"—which were identical. As Hawks told an interviewer at the time of the release of *His Girl Friday:*

> The secret of making movies which have a natural ring . . . is to let the mistakes of rehearsals be apparent in the finished print. . . . If a muffed line, or a carpet flip get a reaction from the players around and the electricians on the set, be sure that you get that same ostensibly unstudied effect in the "take." . . . If my players are good enough—and I try always to get that sort—. . . I let them interpret their scenes in their own way and ad lib if they like, if it helps the plot.[8]

If it helps the plot do what? To seem as if those very characters are generating those very events just then in just that way.

This aesthetic explains the lower voltage (which translates into a lower credibility as well) of the lesser Hawks films—despite their many beauties. *The Dawn Patrol,* which remained one of Hawks's favorite films "for sentimental reasons,"[9] seems one of those. Its story of friendship between two men who must balance their affection for one another with their wartime obligation to fly against death every dawn, its spectacularly beautiful flying sequences, and its symmetrically circular structure of each man's succeeding to the office of flight commander, forced to send friends to their deaths at dawn, are all unmistakable and essential Hawks. But the human center of the film, embodied by Richard Barthelmess and Douglas Fairbanks, Jr., seems empty. The roles could have been played by anybody who would have embodied the contrast of harder and older, sweeter and younger males. Fairbanks never became a major star of the stature of Wayne, Muni, Grant, Bogart, or Clift, while Barthelmess's period of stardom, with a unique star persona, came almost a decade earlier, as the very soft and gentle juvenile of *Way Down East* and *Tol'able David*. When Hawks uses Barthelmess again as Bat Kilgallen in a later aviation film, *Only Angels Have Wings*, he has become the fourth-most-important figure in that narrative structure, a role commensurate with the size of his sound-film personality.

Today We Live suffers from the MGM attempt to stuff Joan Crawford into the guise of a genteel, polite, suffering, stiff-upper-lip member of the British upper class.

> It was again our little love theme about two boys who get together. Well, Metro didn't have a picture for Joan Crawford, so a week before we started they announced to me that she was in the picture.[10]

It was only with great difficulty that Hawks and Faulkner could get Joan Crawford into the picture at all. The first section of the film—the Crawford section—seems as weighted down with MGM's glossy production values as Miss Crawford seems weighted down by lip gloss, mascara, and pancake, the make-up so thick it is a marvel she can keep her eyelids up and her lips off the floor. (No wonder Hawks did not find MGM a very amicable place to work.) Given the essential Hawks equation of star as character as human being, this obvious artificiality strikes at the root of Hawks's narrative credibility. For the same reason, John Wayne's progressively thickening and obvious makeup of *El Dorado* and *Rio Lobo* doesn't do much for his credibility either. Neither the woman (Zita Johann) or friend (Richard Arlen) of *Tiger Shark* can match the vitality and energy of Edward G. Robinson's embodiment of the Ahab-like fisherman—despite the film's careful balancing of the

Hawks claims of love and friendship and its spectacular outdoor tuna-fishing sequences. And the woman between the two soldiers of *The Road to Glory* (June Lang) also lacks both life and depth, although both of the soldiers also remain rather abstract and pale in the film as well, with two coldly theatrical performances by Warner Baxter and Fredric March. Only Lionel Barrymore's caricature of the grotesquely old soldier leaps to life out of the film, and it springs a little too cunningly and ferociously, as cutely self-indulgent a piece of Barrymore's devouring his scenes and the whole film as any in his career.

The less successful Hawks films of the 1950s and 1960s seem afflicted by a sense of human anonymity, the feeling that the characters have been shrunk into anybodies who are nobodies. Hawks found Kirk Douglas too small a personality to carry the narrative responsibility of *The Big Sky:*

> I don't think there was any warmth in the relationship of these two people. . . . I look on Kirk as being one of our great heavies. . . . And when he attempts to be too pleasant or show friendship, it doesn't come off.[11]

It also doesn't come off because Douglas's close friend but rival in love, a familiar Hawks motif, is embodied by the bland and greasy Dewey Martin. Hawks would use Martin again, but in much more thankfully small roles in *Land of the Pharaohs* and *The Thing*. Apparently Hawks wanted Martin in *The Big Sky* to duplicate the sexual resonances and spiritual beauty of Montgomery Clift in *Red River*. Martin spends as much of his two Hawks films as possible with his muscular chest exposed, teasingly covered by a leather vest with a plunging neckline in *Big Sky* (iconographically identical to the vest which Jorge Rivero wears in *Rio Lobo*), openly bare and heavily "bronzed" (*i.e.* greased) in *Land of the Pharaohs* (as if Martin were testing for Steve Reeves's replacement).

Land of the Pharaohs also lacked a human center, its two principal "jerks" impersonated by Jack Hawkins (the distinguished British character actor who could not carry a film as its star) and Joan Collins (a sexy British anybody). Anybody could also have played the roles of the young men and women in *Hatari!* This is, of course, not strictly true, for these young men and women had to be willing and able to play scenes improvisationally during the actual tracking and capturing of elephants, zebra, and rhinos. Those hunting sequences are among the most kinetically exciting, the most visually dazzling, and the most stirringly authentic (with good reason) sequences in the entire work of Howard Hawks; quite simply, they alone justify the making of the film. But when the international assortment of hunters tries to tell the story rather than track the game, they look and sound like anybodies—particularly uncomfortable in the film's English-language dress. For Hawks, the natural sound of talk is a sign of life.

Red Line 7000 contains such an assortment of dull talking anybodies that even after seeing the film six times I cannot pin the names of the characters onto the faces. The film's problem is not only its three conflicting narrative lines—as Hawks himself observes. It is also the spiritual anonymity of all the beings in each of those lines. For what such judgments are worth, *Red Line 7000* is my personal nominee for Hawks's worst film (or least watchable for all but the connoisseur). Despite the rancid Mayo (and Kaye) of *A Song Is Born,* the film contains several spectacular musical sequences (a familiar Hawks strength) with Benny Goodman, Lionel Hampton, Louis Armstrong, Tommy Dorsey, Charlie Barnet, Mel Powell, and the Golden Gate Quartet. Hawks delights in documenting the way that musicians make music— in the same way he documents the ways that people fly planes, catch tuna, drive cattle, chase game. No film with all those musicians can be *all* bad. *Red Line* is close to *all* bad, including (and especially) its musical number, "Wildcat Jones," not only the worst musical sequence in all of Howard Hawks but one of the very worst in anybody's movie anywhere, anytime.

As the discussion of *Red Line* implies, problems with performers lead directly to problems with the narrative itself. The vitality and individuality of the players create the impression that the Hawks narrative, as complexly patterned and symmetrical as it is, has been generated spontaneously by the players-characters rather than being forced upon them. When the players become anonymous, the structural pattern rules their actions rather than their actions' ruling the structural pattern. The result, as in any narrative when character does not determine action, is a loss of probability and credibility.

The first, MGM half of *Today We Live* (the stiff Joan Crawford part of the film) fails to fit its second Hawks-Faulkner half (the vital "men in war" part of the film, with Gary Cooper, Robert Young, Franchot Tone, and a typical Hawks friend, Roscoe Karns).[12] Both *The Criminal Code* and *Ceiling Zero* seem equally frozen by their static narratives (unsuccessfully adapted from stage plays) and leaden performances (by all except Walter Huston and Boris Karloff in the former, James Cagney in the latter). The four separate concerns of *The Big Sky*—the conquering of space and distance, the closeness of two friends, their rivalry in love, and their performing an event which is a chapter in American history—fail to mesh because of the anonymity of the men and the girl (Elizabeth Threatt, one of Hawks's discoveries who did not become a star—for good reason). *The Big Sky* ironically reveals how powerful and effective were the presences of Wayne and Clift in meshing these four identical concerns of *Red River* into a seamlessly single narrative. This lack of human center and formal shape allowed *The Big Sky* to wander and sprawl for over two-and-a-half hours, thirty minutes longer than the distributor, RKO, would permit:

> I've had a little trouble on a couple of pictures they thought were too long. I made the mistake of making them too long and they made the mistake of trying to shorten them.[13]

While the trimming of *Red River* is perhaps its most lamentable rhythmic mistake, the mistakes in the writing and casting of *The Big Sky* seem far more to blame than its cutting. The two central players of *Land of the Pharaohs* fail to weave its two narrative threads—Pharaoh's desire for the pyramid that will make him immortal, his wife's desire for his lucre—into one. The fact that Hawks (and his writers) did not know how a Pharaoh talked probably led to the casting of the stiff but well-spoken Hawkins, an artificial and uncomfortable preference for "classy speech" rather than the casual cadences of a Wayne, Grant, or Bogart.

If *I Was a Male War Bride* has a problem for some (like Pauline Kael), it might also be a similar structural one: its first half (Hawks's own invention) of male-female love as work and conflict not quite meshing tonally with its second farcical half of bureaucratic obstacles and male-female reversals (which came from the original story on which Hawks based his film). But *Male War Bride* rivals the two previous Cary Grant-Howard Hawks comedies in its comic power, synthesizing David Huxley's comic clumsiness and embarrassments in the presence of Susan-Hepburn and Walter Burns's dynamic vocational energy in the presence of Hildy-Russell. Cary Grant (with five films for Hawks between 1938 and 1952) clearly becomes Hawks's own alter ego in this period, just as the aging John Wayne (with five films for Hawks between 1948 and 1970) becomes his alter ego in the next.

The first two sections of *I Was a Male War Bride* rival Hawks's greatest comic work in their structural precision (another temporal compression of day-night-day) and subtextual tension (the explicit verbal warfare between Gates-Sheridan and Henri-Grant concealing their underlying love, fellowship, and teamwork). But the film's final two sections, in which the couple must first transcend the bureaucratic obstacles to their marriage and then find a bed where they can consummate it, lose this compression and tension. The amusing incidents sprawl and wander over a loose succession of days and nights; the tension between the two members of the previously warring team relaxes, to be replaced by their united battle against bureaucratic regulations. In comedies of this type (from *Much Ado About Nothing* to *Man and Superman* to *His Girl Friday*), the most interesting obstacle to a marriage is the internal one—the spiritual blindness of the central couple—not the external one—the social restrictions against their marriage. That is why Shakespeare and Shaw and Hawks postpone the couple's triumph over this internal obstacle until the very end of their very best comedies.

I find my problems with five other Hawks films—*Ball of Fire, Sergeant York, Gentlemen Prefer Blondes, Rio Bravo,* and *El Dorado*—more complicated. These are films that Hawks admired, and that many of those who admire Hawks admire; they are in many ways very admirable films. But for me, these films fall just below Hawks's very greatest work. Obviously, the problem of *Ball of Fire* has nothing to do with its two stars, Gary Cooper and Barbara Stanwyck, who make the two roles of Professor Bertram Potts and Sugarpuss O'Shea completely their own. No other stars, it seems to me, could make more sense of or give more meaning to these two roles and the action which those roles must generate. I have problems with the roles and the actions themselves. And I think Hawks did too.

If Sugarpuss O'Shea (let us pass the name without comment—although the name itself is an obvious comment) is a stripper, why is she singing (dubbed by the voice of either Irene Day or Anita O'Day) with the Gene Krupa orchestra? Hawks certainly knows that if you're "good enough" to be the lead singer with one of the greatest jazz bands of the era (and we are told it is Gene Krupa's orchestra), you don't need to take your clothes off someplace else.* Samuel Goldwyn probably doesn't know (or doesn't care) that jazz singing and stripteasing are not the same job, and the fingerprints of Goldwyn's smeary hand have been smudged all over the film—in its oversized, cavernously huge library where the professors are supposed to work (the set looks left over from the Gothic *The Magnificent Ambersons*); in its rhythm, which feels two or three beats slower than the usual Hawks pace.

Ball of Fire also depicts a kind of life with which Hawks has little sympathy and of which he has little knowledge. While the same might be said of *Bringing Up Baby*, Hawks yanks the professor out of his museum, out of his enclosed and encaged milieu, and shoves him outdoors as soon as he can. In *Ball of Fire*, Hawks drops the lively woman into the stifling library, into the bookish world of the professor. Further, *Ball of Fire* is a "conversion" love story—a woman's coming to think and feel differently about a man and a kind of life from the way she did at the film's beginning when Potts is "that professor jerk." While *Bringing Up Baby* might also seem a "conversion" story, its real action (as the comic psychiatrist articulates) is its overt surfacing of the internal urges which the woman and the professor feel toward one another from their first meeting. Hawks specializes in the surfacing of these internal urges rather than in the converting or reversing of them. Frank Capra is the master of these reversal stories, and for that reason Gary Cooper is the essential Capra actor-character. Cooper is capable of converting anybody—so openly soft, sweet, and spongy on the surface, so vulnerable, so defenseless (despite his size) compared with the harder, more resistant, more defensive surfaces of Grant, Wayne, and Bogart. Cooper does wear his heart on his sleeve, and plucks others' hearts as a result.

Because the vocation of Sugarpuss remains so vague (and vocation is so important to Hawks), because her conversion seems so forced

---

* The Krupa orchestra had recently risen to the height of its popularity with the addition of trumpeter Roy Eldridge and the replacement of vocalist Day by O'Day. In April 1941 Krupa's band was playing its first major engagement in Los Angeles—at the Orpheum Theater downtown, the film capital's most prestigious movie-vaudeville house. Ms. O'Day, however, does not remember singing for Stanwyck (see her autobiography, *High Times Hard Times*, p. 349).

(Stanwyck is most believable as the tough babe who belts the old house-keeper in the kisser), because the life to which she converts is rendered so abstractly and so unsympathetically, and because Cooper is such a sweet simpleton, the film feels as if Hawks was working in a style, a deliberate fable or fairy-tale, that was a bit foreign to him (like *Land of the Pharaohs*); it lacks the texture, drive, and psychological perceptivity of his five greatest comedies. The same kind of conversion, the same sweet actor, and the same fablelike artificiality of working in someone else's pious style seem to infect *Sergeant York*. If *Ball of Fire* was Hawks's Capra comedy, including its Capra-like confession in a dark-ened motel room that parallels an identical confession in an identical place in *It Happened One Night, Sergeant York* was his Ford moral-political-religious allegory of spiritual conversion. Two conversions, ac-tually—first to pacifism, then to militarism—as York becomes the em-bodiment of Divine Will and Historical Inevitability by capturing and killing a passel of Germans in World War I. The film's milieu seems stranded somewhere between the Okies and hillbillies of Ford's *The Grapes of Wrath* and *Tobacco Road;* its title character seems force-fed on the same kinds of books (the Bible and the history of the United States) as Ford's *Young Mr. Lincoln.*

The two women who form the two poles of *Gentlemen Prefer Blondes*—around which both its narrative and its framed spaces pivot—are certainly far from anonymous beings. But almost everyone else in the film is anonymous, especially the males. The only distinctive males in their world of female, sexual energy are the two at the extremes: the repulsively old Sir Francis Beekman (Charles Coburn—just a bit too old and repulsive for this role, and nicknamed, very appropriately, "Piggy") and the perceptive boy-child, Henry Spofford III (played by the perpet-ually precocious George Winslow). A metaphor for the male anonymity which pervades the film is the United States Olympic team, through which Jane Russell strolls and sings, "Is There Anyone Here for Love?" There isn't—not just because the men are too busy flexing their muscles but because there doesn't seem to be anyone there at all. The men have been reduced to a series of anonymous faces, assorted male bodies, and (a familiar Hawks motif) mere moving shadows on the wall of the gym-nasium. Hawks is certainly reversing the sexist cliché in his anonymous handling of all this beefcake; it is Busby Berkeley in sexual reverse. Given Hawks's deliberate sexual reversals in this film and elsewhere, the parody of Berkeley's sexlessly smiling female faces and sexlessly geometricized female limbs may even be intentional. But there is something disturbingly "Hollywood-sterile" about these male bodies, this plethora of well-muscled flesh which is also completely (and repulsively) inhuman.

The two most anonymous and sexless major males in the film are the designated lovers for each of the two ferociously sexy ladies—Tommy Noonan and Elliot Reid. The former is so coyly cute with his woozily blinking eyes, befogged by a mere Monroe kiss (more sexual reversal), you'd like to clout him with a brick. The latter is so morally despicable and so humanly faceless that his comic punishment (stripped of his clothing and physically degraded, like Cary Grant in disguise) seems insufficient; boiling in oil seems more appropriate. The most improbable and incomprehensible element of the narrative is that the two vital women really have any desire or any use for these two faceless, lifeless, charmless, characterless men. Perhaps we must take them as the male equivalents of Ruby Keeler—sexual mannequins dressed as suitors to suit the narrative. Except they can't dance. However, simply to watch the two women devour space with their prowling walks or consume our visual attention at the perpetual center of Hawks's balanced frames is powerful and interesting enough to justify both the making and the frequent viewing of the film.

Rio Bravo is as elegantly structured a story as Hawks ever told— with its precise, chamber-music-like alternations of night followed by day in each of its four parts. It also carefully develops the interrelated Hawks themes of love and friendship as well as love as friendship and friendship as love. Especially charming and perceptive is Chance-Wayne's competence and control in a roomful of men, clumsiness and embarrassment in a room with a woman. A person's commitment to a vocation is again a commitment to a personal definition of honor and integrity as well as an existential assertion of personal meaning and value. The film also sympathizes with those mortal weaknesses which interfere with this assertion of honor, meaning, and integrity. Walter Brennan's embodiment of Stumpy, the crazy-old-cackling-coot friend, is another of his very greatest impersonations. And the film's dynamite climax (I use the term literally—the final gun battle is built around dynamite) provides an explosive release from its previous claustrophobia. *Rio Bravo* is certainly Hawks's most powerful achievement between 1953 and 1970, perhaps his most effective film since *Red River* of 1946-48. My difficulties with this elegant chamber western can be reduced to four words—Dean Martin, Ricky Nelson. I don't know whether I don't believe them because I don't like them or I don't like them because I don't believe them. In truth (and I am speaking of admittedly personal responses here) I never liked them in anything or on anything (with Jerry Lewis, with Ozzie and Harriet, on records, at roasts). In truth, my reactions to both of them in the film have been influenced by my reactions to their general roles and resonances within the culture as a whole.*

It is certainly not difficult to believe that Dean Martin is a drunk (since this is the cultural persona he has so carefully developed and exploited). Hawks confirms that during the shooting Martin spent most of the film hungover in reality—a perfect synthesis of human being and fictional role.[14] But Hawks also observed that there was something easy, something facile, something uncommitted and undemanding about Martin's attitude toward his work.

> Dean's a damn good actor, but he also is a fellow who floats
> through life. He has to be urged. . . . otherwise he won't even
> rehearse some of his shows. He wants to get on and play golf.[15]

This easy "floating through life," Martin's most attractive quality for those who find him attractive, strikes me as a sloppy facility which I sense beneath everything Martin does, including his playing of Dude in *Rio Bravo* (and the refusal to take work seriously is not a virtue in the world of Howard Hawks).[16] Ricky Nelson, on the other hand, seems a blank in the film. Hawks gets him to do as little as possible and to stand as far back in the frame as the narrative and his contract permit. Hawks

---

* In his discussion of *The Awful Truth* as a "comedy of remarriage," Stanley Cavell observes that it is necessary to be able to respond to Irene Dunne's performance in order to respond to the subtler psychological issues of the film (*Pursuits of Happiness*, p. 233). Noting Pauline Kael's inability to respond to Miss Dunne (in Kael's *New Yorker* Profile of Cary Grant), Cavell writes: "Whatever the causes of this curious response, it disqualifies whatever she has to say as a response to *The Awful Truth*." Similarly, my inability to respond to Martin and Nelson probably disqualifies much of my response to the film, so I will not say much about it and refer the reader instead to those who can respond to the two performer-persons.

thought Nelson did quite well; he also took some pride in pointing out that Nelson's mere presence in the film helped it gross "a million dollars more."[17] Hawks's camera views Nelson otherwise, trying to shoot around him as much as possible. As a result, though he plays the kind of role Montgomery Clift created in *Red River,* and though he succeeds in not "annoying the audience" (to use Hawks's advice to John Wayne), Ricky Nelson (like Dewey Martin) isn't Montgomery Clift. *Rio Bravo* cannot have the same impact on a viewer as *Red River* unless one can respond to the Wayne-Brennan-Martin-Nelson foursome with the same enthusiasm and affection as to the Wayne-Brennan-Clift trio in *Red River.*

During the lengthy musical sequence in the jailhouse, Martin sings a crooning, slurring domesticated rendition of the same musical theme that served as the stirring epic song of *Red River;* the very shift of this identical melody from epic chorale ("Settle Down, Little Dogies") to casual pop tune ("Purple Light in the Canyon") seems Hawks's deliberate announcement of his fashioning a more casual, domesticated film out of his formerly epic materials. Immediately following Martin's number, Nelson sings his—"Cindy"—in which he is joined during the choruses by Martin and Stumpy-Brennan (on the harmonica), while the admiring "Papa"—Wayne—looks on. Of course the two songs relate to the men's *esprit* as a group, as a Hawks community, as songs do in so many Hawks films. Of course their song contrasts spiritually with the "death song" sung by their opponents outside the jailhouse, the same song that the Mexican attackers sang before annihilating the defenders inside the Alamo. And of course the two songs show how brilliantly Hawks could make essential narrative sense and significance out of the conflicting contractual demands of Martin and Nelson, who each had to be guaranteed a song (just as he made essential narrative sense and significance by balancing so many frames with both Russell and Monroe in *Gentlemen Prefer Blondes*). I simply wish I did not have to listen to either of these two songs. Although *El Dorado* lacks this particular problem by substituting Robert Mitchum and James Caan for Martin and Nelson, the film also lacks the tightness, the elegance, the symmetry, the complex interrelationship of love and friendship, and the Walter Brennan performance of *Rio Bravo.*[18]

I have been making very fine distinctions between the works of a man who was a master of his art and his craft. Hawks accomplished that greatest work in the two decades of the Studio Era when the making of films was casual and everyday. Hawks enjoyed the many advantages of the studio system—the large permanent staffs of competent craftsmen, the research and legal departments, makeup, set, and costume departments—and few of its disadvantages, because his "track record" had earned him the power to write, cast, shoot, and cut his films as he wished, in the time he needed. Otherwise he walked out—to some other studio. The heads of most studios were happy to deal with Hawks, who developed the properties and shared the costs—and brought them profits in return. Hawks, in turn, knew how to deal with the heads of studios: it was better to "cut them in for 30% and 'have fun' than 10%" and have trouble,[19] since a studio would be a more interested participant in the project if it were a more interested party in the profits. Although films are made by filmmakers they are financed and marketed by and within the existing system of commercial production. Like most great filmmakers—then and now—Hawks converted that existing system into a reasonably functional, workable partner. Hawks learned how and knew how to make films in this era and within this system.

In the new independent era after the war, however, the financing, making, and marketing of individual films became larger, harder, more special, more difficult (as Hawks's production woes with *Red River* indicate). Hawks had to spend more time arranging to make films rather than making them. The "independent" producer-director became terribly dependent on his financial backers, who had raised the money for his specific production.

> Today they want you to stick to a script and the easiest, simplest way for the physical facilities of a studio is the best way to do it.[20]

Hawks never did his best work by sticking to the script and shooting the easiest way. But when money has been invested (usually by a bank) in that specific script, and when people are being paid for their work on that specific film (and not for their work on the entire output of a studio, fifty-two weeks a year), the director must stick to the script and shoot quickly. And there is no other place to go if you walk out. The three late films on which Hawks had the most "fun"—*Rio Bravo, El Dorado,* and the improvisational hunting sequences of *Hatari!,* all of

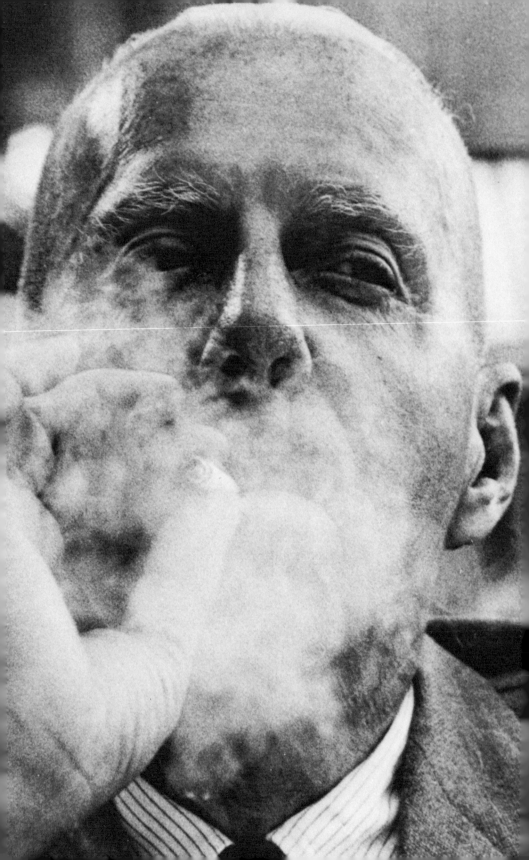

them with John Wayne—were deliberate attempts to get back to the spontaneity of "how we used to make pictures."[21] The greater size of the task of simply getting a film made seemed to reflect itself in the increasing ponderousness and weight of the other films Hawks made in his last two decades. The terrible task of building Pharaoh's immense tomb may have been a deliberate 1955 metaphor for the equally laborious and lugubrious task of making a film in that blockbuster decade.

This added effort and responsibility may well have begun to weigh down Hawks's spirit as well. One of his familiar notions about a vocation is that it represents a circular, repetitive commitment. You don't do a job well by doing it once and having done with it. You do it again and again and again. This repetitive circle, which can seem perpetually exciting and challenging in one's youth, can become vicious and tedious in one's age. The circle itself begins to take its toll. The man performing the task can lose his taste and his zest for doing the job again and again. A friend of mine who worked as an assistant on *Rio Lobo* reported that Hawks seemed impatient, cranky, dissatisfied, disgusted with every setup, every camera angle, impatient with the task and the people before him. That impatience contrasts strikingly with the "perfect gentleman" Christian Nyby describes of two decades earlier. That impatience may also have been a sign of the distastefulness of the vocational circle in which Hawks now found himself. The stars he liked and on whom his stories depended had themselves become too old for his stories—even when he continued to use them (like Wayne).[22] And his eye for new stars faded in the 1950s (*The Big Sky*) and went out altogether (*Hatari!*, *Red Line 7000,* and *Rio Lobo*) after finding Angie Dickinson for *Rio Bravo* (with the sole exception of James Caan). They were all Valerie Whitehouses with scarcely a Lily Garland in the bunch—and like Oscar Jaffe, Hawks was not fully Hawks without some Lily Garland. He had perhaps become bored and bitter. He perhaps wanted to walk out of that now vicious circle altogether.

Even *Rio Lobo* did well enough financially; Hawks probably could have raised the money to make another film if he really wanted to. Like the characters in so many of his films, he said one thing, that he wanted to make another film, but he never actually did. Ironically, *Rio Lobo* went into general release as a second feature on the same bill with that

Howard Hawks in the 1960s

very ponderous Lee Marvin western, *Monte Walsh,* which Hawks refused to make. And *Rio Lobo,* old-fashioned though it was, was commerically successful, especially in Europe, carrying that heavy new-fashioned western on its back as additional commercial freight. The Hawks films of his last two decades convince me that he had become increasingly tired of carrying all that vocational weight and freight.

The aesthetic which Hawks's admirers invoke to explain and even praise the slower rhythms and lower voltages of his late films is that Hawks's films after 1952 are looser and more leisurely—more relaxed and more comfortable creations of an older, more relaxed and comfortable spirit.[23] (Just as John Wayne himself becomes progressively more comfortable in each succeeding Hawks film.) This view—certainly the most effective challenge to the supposition of Hawks's decline—is merely the other side of a coin that is not two-headed. The obverse of loose and leisurely is long and leaden (or "soggy" in Pauline Kael's metaphor).[24] These two antithetical judgments of value, however, share an essential descriptive agreement about Hawks's films after 1952 (which is to say, after Cary Grant)—they differ significantly in their narrative structures, their rhythm and pacing, their spontaneous surprises, and their energetic star performances from the films of his first two decades.

There are other values, of course, which critics might invoke (and indeed have invoked) to question the artistic achievement of either Hawks the younger or Hawks the elder—even granting his undeniable craft and skill at accomplishing the particular narrative and psychological goals he set himself. First, it has been argued that Hawks's vision of the world and the human being's solitary relationship to it necessarily limits his consideration of other important human issues. In particular, Hawks's exclusive interest in solitary men and women who fill up the existential void with their vocational commitment and partnership necessarily excludes the possibility of his examining human action in a universe that is not void but is shaped and filled by certain broader and more traditional sources of human and social meaning. Hawks films take no interest in the home and in the family—two familiar sources of personal and cultural stability which only exist in Hawks's films as metaphors and which can only be applied to his films with the use of quotation marks. A "home" for Hawks is the feeling of spiritual contentment that arises from vocational assertion, while a "family" for Hawks is that small and special community (perhaps as small as two or three) devoted to the same specific vocational task. In truth, the same criticism could be leveled at the works of Hawks's personal friend and spiritual brother, Ernest Hemingway, in whose novels "home" and "family" also exist only in quotation marks. In this flight from family and, more particularly, from the moral and social assumptions of contemporary American society, Hawks and Hemingway are the antistrophe or the recessive to the strophe, the dominant, of a John Ford and a William Faulkner. These antithetical pairs suggest that the conflict of personal assertion and communal commitment is one of the central American cultural issues of this century.[25]

The preference of John Ford to Howard Hawks is one practical and familiar consequence of Hawks's "limited" view.[26] But then Ford is necessarily "limited" by his inability to depict, as Hawks can, solitary men and women in their struggle for spiritual fulfillment and assertion of existential meaning through vocational accomplishment. Hawks—like Hemingway and unlike Ford—defines life by the presence of death. Any clear and powerful vision of human experience necessarily limits the artist's ability to envision its opposite. To prefer Ford's examinations of home, family, and country to Hawks's examinations of work, honor, and partnership is a matter of moral conviction and personal belief. It is an issue that can be debated only on ethical rather than aesthetic grounds, that cannot be affirmed or denied by references to narrative structures, frames of film, the performances of players, or the handling of physical objects. That feminist and gay film critics are extremely receptive to Hawks's films—despite his candid rejection of their views—indicates the parallel moral sympathies of these widely divergent people who define home, family, and country in opposition to their most familiar, mainstream senses.[27]

True enough, although Hawks fills his films with perceptive cultural paradoxes, his works lack a conscious and systematic critique of the political and economic structures which shape the lives of his characters and control the flow of his narratives. Hawks presents his cultural paradoxes—his scrambling the familiar paradigms of male and female, hard and soft, thought and feeling, work and play, love and friendship—as eternal ironies, suggesting the "idealist" (in Marxist terminology) presumption that such paradoxes are inevitable ironies and ineradicable confusions, arising from the nature of human existence itself. Hawks notes the simplistic inadequacies of these cultural clichés without tracing their origins or attributing their existence to the political and economic interests of the ruling ideology. Hawks merely replaces one idealist myth—that men and women are inherently different and unequal—with another—that men and women are paradoxically alike and equal. And there are any number of other idealist-capitalist myths in Hawks's films which are neither ironic nor paradoxical: the myth of individuality and of individualist assertion; the myth of leadership and, consequently, of followership; the myth of private property as a religious right (and rite) and of the financial transaction as a code of honor.

In Hawks's defense, of course, it must be quickly conceded that he was not a Marxist, that his audiences not only were not interested in such a cultural critique but had no perception that such a critique was even possible (much less desirable), and that the very perception of this possibility for film art as conscious cultural critique would need to await the 1960s and Godard (and the application of Brecht's theatre theories to film).[28] For the Marxist, Hawks's films might be most interesting for their internal contradictions—their contentment with certain cultural myths (say, the myth of leadership) and their dissatisfaction with others (say, the myth that men belong in the world and women belong in the kitchen).

Further, Hawks's films reveal no interest in the parallel modernist critique of artistic illusion and illusionism. The Hawks frame is transparent, permitting an undisturbed view of the people, places, and events within it, making his world seem both natural and inevitable, somehow generating itself spontaneously rather than generated by the constraints and constructs of art. This commitment to the illusion of reality in Hawks's films—and almost all Hollywood films of the 1930s and 40s—seems anachronistic to many modernist critics, a preference for the realistic narrative style of pre-twentieth-century fiction and for the realist pictorial style of pre-twentieth-century painting.[29] To criticize Hawks's films—or any Hollywood movies—for their realism is probably to apply a false and facile historical analogy. The popular arts have never abandoned realism (hence their popularity). Not even all the serious arts abandoned realism in the early twentieth century. Some of them—like the novel—have steadily returned to realist mimetic assumptions in the last four decades. Others—like the drama—never abandoned realism at all (especially in America) except for the occasional modernist experiment.

The apparent artlessness and naturalness of the Hawks film world is, paradoxically, the ultimate aspiration of its art—to make the absolutely artificial world of patterned human action seem absolutely natural and accidental. The transparent naturalness of Hawks's images (and those of other Hollywood movies of this period) convinces us of the absolute easiness of such an art—not art at all but life itself, *sui generis,* "fully sprung." [30] This transparency is the ultimate art that conceals art, the perfect art of the easy and artless. If Hawks's films of the 1950s and 60s reveal a decline in their art, it may result not only from the fact that he himself was aging and the old industrial system of production with which he was familiar had disappeared; the very stylistic assumption of an artless art of film was itself in decline—crumbling under the modernist pressures of the films from abroad. Hawks may well have been the most perfectly artful of any Hollywood director at achieving its aesthetic, so perfect at convincing the audience of the artlessness of his art that the artist literally disappeared for every contemporary commentator—only to be discovered by a later generation of critics and theorists as the creator of his world. His actors spontaneously seem to embody the film's characters, his narratives seem to flow spontaneously according to the conventions of their genres, and everything in the Hawks frame seems accidental and unmotivated, like the supply wagon and the hanging lamp that just happen to get into the frame so the actors can accidentally bump into them. The apparent ease and accident of Hawks's stories is the ultimate artistic ruse which allows his monuments of artifice to masquerade as accidental chronicles of fictionalized life.

Like Vashtar's tomb for Pharaoh, Hawks's films will serve as both his and their own monument and testament. It may seem trivial to conclude that Hawks films were great when they accidentally seemed to get great stars in great stories, for Pauline Kael demeaned Hawks's claim to artistic integrity on this very ground in her initial attack on the *auteur* theory.[31] But there was no luck or chance in this union of star, style, and story. Hawks selected the stories for the stars and the stars for the stories. The psychological and moral principles which those stars embodied became one with the characters they played, and the revelation of those underlying psychological and moral attributes became the structural goal of those stories. That revelation, foreshadowed by both our knowledge of the stars' qualities and our perceptions of their resonances through the little bits of physical data which Hawks and his

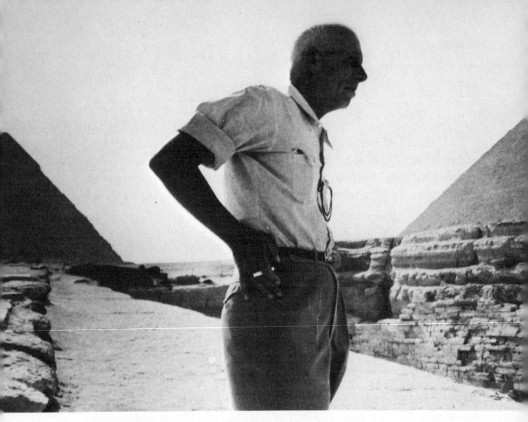

Hawks on location for *Land of the Pharaohs*

stars allowed us to see without their knowing it, became the overall strategy of the entire story. Hawks's camera allowed us to observe that physical data, allowed us to make proper inferences from it, always guaranteeing our making the right inference (by his careful handling of point-of-view) but never explicitly confirming the rightness of the inference until the reward of the story's climax—when the stars' personalities, the narrative's structure, and the audience's inferences become one.

At the end of *Land of the Pharaohs*, one of the newly freed slaves, departing Egypt, looks back on Pharaoh's huge pyramid and addresses a question to Vashtar, its architect. The question and its elliptical answer could well serve as Hawks's own epitaph:

"Will he be remembered?"
"He built better than he knew."

Notes

CHAPTER 1: LIFE AND WORK, STORIES AND MACHINES

1. Howard Hawks, unpublished interview with Winston S. Sharples, Jr., Palm Springs, California, July 27, 1977. Collected with the Papers of Howard W. Hawks, Harold B. Lee Library of Brigham Young University, part I, p. 12 (hereafter referred to as Sharples Interview).

2. Howard Hawks, an interview with Joseph McBride for the Directors' Guild of America, October 21–23, 1977. Private publication of the Directors' Guild, p. 2 (hereafter referred to as DGA Interview).

3. Ibid., p. 7.

4. Ibid., p. 26.

5. Ibid.

6. See Bruce Kawin, *Faulkner and Film* (New York, 1977).

7. Sharples Interview, Part II, pp. 12–13.

8. Ibid., p. 28.

9. Ibid.

10. Ibid., Part I, pp. 5–6.

11. Ibid., Part II, p. 7.

12. Howard Hawks, "Gunplay and Horses," an interview with David Austen, *Films and Filming* 15 (October 1968): 25.

13. Sharples Interview, Part II, p. 11.

14. Both of these Faulkner scripts can be found in Hawks's papers at Brigham Young (Box 5, Folder 9; Box 8, Folders 4–7). So can the script for a third film which Hawks wanted to make for Fox, *Morningstar,* by Robert Carr, which Zanuck also rejected (Box 9, Folder 9). Zanuck rather thoughtfully outlines his difficulties with these scripts in a letter dated January 25, 1951 (Box 5, Folder 8). Both the respectful tone and the relevant criticism of this letter contradict the familiar stereotype of the vulgar and stupid movie mogul.

15. See Kawin, *Faulkner and Film,* pp. 1–2.

16. Ibid., p. 76.

17. Ibid., pp. 77–78.

18. See Ben Hecht, *A Child of the Century* (New York, 1954), pp. 396, 482.

19. DGA Interview, p. 20.

20. Christian Nyby, second tape of responses to author's questions, January 1981 (hereafter referred to as Second Nyby Tape).

21. See Joseph McBride, "Hawks," *Film Comment* 14, no. 2 (March 1978): 41.

22. Second Nyby Tape.

23. Ibid.

24. See *Look,* November 14, 1944, p. 64; Rosalind Russell, *Life Is a Banquet* (New York, 1977), p. 87; and Lauren Bacall, *By Myself* (New York, 1978), pp. 100–164.

25. McBride, "Hawks," p. 39.

26. Second Nyby Tape.

27. Hawks recounts this story in the Sharples Interview, Part I, pp. 17–19.

28. Sharples Interview, Part I, p. 22.

29. This account of Hawks's fatal accident and final days is indebted to Joseph McBride's obituary and reminiscence, "Hawks."

30. In addition to Wood's study, *Howard Hawks* (London, 1968), there is an uneven collection of critical essays in Joseph McBride, ed., *Focus on Howard Hawks* (Englewood Cliffs, N.J., 1972); John Belton's efficient introductory study, *Howard Hawks, Frank Borzage, Edgar G. Ulmer* (New York, 1974); Donald Willis's flimsy summary, *The Films of Howard Hawks* (Metuchen, N.J., 1975); and the recently published collection of Hawks's interviews, edited by Joseph McBride, *Hawks on Hawks* (Berkeley and Los Angeles, 1982).

31. *Focus!* 1 (Chicago; n.d.).

32. Joseph McBride refers to François Truffaut's paralleling game-tracking and filmmaking in *Hatari!* (DGA Interview, p. 6). But I will demonstrate the identical vocational parallels in many Hawks films.

33. See Leo Braudy, *The World in a Frame* (Garden City, N.Y., 1976), pp. 104ff.

CHAPTER 2: *AUTEUR* OR STORYTELLER

1. DGA Interview, p. 3.

2. Howard Hawks, "An Interview with Howard Hawks," by Naomi Goodwin and Michael Wise, *Take One* 3, no. 8 (Nov.–Dec. 1971): (hereafter referred to as Goodwin-Wise Interview).

3. Howard Hawks, Interview by Jacques Rivette and François Truffaut originally published in *Cahiers du Cinéma,* translated and published in *Interviews with Film Directors,* edited by Andrew Sarris (New York, 1967), p. 189 (hereafter referred to as *Cahiers* Interview).

4. Ibid., p. 195.

5. The original and most extreme statement of *auteur* intentions can be found in Andrew Sarris's major essay, "Notes on the Auteur Theory in 1962," collected in Gerald Mast and Marshall Cohen, eds., *Film Theory and Criticism: Introductory Readings,* 2nd ed. (New York, 1979), pp. 650–65. Later Sarris writings, particularly the introductory essay to his *The American Cinema* (New York, 1968), have pulled back from many of his most provocative claims.

6. Several Howard Hawks interviews contain his insistence that Christian Nyby directed *The Thing.* Hawks produced the film, helped shape the script, and advised Nyby repeatedly on how he might handle scenes (as any creative

producer might). Christian Nyby, in a personal tape-recorded interview with the author in May 1980, makes the same claim: he discussed script and shots with Hawks but he himself directed every scene of the film. The relevance of such controversy to a discussion of Howard Hawks is not to attempt to determine exactly who directed what. The collaboration of Nyby and Hawks on *The Thing* reveals that the separation of script and film, directing and producing, cannot be maintained in evaluating Hawks's work. Hawks did not simply direct any of his major films. But if he had directed *The Thing,* the film might not only have shown traces of Hawks's structure and themes; it might also have been a lot more energetic and spontaneous than it turned out to be.

7. John Belton, "Hawks and Co." in *Focus on Howard Hawks,* p. 108.

8. Wayne C. Booth, *The Rhetoric of Fiction* (Chicago, 1960), pp. 3–20.

9. As quoted in Elder Olson, *Tragedy and the Theory of Drama* (Detroit, 1961), p. 158.

CHAPTER 3: STORIES AND MOVIES

1. Howard Hawks, "Interview" by Peter Bogdanovich, *Movie 5* (December 1962): 8 (hereafter referred to as Bogdanovich Interview).

2. Howard Hawks, "Man's Favorite Director: Interview," *Cinema 1* (November–December 1963): 10 (hereafter referred to as *Cinema* Interview).

3. *Cahiers* Interview, pp. 191–92.

4. DGA Interview, p. 9.

5. *Cinema* Interview, p. 10. Stephen Heath also attacks the simple distinction between subjective and omniscient point-of-view in cinema, which "depends on an overlaying of first and third person modes." In "Narrative Space," *Screen* 17, no. 3 (Autumn 1976): 94. Seymour Chatman makes a similar claim in *Story and Discourse: Narrative Structure in Fiction and Film* (Ithaca, N.Y., 1978). Such attacks on the simple notion of "objective" point-of-view in the cinema as Heath's, Chatman's, and my own reveal an impatience with the reigning imprecision of both thinking and terminology related to this matter.

6. *Cahiers* Interview, p. 195.

7. Andrew Sarris, *The American Cinema,* p. 55.

8. Stephen Heath, in "Narrative Space," provides a very effective introduction to the controversy of two- and three-dimensionality in cinema space by drawing upon the three major theories which have addressed this issue: Rudolph Arnheim's *Film as Art,* Noel Burch's *Theory of Film Practice,* and Jean Mitry's *Esthetique et psychologie du cinéma.*

9. Stanley Cavell, in *The World Viewed* (New York, 1971), makes much of this fact in distinguishing a photograph, which is *of* the world, from a painting, which *is* a self-contained world. While it makes no sense to ask what lies beyond the frame of a painting, it makes perfect sense to ask this of a photograph since the question has an answer.

10. Sharples Interview, Part II, p. 5.

11. Ibid., p. 6.

12. DGA Interview, p. 29.

13. Goodwin-Wise Interview, p. 21.

14. Erwin Panofsky, "Style and Medium in the Motion Pictures," in Mast and Cohen, *Film Theory and Criticism,* p. 257.

15. Cavell, *The World Viewed,* pp. 25–29.

16. Goodwin-Wise Interview, p. 20.

17. *Cinema* Interview, p. 11.

18. Letter from Howard Hawks to Jack L. Warner, December 18, 1945. In the Papers of Howard W. Hawks at the Harold B. Lee Library of Brigham Young University, Box 3, Folder 7.

19. *New York Times,* December 28, 1977, Section D, p. 14.

20. The scripts for these three films—in original and revised versions, including Hawks's own pencilled emendations in the margins—can be found in the collection of Hawks's papers at Brigham Young University. Unfortunately, many of Hawks's private papers—scripts and correspondence—were destroyed by a fire in his garage or by exposure to weather before he donated them to Brigham Young. This collection of his papers is therefore spotty—but there is particularly good coverage of the period 1940–1952. Any number of other Hawks stories may have evolved in this same way, but solid evidence exists to support the claim for these three films.

21. Second Nyby Tape.

22. Hawks's use of these cards was described to me by Christian Nyby, in tape-recorded answers to the author's questions, May 1980 (hereafter referred to as First Nyby Tape).

23. DGA Interview, p. 3.

24. *Cinema* Interview, p. 32.

CHAPTER 4: STORIES AND VALUES

1. DGA Interview, p. 14.

2. Goodwin-Wise Interview, p. 23.

3. Bogdanovich Interview, p. 15.

4. *Cahiers* Interview, p. 191.

5. Hawks receives no screen credit for his work on this film, but he may have continued to help Lasky with stories at Paramount even after he began directing films at Fox. Hawks has repeatedly spoken of his contribution to *Underworld.* His personal copies of *Morocco* and *Shanghai Express,* are in the Brigham Young collection of his papers (Box 9, Folder 11; Box 13, Folder 1), suggesting that he must have had something to do with those two films. Perhaps Paramount retained Hawks expressly to help with the Sternberg projects, or perhaps he had already begun to work informally with Jules Furthman, as he would do—formally and informally—for almost three decades.

CHAPTER 5: DANGEROUS PROFESSIONS

1. Goodwin-Wise Interview, p. 24.

2. *Cahiers* Interview, p. 190.

3. See Robin Wood, *Howard Hawks* (London, 1968), pp. 58–68.

4. He repeats the preference in one of his final interviews, the DGA Interview, p. 24.

5. Two copies of the script, one marked "first draft," one marked "revised," can be found in the Papers of Howard W. Hawks at the Harold B. Lee Library of Brigham Young University (Box 12, Folders 5, 6). All references to the script of *Scarface* are to one or both of these two manuscripts. Hawks comments on the added scene in the newspaper publisher's office: "The scene with the publisher was shot by somebody else and whoever did it did a stupid job." (Personal letter from Howard Hawks to John Belton, June 5, 1974.)

6. DGA Interview, p. 24.

7. McBride Interview, p. 21.

8. DGA Interview, p. 28.

9. Ibid., p. 24.

10. Martin Quigley, *Decency in Motion Pictures* (New York, 1937), p. 39.

11. Most of the Hawks interviews contain references to this intention. For example, Hawks describes his telling Ben Hecht the idea for the film: " 'Well, Ben, I've got an idea about a Borgian family living in Chicago today; see, our Borgia is Al Capone and his sister does the same incest thing.' " DGA Interview, p. 24.

12. DGA Interview, p. 27.

13. Goodwin-Wise Interview, p. 20.

14. "When you use close-ups sparingly, the public realizes that they are important." *Cahiers* Interview, p. 195.

15. Sharples Interview, Part II, p. 26.

16. Bogdanovich Interview, p. 9.

17. One member of the audience during the DGA Interview felt the change was "very abrupt; it's very hard to go with that change" (p. 27). The "change" can only seem "abrupt" if one sees it as a change rather than an evolution, and if one assumes that stories make such developments "non-abrupt" by explicating them verbally. Hawks does not believe that psychology—in either life or art—works that way.

18. Censorship boards in some states even required a weaker ending "in which Tony was tried and hung at the end" (Hawks's letter to Belton, June 5, 1974). Because Muni was not available for retakes, Hawks used a double for Tony on the gallows.

19. A copy of "Plane Four from Barranca," dated September 9, 1938, received and registered by the Academy of Motion Pictures Arts and Sciences, September 22, 1938, 4:48 P.M., can be found in the Hawks papers at Brigham Young (Box 10, Folder 5). All references to the story fragment are to this manuscript copy.

20. *New York Times,* May 12, 1939, section 2, p. 25.
21. Sharples Interview, Part II, p. 27.
22. DGA Interview, p. 4.
23. Goodwin-Wise Interview, p. 23.
24. DGA Interview, p. 19.
25. Howard Hawks, in an interview with Alex Ameripoor and Donald Willis, August 14, 1974. Published in Donald C. Willis, *The Films of Howard Hawks* (Metuchen, N.J., 1975), p. 201 (hereafter referred to as Willis Interview).
26. For this description of the visual groupings in the scene I am indebted to a seminar presentation by Mark Kay at the University of Chicago, Autumn 1979.
27. Sharples Interview, Part I, p. 3.
28. No such phrase can be found in *Bartlett's,* or in Concordances to either the Bible or Shakespeare. Todd McCarthy, who is working on a biography of Hawks, also has no idea about the source of the quotation. It occurred to me that the line may derive from some far less literary source: perhaps a training manual or some other book familiar only to fliers.

CHAPTER 6: COMEDIES OF YOUTH AND AGE

1. *Cahiers* Interview, p. 193.
2. Ibid., p. 195.
3. Sharples Interview, Part I, p. 21.
4. For a definition of comic tone and structure, see Gerald Mast, *The Comic Mind,* 2nd ed. (Chicago, 1979), pp. 3–13.
5. Cavell's discussions of *Bringing Up Baby* can be found in several places: most fully in "Leopards in Connecticut," *Georgia Review,* 30, No. 2 (Summer 1976): 233–92.
6. Robin Wood, *Howard Hawks,* p. 68.
7. Donald C. Willis, *The Films of Howard Hawks* (Metuchen, N.J.: 1975), pp. 22–25. This book is an example of how bad a "film book" can be, a parade of the author's opinions unsupported by critical argument and a theory of value. Although I agree with many of his opinions, perhaps more often than with those of Robin Wood (for example, Willis, like myself, considers *Red River,* not *Rio Bravo,* Hawks's genre masterpiece), there is something far less useful and interesting about mere opinion as opposed to Wood's stronger sense of argument.
8. See the *Cahiers* Interview, p. 191.
9. "Circles and Squares," reprinted in Mast and Cohen, *Film Theory and Criticism,* p. 679.
10. I treat *I Was a Male War Bride* in *The Comic Mind,* pp. 257–59.
11. In Cavell, "Leopards in Connecticut," p. 250.
12. Sharples Interview, Part I, p. 4.
13. Willis Interview, pp. 199–200.

14. See the Bogdanovich Interview, p. 11.

15. For this reference to Rodin and for many other observations about the film's sexual puns and suggestions, I am indebted to Stanley Cavell's "Leopards in Connecticut."

16. In the *Cahiers* interview (p. 194) Hawks refers to his own nervous playing with his key chain, a mania which he finds both perfectly normal and quite idiosyncratic at the same time—depending upon how you look at the action. This consciousness of his playing with a material object shows how conscious that method is in his films—for example, Johnny Lovo's saltshaker.

17. In his essay, "The Virtues and Limitations of Montage," in *What Is Cinema?*, vol. I (Berkeley and Los Angeles, 1967), pp. 41–52.

18. The script of *Monkey Business,* titled "Darling I Am Growing Younger," exists in two forms: First Draft Revised, dated February 6, 1952, and Revised on Set, n.d. Both scripts are part of the collection of the Papers of Howard W. Hawks in the Harold B. Lee Library of Brigham Young University (Box 7, Folders 6, 7). All references to the script of *Monkey Business* are to these two manuscripts.

19. Sharples Interview, Part II, p. 23.

20. Ibid.

21. Ibid., pp. 23–24.

22. *Cahiers* Interview, p. 191.

23. The opinion of both Robin Wood, *Howard Hawks,* p. 78, and John Belton, *"Monkey Business," Film Heritage* 6, no. 2 (Winter 1970–71): 19–26.

24. In Cavell, "Leopards in Connecticut." This subgenre, the comedy of remarriage, is the topic of Cavell's recent book, *Pursuits of Happiness* (Cambridge, Mass., 1981), which links seven major screwball comedies (two of them by Hawks) within such a tradition.

25. John Belton (in a personal note to the author) believes it to be Hawks's voice. But it sounds very professionally trained to me—like that of a professional radio announcer. And would the Screen Actors' Guild allow the director to speak on a film's sound track, even as a joke, without joining the union? Certainly the voice is supposed to seem as if it belongs to the film's director, whether it literally does or not.

CHAPTER 7: TWO HECHT-MacARTHUR PLAYS INTO HOWARD HAWKS FILMS

1. *Cinema* Interview, p. 12.

2. Goodwin-Wise Interview, p. 23.

3. *Cinema* Interview, p. 11.

4. Willis Interview, p. 205.

5. Ibid., p. 206.

6. Cited in John Belton, *Howard Hawks, Frank Borzage, and Edgar G. Ulmer,* p. 25.

7. See the section on Hawks in Lauren Bacall, *By Myself* (New York, 1977), pp. 100–164.

8. *Twentieth Century* as a play has a rather checkered theatrical history. Hecht and MacArthur were called in to salvage an originally serious and melodramatic play based on the Svengali legend—*Napoleon of Broadway* by Bruce Charles Mulholland. Hecht and MacArthur turned this fussy study of a Broadway martinet into the comic study of egomania, *Twentieth Century,* which opened on Broadway on December 29, 1932.

9. This distinction between the "narrative mode" and the "dramatic mode" comes from Aristotle's *Poetics:* the mimetic differences he draws between the epic and the drama. That narrative film occupies a position between these two "modes" makes it suitable for adapting both plays and stories. Indeed, the question, Is a film more like a play or a novel? has no very precise or satisfactory answer. I argue this position most fully in *Film/Cinema/Movie* (New York, 1977), p. 18, and in "Literature and Film," an essay to be included in *Interrelations of Literature,* a collection of essays comparing literature with the other arts to be published by the Modern Language Association sometime in 1982.

10. Hawks's appeal to feminist critics can be seen in Marjorie Rosen, *Popcorn Venus* (New York, 1973), pp. 199, 229–30; in Molly Haskell, *From Reverence to Rape* (New York, 1973), pp. 208–14; and in Naomi Wise, "The Hawksian Woman," *Take One* 3, no. 3 (January–February, 1971): 17–19. That same issue (pp. 19–20) contains a brief response by Leigh Brackett, the woman script writer who worked with Hawks on many films.

11. Bogdanovich Interview, p. 13.

12. Ben Hecht, *A Child of the Century* (New York, 1954), p. 498.

13. Several drafts of the script of *His Girl Friday* can be found in the collection of Howard Hawks's papers in the Harold B. Lee Library of Brigham Young University (Box 7, Folder 6). All references will be to these different versions of the script. Without any question, this script, more than any other in the Hawks archive, reveals the greatest amount of tampering, revision, and scribbled dialogue in pencil. There are two drafts, original and revised, on white paper, revised pages of dialogue on yellow paper, and numerous pencilled revisions, in both shorthand and longhand, which Hawks himself scrawled all over the pages. The density of these pencilled revisions supports many of the stories about the making of the film (for example in Rosalind Russell's autobiography, *Life Is a Banquet* [New York, 1977], pp. 87–91) as a very free-spirited, wildly improvisational undertaking.

14. This improvisational line may have been contributed specifically by Rosalind Russell or her gag writer. In *Life Is a Banquet,* p. 90, Ms. Russell claims that she had difficulty keeping pace with the constant improvising on the set, so she hired a gag writer to provide her with lines she could toss into the improvisational melee. This particular line, with its combination of journalistic and vulgar anatomical reference, does not exist in any script of the film, not even in Hawks's handwriting.

15. For many of these signs of Hildy's defeat I am indebted to the seminar presentation of Andrea Staskowski at the University of Chicago, Autumn 1979.

CHAPTER 8: FROM HEMINGWAY AND CHANDLER
TO BOGART-BACALL AND HAWKS

1. DGA Interview, p. 21.
2. *Cinema* Interview, p. 11.
3. Goodwin-Wise Interview, p. 22.
4. DGA Interview, p. 31.
5. Ibid., p. 21.
6. *Cahiers* Interview, p. 193.
7. All quotations and references are to the Scribner's edition of *To Have and Have Not* (New York, 1970; original edition, 1937).
8. The scripts of *To Have and Have Not* can be found in the Papers of Howard W. Hawks at the Harold B. Lee Library of Brigham Young University. The earliest script is dated November 22, 1943, and attributed to Jules Furthman (Box 14, Folder 3). The second script (n.d.) is ascribed to Furthman, revised by Cleve F. Adams (Box 14, Folder 4). The Hawks collection also includes several scenes used for the screen tests, among them the famous "whistle scene" and a test scene for the Cuban revolutionaries (Box 14, Folder 5). Even during screen tests, just before production, the film was still set in Cuba. All references to the film's scripts are to these documents. A transcription of the film's dialogue and a description of its action, edited by Bruce Kawin, has recently been published (Madison, Wisc., 1980). Kawin's introductory essay provides a superb detailing of the project's background and evolution.
9. *New York Times,* October 12, 1944, p. 24.
10. Christian Nyby, who edited the film, does not recall any governmental pressure to shift the film's setting from Cuba. He suspects that the studio's publicity department may have fed such stories to the press to publicize the production (Second Nyby Tape). It is difficult to explain, however, the existence of so many Havana-based scripts; one week before shooting began Hawks was still running screen tests for the Cuban bank robbers. (The pieces of script and the shooting logs for those tests can be found in the Hawks papers at Brigham Young.) Either the shift from Havana to Martinique was a sudden, unprovoked inspiration on somebody's part—Hawks, Furthman, Faulkner, or someone at Warners—or government pressure forced the shift of setting, as reported in the *New York Times* (even if the studio's publicity department spiced up the account a bit). The most likely explanation is that there was some outside pressure during the wartime period when the film industry (Warner Bros. especially) and the government strived to work so closely. Unfortunately, no one asked Hawks about his shift of setting while he was alive, apparently because no one knew about it.
11. DGA Interview, p. 21.
12. Robert Richardson, *Literature and Film* (Bloomington, Ind., 1969), p. 48.
13. John Brades, *"The Big Sleep," Film Heritage* 5, no. 4 (Summer 1970): 13.

14. Sharples Interview, Part I, p. 32.

15. Ibid.

16. John Cawelti's essay, *"Chinatown* and Generic Transformation in Recent American Films," (in Mast and Cohen, *Film Theory and Criticism,* pp. 559–79) contains a useful enumeration of the most common characteristics of the detective-mystery genre.

17. All citations refer to the Vintage edition of *The Big Sleep* (New York, 1976; originally published, 1939).

18. See the DGA Interview, pp. 29–30. With all the interest in the "horse-racing" scene, *The Big Sleep*'s sequel to *To Have and Have Not*'s "whistle scene," no one seems to realize that this earlier scene was added at the same time. The fact that the film was shown to servicemen in 1945, before these two scenes were shot, accounts for the existence of different prints of the film today. For a fuller discussion of alternate versions of Hawks's films, see the note to the next chapter on the alternate versions of *Red River.*

19. John Brades, *"The Big Sleep,"* p. 12.

20. First Nyby Tape. At least a half-dozen of Hawks's interviews also contain variations on this same tale.

21. There are three scripts in the Hawks papers at Brigham Young. The first, by William Faulkner and Leigh Brackett, is dated September 11, 1944 (Box 3, Folder 8). The second, by Faulkner and Brackett, is dated September 26, 1944 (Box 3, Folder 9). The third is a "Cutter's Script," dated March 16, 1945 (Box 4, Folder 1). The cutter's script is a script designed for use by the editor (for this film, Christian Nyby), after the film has been shot, so he knows precisely which scenes belong where in the film's overall continuity. It is not surprising for a cutter's script to contain scenes which the final film does not (these scenes would have been shot but then removed from the film in cutting it). But the cutter's script of *The Big Sleep* lacks two scenes that exist in the film: Marlowe's bringing Carmen home from Geiger's and the "horse-racing" scene in the restaurant. This evidence makes it probable that these two scenes were shot after the film's original continuity had been forged from all those scenes which were already shot.

22. I am indebted for many of these points about the details which Hawks preserves from Chandler's novel, while omitting their explanations, to the Bachelor's essay of Thomas Ryan, the University of Chicago, August 15, 1980.

23. There are two letters in the Hawks papers at Brigham Young from Joseph Breen to Howard Hawks, dated September 27 and 29, 1944 (Box 4, Folder 3). Breen's office was worried in particular about Carmen's "depravity." They also commented that there was too much drinking throughout the film and asked Hawks to eliminate as much of it as possible. Hawks claims that the suggestion for his final scene came from Breen's Office. "The end of the story was done by the censors. They said, 'Howard you can't get away with this,' and I said, 'Okay, you write a scene for me.' They wrote the scene where he sent a fellow out the door" (DGA Interview, p. 31). This claim seems both curious and fuzzy. The script of September 26 already "sent a fellow out the

door," except the fellow was Carmen. Maybe the Breen Office suggested machine-gunning Carmen, and Hawks modified the suggestion so that the bullets from Mars's own men cut down their boss.

24. Goodwin-Wise Interview, p. 22.

25. The 1945 Armed Forces release print apparently contained this one scene with the district attorney, but Hawks cut it when he added the two scenes for Marlowe and Vivian.

26. See the DGA Interview, pp. 29–30.

27. *Cinema* Interview, p. 11.

28. In the revised script, Marlowe was to grind the white queen, which had fallen from the chessboard to the floor, into his carpet. Hawks removed this fancy symbol, which Bruce Kawin attributes to Faulkner (see *Faulkner and Film* [New York, 1977], pp. 117–20), obviously because it was so preciously arty and fancy. Although Kawin told Hawks that he thought eliminating the symbol ruined the scene, Hawks replied that Kawin didn't understand the movie. Hawks had refused to use such purely commentative symbols since the exuberantly youthful "World Is Yours" of *Scarface*.

CHAPTER 9: THE GENRE EPIC

1. Willis Interview, p. 207.

2. Goodwin-Wise Interview, p. 21.

3. DGA Interview, p. 18.

4. Howard Hawks, untranslated interview in *Cahiers du Cinéma* 192 (July–August 1967). Reprinted in Jean A. Gili, *Howard Hawks* (Paris, 1971), p. 116. Translation mine.

5. A copy of these subpoenae can be found in the Papers of Howard W. Hawks at the Harold B. Lee Library of Brigham Young University (Box 10, Folders 13, 14).

6. The story of this threatened injunction will be told in the note to this chapter. The information comes from the First Nyby Tape.

7. Gili, *Howard Hawks,* prefers *Rio Bravo* to *Red River* for its humor. I'm not sure he heard or understood the humor of *Red River*—for example, the comic battle between the singular "tooth" and plural "teeth" in Quo's arguments with Groot.

8. See the Willis Interview, p. 202. One of the interviewers finds the music "too loud."

9. Howard Hawks, "Gunplay and Horses," an interview with David Austen, *Films and Filming* 15 (October 1968): 25.

10. First Nyby Tape.

11. There is a letter in the Hawks papers at Brigham Young requesting the *Post* to use "Red River" rather than "The Chisholm Trail" (Box 10, Folder 13). There is no answer to that letter, but when the story appeared it was not called "Red River." Interestingly, there was pressure on Hawks to use some title other

than *Red River*. Hawks resolutely stuck to it, although no one could see the relevance of the title to the story. I will develop this relevance in due course.

12. DGA Interview, p. 1.

13. Goodwin-Wise Interview, p. 22.

14. DGA Interview, p. 16.

15. The script of *Red River*, heavily annotated with Hawks's pencilled emendations, is collected in the Hawks papers at Brigham Young (Box 10, Folders 15, 16; Box 11, Folders 1, 2). All references to the film's script are to that copy.

16. Chase's views can be found in his interview in *Film Comment* 6, no. 4 (Winter 1970–71): 40–42; Nyby's on the First Nyby Tape.

17. When Hawks was asked about the "homosexual subtext" in his films, his answer was: "That's a god-damn silly statement to make." See Joseph McBride, "Hawks," *Film Comment* 14, no. 2 (March 1978): 39. But the fact that Hawks consistently uses these young, beautiful men, these "pretty boys," and that there are no words in the English language for such men other than beautiful and pretty, which are almost exclusively applied to descriptions of women, indicate that Hawks is playing with a culturally atypical and elusive sense of maleness that might suggest a "gay subtext."

18. The Borden Chase story has never been reprinted. All references, therefore, are to those six consecutive issues of *The Saturday Evening Post*, December 7, 1946, through January 11, 1947.

19. Hawks repeatedly crossed out Chase's lengthy explanations of motivation and feeling, pencilling in his understated verbal ellipses in their place. The kind of dialogue Hawks eliminated can be heard in Anthony Mann's *Winchester 73*, Chase's next screenplay, in which characters perpetually overexplain their feelings and intentions.

20. First Nyby Tape. The narrative symmetries of *Red River* seem especially Furthman-like.

21. Borden Chase himself is one of those who finds the film's ending preposterous (*Film Comment* interview). It is no more preposterous than the one he wrote for his story. And, given Hawks's rather thorough rejection and revision of Chase's original script, his opinion may merely imply sour grapes.

22. Contrary to certain suspicions, Hawks liked the score of *Red River*. In the Willis Interview, p. 202, he says, "Now, the picture you're going to see [*Red River*] has a really good score."

23. Goodwin-Wise Interview, p. 21.

24. Second Nyby Tape.

25. Willis Interview, p. 207.

26. Ibid.

27. Bogdanovich Interview, p. 15.

28. Ibid.

29. John Belton (in a personal note to the author) points out that Cooper was originally asked to play Dunson. Whatever the advantages of such a choice, the film that resulted would have never been the same.

30. See the untranslated *Cahiers du Cinéma* interview, reprinted in Gili, *Howard Hawks,* pp. 115–16.

31. John Belton carefully analyzes this leftward consistency *(Howard Hawks, Frank Borzage, Edgar Ulmer* [New York, 1974], pp. 37–42).

32. Robert Scholes and Robert Kellogg, *The Nature of Narrative* (New York, 1966), pp. 12–15.

33. First Nyby Tape.

34. DGA Interview, p. 17.

35. There is an interoffice memorandum to Hawks from Charles K. Feldman, the vice-president of Monterrey Productions at the time, dated July 22, 1947, suggesting these (and many other) alternate titles (in the Hawks papers at Brigham Young [Box 11, Folder 4]).

36. First Nyby Tape.

37. First Nyby Tape. Chris Nyby claims that when Hawks gave him the written passages which make these narrative transitions, they were very short— only the essential phrases of narrative information. The list of these passages also exists in the Hawks papers at Brigham Young (Box 11, Folder 2), and these transitional passages were indeed only a sentence each. Nyby realized, of course, that these single sentences could not fill up an entire page of a handwritten history book. So Nyby and his wife invented the surrounding text to fill up each page.

38. David Shepard, director of Special Projects at the Directors' Guild of America, wrote me of a conversation with Hawks about the two versions of *Red River* (letter dated April 28, 1980): "In 1977, he did not seem to have strong feelings about the two versions of *Red River,* although his feelings about the changes he was forced to make in *Scarface* were not much mellowed by time."

39. The opinion of John Belton, the only critic I know to have discussed the two versions of the film in print (a column of queries in "Cinemarginalia," *Thousand Eyes Magazine,* October 1974). For me, the gain of that voice accompanies too many losses. Belton also notes that the Voice Version eliminates several process shots that use an obvious and fake rear projection, which violates the film's stunning visual realism. Here, I certainly agree and wish those few disturbing shots were gone. But I'm unwilling to lose so much that is essential to the film for a few uncomfortable seconds.

40. This is what Hawks told Christian Nyby (First Nyby Tape). The story of Howard Hughes's cutting of the film's final scene also comes from the First Nyby Tape. He was in a unique position to tell this story. The quotations all come directly from Nyby's recitations on the tape.

41. Personal letter from Hawks to John Belton, June 5, 1974. Belton believes this decision on Hawks's part reveals his preference. But Hawks may have simply been making the sensible business decision, particularly since by 1950 he was back again distributing films through Hughes's RKO Company.

42. John Belton (in a personal note to the author) wonders about the possibility of making a composite version of the film which would retain the Bren-

nan narration but restore the final gun battle (and several other scenes) to their original form. Such composite texts are common enough in literary study, where scholars choose between variants in an A text and a B text to produce the editor's version of the "best" artistic work of Shakespeare or Chaucer. It will probably be another century before film scholars gain the legal right (because existing copyrights must first expire) and cultural power to establish such authorized texts. Recent attempts to establish authorized texts for films in the public domain, for example, Von Stroheim's *Foolish Wives,* have gained only limited, scholarly acceptance. Most audiences still see the bowdlerized versions. On the other hand, the existing prints of *Grand Illusion* and *Rules of the Game* could be entirely constructed in this manner because Jean Renoir was alive to supervise and authorize the reconstructions.

CHAPTER 10: THE VALUE OF THE STORIES

1. Willis Interview, pp. 203–4.
2. Goodwin-Wise Interview, pp. 23–24.
3. Sharples Interview, Part II, p. 24.
4. Willis Interview, p. 204.
5. DGA Interview, p. 9.
6. Hawks's criticism of Ginger Rogers in *Monkey Business* has been cited already. The dissatisfactions with Kirk Douglas and Dewey Martin in *The Big Sky* can be found in the Sharples Interview (Part II, p. 26) and in the Bogdanovich Interview. Several interviews find fault with the inability of anyone in *Hatari!* to "stand up to" John Wayne and the paucity of that film's narrative as a result.
7. DGA Interview, p. 6.
8. The quotation is from an article by Irene Thirer, "Screen Views and News: Howard Hawks Discloses His Secret for Realism in Films." The article is in the Howard Hawks file at the Lincoln Center Library of the Performing Arts, New York City. No specific source or date of the article is cited.
9. *Cahiers* Interview, p. 196.
10. Bogdanovich Interview, p. 10.
11. Ibid., p. 16.
12. A recent article by Peter Hogue, "Hawks and Faulkner: *Today We Live,*" *Literature/Film Quarterly* 9, no. 1 (1981): 51–58, carefully shows how Hawks and Faulkner attempted to fashion a coherent narrative from these impossible materials.
13. Howard Hawks, "Do I Get To Play the Drunk This Time: An Encounter with Howard Hawks," Interview by Joseph McBride and Michael Wilmington, *Sight and Sound* 40 (Spring 1971): 99.
14. See the DGA Interview, p. 11.
15. Ibid.
16. In his attack on Hawks in general and *Rio Bravo* in particular, Raymond Durgnat also finds Dean Martin's performance inadequate ("Durgnat vs.

Paul," *Film Comment* 14, no. 2 [March 1978]: 66). Although I disagree with Durgnat's general indictment of Hawks, his response shows, I think, that you have to like Martin to like *Rio Bravo* and that it is difficult for some to like Martin.

17. Willis Interview, p. 197.

18. The case for *Rio Bravo* and *El Dorado* has been most effectively made by Robin Wood (in *Howard Hawks,* pp. 32–57, 152–62 and *"Rio Bravo," Movie* 5 [December, 1962], 26–28) and by John Belton (in *Hawks, Borzage, Ulmer,* pp. 44–49, 54–60). I do not believe these films to be as good as they do—not that I disagree with the arguments they make, but I cannot be convinced by arguments they do not make: the problems of performance, character, and energy in *Rio Bravo,* the dissipation of narrative concentration, and the even greater reduction of energy in *El Dorado.*

19. Howard Hawks, "Gunplay and Horses," an interview with David Austen, *Films and Filming* 15 (October 1968): 26.

20. Bogdanovich Interview, p. 17.

21. Ibid.

22. See Joseph McBride's obituary tribute, "Hawks," *Film Comment* 14, no. 2 (March, 1978): 36ff.

23. See William Paul, "Hawks vs. Durgnat," *Film Comment* 14, no. 1 (Jan.–Feb. 1978): 68ff.

24. Pauline Kael, "Circles and Squares," in Mast and Cohen, *Film Theory and Criticism,* p. 677.

25. A chapter of Paul Seydor's *Peckinpah: The Western Films* (Champaign-Urbana, 1980), entitled "The Masculine Principle in American Art and Expression," provides a superb historical summary of this very opposition.

26. Peter Wollen ultimately prefers Ford to Hawks for this reason. In *Signs and Meaning in the Cinema* (Bloomington, Ind., 1972), p. 102.

27. Hawks's feminist admirers have been cited in an earlier chapter. Robin Wood's "Responsibilities of the Gay Film Critic," *Film Comment* 14, no. 1 (Jan.–Feb. 1978): 12ff, assesses his present responses to Hawks and Ingmar Bergman, about both of whom he had written books before he "came out." Wood finds Hawks far more relevant to gay issues than Bergman. In his Hawks obituary-reminiscence, Joseph McBride also notes Hawks's appeal to the gay sensibility.

28. One of the young Brecht's statements sounds surprisingly close to Hawks, however—a statement conveniently overlooked by Marxist-Brechtian critics and unfortunately ignored by many Marxist-Brechtian filmmakers: *"Nobody who fails to get fun out of his activities can expect them to be fun for anybody else"* (Brecht's italics). In Bertolt Brecht, *Brecht on Theatre,* trans. John Willett (London, 1964), p. 7. A very good summary of the Brechtian-modernist-materialist critique of film can be found in Peter Wollen, "Ontology and Materialism in Film," *Screen* 17, no. 1 (Spring 1976): 7–23.

29. Examples of the modernist prejudice against realist Hollywood movies can be found in Robert Richardson, *Literature and Film* (Bloomington, Ind., 1969) and Keith Cohen, *Film and Fiction* (New Haven, Conn., 1979). Both

critics assume the modernist norm for twentieth-century fiction and either disparage or simply ignore any film storytelling that does not accept the same norm.

30. In the first chapter of *The World Viewed* (New York, 1971), Stanley Cavell describes his surprise when first encountering the *auteur* theory, for he previously accepted these films as creatorless, believing they "sprang full grown" (p. 7) from the Hollywood world itself. Cavell claims that most film audiences accepted those films exactly that way in the 1930s and 40s, and were expected to do so. Hawks, the most invisible master of that aesthetic, would therefore be its most complete embodiment precisely because of his invisibility.

31. Pauline Kael, "Circles and Squares," p. 677: "When he has good material, he's capable of better than good direction . . . with help from the actors he can jazz up ridiculous scripts."

Bibliography

BOOKS ON HAWKS

Belton, John. *The Hollywood Professionals* (volume 3): *Howard Hawks, Frank Borzage, Edgar G. Ulmer.* New York: A. S. Barnes, 1974.

Gili, Jean A. *Howard Hawks.* Paris: Editions Seghers, 1971.

McBride, Joseph, ed. *Focus on Howard Hawks.* Englewood Cliffs, N.J.: Prentice-Hall, 1972.

_____. *Hawks on Hawks.* Berkeley and Los Angeles: University of California Press, 1982.

Missiaen, Jean-Claude. *Howard Hawks.* Paris: Editions Universitaires, 1966.

Willis, Donald C. *The Films of Howard Hawks.* Metuchen, N.J.: Scarecrow Press, 1976.

Wood, Robin. *Howard Hawks.* London: Secker and Warburg, 1968.

INTERVIEWS WITH HAWKS (in chronological order)

Becker, Jacques, Jacques, Rivette, and François Truffaut. "Interview with Howard Hawks," *Cahiers du cinéma* 56 (Feb. 1956), translated into English and published in Andrew Sarris, ed., *Interviews with Film Directors.* New York: Bobbs-Merrill, 1967, pp. 186–96.

Bogdanovich, Peter. "Interview," *Movie* 5 (Dec. 1962), pp. 8–18.

"Man's Favorite Director," *Cinema* 1 (Nov.–Dec. 1963), pp. 10–12, 31–32.

Austen, David. "Gunplay and Horses," *Films and Filming* 1 (Oct. 1968), pp. 25–27.

McBride, Joseph, and Michael Wilmington. "A Discussion with the Audience of the 1970 Chicago Film Festival," in Joseph McBride, ed., *Focus on Howard Hawks,* pp. 14–26.

_____. "Do I Get To Play the Drunk This Time? An Encounter with Howard Hawks," *Sight and Sound* 40, no. 2 (Spring 1971), pp. 97–100.

Goodwin, Michael, and Naomi Wise. "An Interview with Howard Hawks," *Take One* 3, no. 8 (July–Aug. 1971), pp. 19–25.

Ameripoor, Alex, and Don Willis. "Howard Hawks: An Interview [August 14, 1974]," in Donald C. Willis, *The Films of Howard Hawks,* pp. 196–209.

Lehman, Peter, and Staff. "Howard Hawks: A Private Interview," *Wide Angle* 1, no. 2 (Summer 1976), pp. 28–57.

Sharples, Winston S., Jr. Unpublished interview [July 27, 1977]. In the papers of Howard Winchester Hawks, Harold B. Lee Library, Brigham Young University, Box 1, Folder 13.

McBride, Joseph. Unpublished interview, for the Directors' Guild of America, Laguna Conference, October 21–23, 1977.

GENERAL ARTICLES ON HAWKS (in English)

"Ace Director at Pinnacle in Films," *Literary Digest* 121 (Feb. 15, 1936), p. 24.

Belton, John. "Hawks and Co.," in Joseph McBride, ed., *Focus on Howard Hawks,* pp. 94–108.

"Best Dressed Woman," *Time* 47 (Jan. 6, 1947), p. 38.

Brackett, Leigh. "A Comment on the Hawksian Woman," *Take One* 3, no. 8 (July–Aug. 1971), pp. 17-20.

Durgnat, Raymond. "Durgnat vs. Paul: Last Round in the Great Hawks Debate," *Film Comment* 14, no. 2 (March–April 1978), pp. 64–68.

————. "Hawks Isn't Good Enough," *Film Comment* 13, no. 3 (July–Aug. 1977), pp. 8–19.

Dyer, Peter John. "Sling the Lamps Low," in Joseph McBride, ed., *Focus on Howard Hawks,* pp. 78–93.

Farber, Manny. "Howard Hawks," in Joseph McBride, ed., *Focus on Howard Hawks,* pp. 28–34.

————. "Howard Hawks and the Action Film," in Leo Braudy and Morris Dickstein, eds., *Great Film Directors.* New York: Oxford University Press, 1978, pp. 437–44.

Giannetti, Louis. "Howard Hawks," in *Masters of the American Cinema,* Englewood Cliffs, N.J.: Prentice-Hall, 1981, pp. 184–204.

Kasindorf, Martin. "The Hawk," *Newsweek* 77 (Feb. 8, 1971), pp. 96, 98.

Langlois, Henri. "The Modernity of Howard Hawks," in Joseph McBride, ed., *Focus on Howard Hawks,* pp. 65–69.

Mast, Gerald. "Howard Hawks," in *The Comic Mind: Comedy and the Movies,* 2nd ed. Chicago: University of Chicago Press, 1979, pp. 250–59.

McBride, Joseph. "Introduction" to *Focus on Howard Hawks,* pp. 1–7.

————. "Hawks," *Film Comment* 14, no. 2 (March–April 1978), pp. 36–41.

Obituary. *The New York Times,* Dec. 28, 1977, section D, p. 14.

Paul, William. "Paul vs. Durgnat," *Film Comment* 14, no. 1 (Jan.–Feb. 1978), pp. 68–71.

Peary, Gerald, and S. Groash. "Hawks at Warner Bros.: 1932," *Velvet Light Trap* 1 (June 1971).

Perkins, V. F. "Comedies," *Movie* 5 (Dec. 1962), pp. 21–22.

Rivette, Jacques. "The Genius of Howard Hawks," in Joseph McBride, ed., *Focus on Howard Hawks,* pp. 70–77. And in Leo Braudy and Morris Dickstein, eds. *Great Film Directors,* pp. 445–51.

_____. "Rivette on Hawks," *Movie* 5 (Dec. 1962), pp. 19–20.

Sarris, Andrew. "The World of Howard Hawks," in Joseph McBride, ed., *Focus on Howard Hawks,* pp. 35–64.

"Slim Hawks Voted Best-Dressed Woman," *Life* 22 (Jan. 20, 1947), pp. 67–71.

Wellman, William, Jr. "Howard Hawks: The Distance Runner," in Joseph McBride, ed., *Focus on Howard Hawks,* pp. 8–12.

Wise, Naomi. "The Hawksian Woman," *Take One* 3, no. 3 (Jan.–Feb. 1971), pp. 17–29.

Wollen, Peter. "The Auteur Theory," in Gerald Mast and Marshall Cohen, eds., *Film Theory and Criticism: Introductory Readings,* 2nd ed. New York: Oxford University Press, 1979, pp. 680–91.

Wood, Robin. "Responsibilities of the Gay Film Critic," *Film Comment* 14, no. 1 (Jan.–Feb. 1978), pp. 12–18.

_____. "Who the Hell Is Howard Hawks?" *Focus!* 1 and 2 (1967), pp. 3–6; 8–18.

EXTENDED DISCUSSION OF INDIVIDUAL FILMS

AIR FORCE
   Crichton, Kyle. "Director Hawks Makes His Greatest Movie: *Air Force,*" *Colliers,* Jan. 16, 1943, pp. 36ff.

THE BIG SKY
   Alpert, Hollis. "In the Land of the Blue Teal Eye," *Saturday Review* 35 (Aug. 16, 1952), pp. 28–29.
   "The Big Sky," *Films in Review* 3, no. 7 (Aug.–Sept. 1952), p. 357.

THE BIG SLEEP
   Brades, John. "The Big Sleep," *Film Heritage* 5, no. 4 (Summer 1970), pp. 7–15.
   Davis, Paxton. "Bogart, Hawks, and *The Big Sleep* Revisited—Frequently," *Film Journal* 1, no. 2 (Summer 1971), pp. 3–9.
   Gregory, Charles. "Knight Without Meaning?: Marlowe on the Screen," *Sight and Sound* 40, no. 3 (Summer 1973), pp. 155–59.
   McConnell, Frank. *Storytelling and Mythmaking: Images from Film and Literature.* New York: Oxford University Press, 1979, pp. 144–50.
   Monaco, James. "Notes on *The Big Sleep*—Thirty Years After," *Sight and Sound* 44, no. 1 (Winter 1975), pp. 34–38.

BRINGING UP BABY
   Cavell, Stanley. "Leopards in Connecticut," in *Pursuits of Happiness: The Hollywood Comedy of Remarriage.* Cambridge, Mass.: Harvard University Press, 1981, pp. 113–32.

THE CROWD ROARS
   Peary, Gerald. "Fast Cars and Women," in Joseph McBride, ed., *Focus on Howark Hawks,* pp. 109–17.

EL DORADO

Bogdanovich, Peter. *"El Dorado,"* in Joseph McBride, ed., *Focus on Howard Hawks,* pp. 147–49.

Ehrenstein, David. *"El Dorado," Medium* 1, no. 3 (Winter 1967–68).

Farber, Steven. *"El Dorado," Film Quarterly* 21, no. 1 (Fall 1967), pp. 58–59.

Gillett, John. *"El Dorado," Sight and Sound* 36, no. 3 (Summer 1967), p. 148.

Sarris, Andrew. *"El Dorado,"* in *Confessions of a Cultist,* New York: Simon and Schuster, 1970, pp. 299–302.

GENTLEMEN PREFER BLONDES

Shivas, Mark. "Blondes," *Movie* 5 (Dec. 1962), pp. 23–24.

Teple, James R. *"Gentlemen Prefer Blondes," Films in Review* 4, no. 7 (Aug.–Sept. 1953), p. 365.

HATARI!

Bogdanovich, Peter. *"Hatari!," Film Culture* 25 (Summer 1962), pp. 24–25.

Perkins, V. F. *"Hatari!," Movie* 5 (Dec. 1962), pp. 28–30.

HIS GIRL FRIDAY

Campbell, Marilyn. *"His Girl Friday:* Production for Use," *Wide Angle* 1, no. 2 (Summer 1976), pp. 22–27.

Cavell, Stanley. "Counterfeiting Happiness," in *Pursuits of Happiness,* pp. 163–87.

I WAS A MALE WAR BRIDE

Belton, John. *"I Was a Male War Bride," The Velvet Light Trap* 3 (Winter 1971–72).

MAN'S FAVORITE SPORT?

Haskell, Molly. *"Man's Favorite Sport?*—Revisited," in Joseph McBride, ed., *Focus on Howard Hawks,* pp. 135–38.

Sarris, Andrew. *"Man's Favorite Sport?"* in *Confessions of a Cultist,* New York: Simon and Schuster, 1970, pp. 128–29.

MONKEY BUSINESS

Belton, John. *"Monkey Business," Film Heritage* 6, no. 2 (Winter 1970–71), pp. 19–26.

THE OUTLAW

Bazin, André. *"The Outlaw,"* in *What is Cinema?,* vol. II. Translated by Hugh Gray. Berkeley and Los Angeles: University of California Press, 1971, pp. 163–68.

RED LINE 7000

Thompson, Richard. "Hawks at 70," in Joseph McBride, ed., *Focus on Howard Hawks,* pp. 139–46.

RED RIVER

McConnell, Frank. *Storytelling and Mythmaking,* pp. 98–104.

RIO BRAVO

Jameson, Richard T. "Talking and Doing in *Rio Bravo," The Velvet Light Trap* (Spring 1974), pp. 26–30.

"Movie Discoverer's Latest Find," *Life* 45 (Nov. 17, 1958), pp. 163ff.

Wood, Robin. *"Rio Bravo," Movie* 5 (Dec. 1962), pp. 25–27.

RIO LOBO

Astruc, Alexander. "A Massacre in Sequence: *Rio Lobo* by Howard Hawks," *Wide Angle* 1, no. 2 (Summer 1976), pp. 7–9.

Ford, Greg. "Mostly on *Rio Lobo,*" in Joseph McBride, ed., *Focus on Howard Hawks,* pp. 150–62.

TODAY WE LIVE

Hogue, Peter. "Hawks and Faulkner: *Today We Live," Literature/Film Quarterly* 9, no. 1 (Jan. 1981), pp. 51–58.

TO HAVE AND HAVE NOT

Kawin, Bruce, ed. *To Have and Have Not.* Madison: University of Wisconsin Press, 1980. Introductory essay and transcription of the complete screenplay.

Wood, Robin. "To Have (Written) and Have Not (Directed): Reflections on Authorship," *Film Comment* 9, no. 3 (May–June 1973), pp. 30–35.

BOOKS WITH REFERENCES TO HAWKS

Bacall, Lauren. *By Myself.* New York: Knopf, 1978, pp. 100–164.

Baker, Carlos, *Ernest Hemingway: A Life Story.* New York: Scribner's, 1969, pp. 368, 454.

Faulkner, John. *My Brother Bill: An Affectionate Remembrance.* New York: Trident, pp. 224–25.

Haskell, Molly. *From Reverence to Rape: The Treatment of Women in the Movies.* New York: Holt, Rinehart, 1974, pp. 15–18, 134–39, 208–13.

Hecht, Ben. *A Child of the Century.* New York: Simon and Schuster, 1954, pp. 396, 482.

Hemingway, Gregory. *Papa: A Personal Memoir.* New York: Houghton Mifflin, 1976, p. 46.

Kawin, Bruce F. *Faulkner and Film.* New York: Ungar, 1977, pp. 1–5, 72–100, 108–25, 144–60.

Mast, Gerald. *A Short History of the Movies.* 3rd edition. Chicago: University of Chicago Press, 1981, pp. 244–49.

Rosen, Marjorie. *Popcorn Venus: Women, Movies, and the American Dream.* New York: Coward-McCann, 1975, pp. 199, 229–30.

Russell, Rosalind. *Life Is a Banquet,* with Chris Chase. New York: Random House, 1977, pp. 87–93.

Sarris, Andrew. *The American Cinema: Directors and Directions 1929–1968.* New York: Dutton, 1968, pp. 52–56.

Filmography

FILMS PRODUCED AND/OR DIRECTED (in whole or in part) BY HAWKS

Principal Production Credits

Explanation of symbols:
   dir: directed by; *prod:* produced by; *sc:* screenplay credited to (the least reliable credit for any film); *ph:* photographed by; *mus:* musical score by; *ed:* edited by; *des:* designed by.

   BYU: indicates script and/or other production materials can be found in the collection of Hawks Papers at the Harold B. Lee Library of Brigham Young University; Box and Folder numbers indicated.

1926   **The Road to Glory** (Fox)
        dir: Hawks; *prod:* William Fox; *sc:* L. G. Rigby; *ph:* Joseph August.

       Fig Leaves (Fox)
        dir: Hawks; *prod:* William Fox; *sc:* Hope Loring, Louis D. Lighton; *ph:* Joseph August; *ed:* Rose Smith; *des:* William S. Darling, William Cameron Menzies.

1927   **The Cradle Snatchers** (Fox)
        dir: Hawks; *prod.:* William Fox; *sc:* Sarah Y. Mason, after the play by Russell Medcraft and Norma Mitchell; *ph:* L. William O'Connell.

       Paid to Love (Fox)
        dir: Hawks; *prod:* William Fox; *sc:* William M. Counselman, Seton I. Miller, Benjamin Glazer, from a story by Harry Carr; *ph:* L. William O'Connell; *ed:* Ralph Dixon; *des:* William S. Darling.

1928   **A Girl in Every Port** (Fox)
        dir: Hawks; *prod:* William Fox; *sc:* Seton I. Miller, Reginald Morris, William Tommel; *ph:* L. William O'Connell, R. J. Becquist; *ed:* Ralph Dixon; *des:* William S. Darling. **BYU:** Box 6, Folders 8–12.

Fazil (Fox)
> *dir:* Hawks; *prod:* William Fox; *sc:* Seton I. Miller, Philip Klein, after a play by Pierre Frondaie; *ph:* L. William O'Connell; *ed:* Ralph Dixon.

The Air Circus (Fox)
> *dir:* Hawks, Lewis B. Seiler; *prod:* William Fox; *sc:* Seton I. Miller, Norman Z. McLeod, Hugh Herbert [dialogue]; *ph:* Don Clarke; *ed:* Ralph Dixon.

1929 **Trent's Last Case** (Fox)
> *dir:* Hawks; *prod:* William Fox; *sc:* Scott Darling, Beulah Marie Dix, after a story by E. C. Bentley; *ph:* Harold Rosson.

1930 **The Dawn Patrol** (First National)
> *dir:* Hawks; *prod:* Hal B. Wallis; *sc:* Hawks, Seton I. Miller, Dan Totheroh, after "The Flight Commander" by John Monk Saunders; *ph:* Ernest Haller; *mus:* Leo F. Forbstein; *ed:* Ray Curtis; *des:* Jack Okey. **BYU:** Box 5, Folder 4.

1930– **Scarface** (United Artists)
32
> *dir:* Hawks; *prod:* Hawks, Howard Hughes; *sc:* Ben Hecht, Seton I. Miller, John Lee Mahin, William R. Burnett, after "Scarface" by Armitage Trail; *ph:* Lee Garmes, L. William O'Connell; *mus:* Adolph Tandler, Gus Arnheim; *ed:* Edward Curtis, Douglass Biggs; *des:* Harry Olivier. **BYU:** Box 12, Folders 4–6.

1931 **The Criminal Code** (Columbia)
> *dir:* Hawks; *prod:* Hawks, Harry Cohn; *sc:* Seton I. Miller, Fred Niblo, Jr., after the play by Martin Flavin; *ph:* James Wong Howe, L. William O'Connell; *ed:* Edward Curtis.

1932 **The Crowd Roars** (Warner Bros.)
> *dir:* Hawks; *prod:* Hawks, Bryan Foy; *sc:* Hawks, Seton I. Miller, Kubec Glassman, John Bright, Niven Busch; *ph:* Sidney Hickox; *mus:* Leo F. Forbstein; *ed:* John Stumar, Thomas Pratt; *des:* Jack Okey.

Tiger Shark (First National)
> *dir:* Hawks; *prod:* Hawks, Bryan Foy; *sc:* Wells Root, after "Tuna" by Houston Branch; *ph:* Tony Gaudio; *mus:* Leo F. Forbstein; *ed:* Thomas Pratt; *des:* Jack Okey.

1933 **Today We Live** (MGM)
> *dir:* Hawks; *prod:* Hawks; *sc:* Edith Fitzgerald, Dwight Taylor, William Faulkner, after "Turn About" by Faulkner; *ph:* Oliver T. Marsh; *ed:* Edward Curtiss. **BYU:** Box 13, Folders 9–11.

The Prize Fighter and the Lady (MGM)
> *dir:* Hawks [uncredited], W. S. Van Dyke; *sc:* based on a story by Frances Marion.

1934 **Viva Villa!** (MGM)
> *dir:* Hawks, Jack Conway; *prod:* David O. Selznick; *sc:* Hawks, Ben Hecht, after the book by Edgcumb Pinchon and O. B. Stade; *ph:* James Wong Howe, Charles G. Clarke; *mus:* Herbert Stothart; *ed:* Robert J. Kern; *des:* Edwin B. Willis, Harry Olivier.

Twentieth Century (Columbia)
> *dir:* Hawks; *prod:* Hawks; *sc:* Ben Hecht, Charles MacArthur, after their comedy adapted from "Napoleon of Broadway" by Charles Bruce Mulholland; *ph:* Joseph Walker, Joseph August; *ed:* Gene Havlick; **BYU:** Box 14, Folder 10.

1935 **Barbary Coast** (United Artists/Goldwyn Productions)
> *dir:* Hawks; *prod:* Samuel Goldwyn; *sc:* Ben Hecht, Charles MacArthur, Edward Chodorov; *ph:* Ray June; *mus:* Alfred Newman; *ed:* Edward Curtiss; *des:* Richard Day.

Ceiling Zero (First National)
> *dir:* Hawks; *prod:* Hawks, Harry Joe Brown; *sc:* Frank Wead, after his play; *ph:* Arthur Edeson; *mus:* Leo F. Forbstein; *ed:* William Holmes; *des:* John Hughes. **BYU:** Box 4, Folder 10.

1936 **The Road to Glory** (Twentieth Century-Fox)
> *dir:* Hawks; *prod:* Darryl F. Zanuck; *sc:* Joel Sayre, William Faulkner, after the film *Le Crois de bois*; *ph:* Gregg Toland; *mus:* Louis Silvers; *ed:* Edward Curtiss; *des:* Thomas Little, Hans Peters.

Come and Get It (United Artists/Goldwyn Productions)
> *dir:* Hawks, William Wyler; *prod:* Merritt Hulburd; *sc:* Jules Furthman, Jane Murfin, Robert Wyler, after the novel by Edna Ferber; *ph:* Gregg Toland, Rudolph Maté; *mus:* Alfred Newman; *ed:* Edward Curtiss.

1938 **Bringing Up Baby** (RKO)
> *dir:* Hawks; *prod:* Hawks; *sc:* Dudley Nichols, Hagar Wilde, after a story by Wilde; *ph:* Russell Metty; *mus:* Roy Webb; *ed:* George Hively; *des:* Darrell Silvera, Van Nest Polglase, Perry Ferguson.

1939 **Only Angels Have Wings** (Columbia)
> *dir:* Hawks; *prod:* Hawks; *sc:* Hawks, Jules Furthman; *ph:* Joseph Walker; *mus:* Dimitri Tiomkin; *ed:* Viola Lawrence; *des:* Lionel Banks. **BYU:** Box 10, Folders 5–7.

1940 **His Girl Friday** (Columbia)
> *dir:* Hawks; *prod:* Hawks; *sc:* Charles Lederer, after the play "The Front Page" by Ben Hecht and Charles MacArthur; *ph:* Joseph

Walker; *mus:* Morris Stoloff; *ed:* Gene Havlick; *des:* Lionel Banks. BYU: Box 7, Folders 6–7.

1941 **The Outlaw** (RKO)

dir: Hawks, Howard Hughes; *prod:* Hughes; *sc:* Jules Furthman; *ph:* Gregg Toland; *mus:* Victor Young; *ed:* Wallace Grissell.

Sergeant York (Warner Bros.)

dir: Hawks; *prod:* Jesse L. Lasky, Hal B. Wallis; *sc:* Abem Finkel, Harry Chandler, Howard Koch, John Huston, after *The War Diary of Sergeant York,* edited by Sam Cowan, *Sergeant York and His People,* by Sam Cowan, and *Sergeant York, Last of the Long Hunters,* by Tom Skeyhill; *ph:* Sol Polito; *mus:* Max Steiner; *ed:* William Holmes; *des:* Fred McLean, John Hughes. BYU: Box 12, Folders 7–8.

Ball of Fire (RKO/Goldwyn Productions)

dir: Hawks; *prod:* Samuel Goldwyn; *sc:* Billy Wilder, Charles Brackett, after "From A to Z" by Wilder and Thomas Monroe; *ph:* Gregg Toland; *mus:* Alfred Newman; *ed:* Daniel Mandell; *des:* Perry Ferguson. BYU: Box 2, Folder 9.

1943 **Air Force** (Warner Bros.)

dir: Hawks; *prod:* Hawks, Hal B. Wallis; *sc:* Dudley Nichols; *ph:* James Wong Howe; *mus:* Franz Waxman; *ed:* George Amy; *des:* Walter F. Tilford, John Hughes. BYU: Box 2, Folder 7.

Corvette K-225 (Universal)

dir: Richard Rossen; *prod:* Hawks; *sc:* Lt. John Rhodes Sturdy; *ph:* Tony Gaudio, Harry Perry; *mus:* David Buttolph; *ed:* Edward Curtis; *des:* Russell Gausman, A. J. Gilmore, John B. Goodman, Robert Boyle. BYU: Box 4, Folders 13–14.

1944 **To Have and Have Not** (Warner Bros.)

dir: Hawks; *prod:* Hawks; *sc:* Jules Furthman, William Faulkner, after the novel by Ernest Heminway; *ph:* Sidney Hickox; *mus:* Leo F. Forbstein, Hoagy Carmichael, Johnny Mercer; *ed:* Christian Nyby; *des:* Casey Roberts, Charles Novi. BYU: Box 14, Folders 1–9.

1946 **The Big Sleep** (Warner Bros.)

dir: Hawks; *prod:* Hawks; *sc:* William Faulkner, Leigh Brackett, Jules Furthman, after the novel by Raymond Chandler; *ph:* Sidney Hickox; *mus:* Max Steiner; *ed:* Christian Nyby; *des:* Fred McLean, Carl Jules Weyl. BYU: Box 3, Folders 7–9; Box 4, Folders 1–6.

1948 **Red River** (United Artists/Monterey Productions)

dir: Hawks; *prod:* Hawks; *sc:* Borden Chase, Charles Schnee, after "The Chisholm Trail" by Chase; *ph:* Russell Harlan; *mus:* Dimitri

Tiomkin; *ed:* Christian Nyby; *des:* John Datu Arensma. **BYU:** Box 10, Folders 13–16; Box 11, Folders 1–15.

A Song Is Born (RKO/Goldwyn Productions)

    dir: Hawks; *prod:* Samuel Goldwyn; *sc:* Harry Tugend, based on the film *Ball of Fire; ph:* Gregg Toland; *mus:* Emil Newman, Hugo Friedhofer, Don Raye, Gene DePaul; *ed:* Daniel Mandell; *des:* Julia Heron, George Jenkins, Perry Ferguson. **BYU:** Box 13, Folder 3.

1949 **I Was a Male War Bride** (Twentieth Century-Fox)

    dir: Hawks; *prod:* Sol C. Siegel; *sc:* Charles Lederer, Leonard Spigelgass, Hagar Wilde, after the novel by Henri Rochard; *ph:* Norbert Brodine, Osmond H. Borradaille; *mus:* Cyril Mockridge; *ed:* James B. Clark; *des:* Thomas Little, Lyle R. Wheeler, Albert Hogsett.

1951 **The Thing** (RKO/Winchester Productions)

    dir: Christian Nyby; *prod:* Hawks; *sc:* Hawks, Charles Lederer, after the story by John Wood Campbell, Jr., "Who Goes There?"; *ph:* Russell Harlan; *mus:* Dimitri Tiomkin; *ed:* Roland Cross; *des:* Darrell Silvera, Wiliam Stevens, Albert S. D'Agostino, John Hughes. **BYU:** Box 13, Folders 6–8.

1952 **The Big Sky** (RKO/Winchester Productions)

    dir: Hawks; *prod:* Hawks; *sc:* Dudley Nichols, after the novel by A. B. Guthrie, Jr.; *ph:* Russell Harlan; *mus:* Dimitri Tiomkin; *ed:* Christian Nyby; *des:* Darrell Silvera, Albert S. D'Agostino, William Stevens, Perry Ferguson. **BYU:** Box 2, Folder 19; Box 3, Folders 1–6.

O'Henry's Full House—"The Ransom of Red Chief" (Twentieth Century-Fox)

    dir: Hawks; *prod:* André Hakim; *sc:* Nunnally Johnson, after the story by O'Henry; *ph:* Milton Krasner; *mus:* Alfred Newman; *des:* Chester Goce. **BYU:** Box 10, Folders 11–12.

Monkey Business (Twentieth Century-Fox)

    dir: Hawks; *prod:* Sol C. Siegel; *sc:* Ben Hecht, I. A. L. Diamond, Charles Lederer, after a story by Harry Segall; *ph:* Milton Krasner; *mus:* Leigh Harline; *ed:* William B. Murphy; *des:* Thomas Little, Walter M. Scott, Lyle R. Wheeler, George Patrick. **BYU:** Box 9, Folders 6–7.

1953 **Gentlemen Prefer Blondes** (Twentieth Century-Fox)

    dir: Hawks; *prod:* Sol C. Siegel; *sc:* Charles Lederer, after the musical comedy by Anita Loos and Joseph Fields; *ph:* Harry J. Wild; *mus:* Jule Styne, Leo Robin, Hoagy Carmichael, Harold Adamson;

ed: Hugh S. Fowler; *des:* Claude Carpenter, Lyle R. Wheeler, Joseph C. Wright. BYU: Box 6, Folders 5–6.

1955   **Land of the Pharaohs** (Warner Bros./Continental Productions)
dir: Hawks; *prod:* Hawks; *sc:* William Faulkner, Harry Kurnitz, Harold Jack Bloom; *ph:* Russell Harlan, Lee Garmes; *mus:* Dimitri Tiomkin; *ed:* V. Sagovsky, Rudi Fehr; *des:* Alexandre Trauner. BYU: Box 8, Folder 3.

1959   **Rio Bravo** (Warner Bros./ Armada Productions)
dir: Hawks; *prod:* Hawks; *sc:* Jules Furthman, Leigh Brackett, after the story by B. H. Campbell; *ph:* Russell Harlan; *mus:* Dimitri Tiomkin, Paul Francis Webster; *ed:* Folmar Blangsted; *des:* Ralph S. Hurst, Leo F. Kuter. BYU: Box 12, Folder 1.

1962   **Hatari!** (Paramount/Malabar Productions)
dir: Hawks; *prod:* Hawks; *sc:* Harry Kurnitz, Leigh Brackett; *ph:* Russell Harlan; *mus:* Henry Mancini, Johnny Mercer, Hoagy Carmichael; *ed:* Stuart Gilmore; *des:* Hal Pereira, Carl Anderson. BYU: Box 7, Folders 2–5.

1964   **Man's Favorite Sport?** (Universal/Gibraltar and Laurel Productions)
dir: Hawks; *prod:* Hawks; *sc:* John Fenton Murray, Steve McNeil, after the story by Pat Frank, "The Girl Who Almost Got Away"; *ph:* Russell Harlan; *mus:* Henry Mancini, Johnny Mercer; *ed:* Stuart Gilmore; *des:* Robert Priestly, Alexander Golitzen, Tambi Larsen. BYU: Box 9, Folders 3–4.

1965   **Red Line 7000** (Paramount/Laurel Productions)
dir: Hawks; *prod:* Hawks; *sc:* Hawks, George Kirgo; *ph:* Milton Krasner; *mus:* Nelson Riddle, Hoagy Carmichael, Harold Adamson, Carol Connors; *ed:* Stuart Gilmore, Bill Brame; *des:* Hal Pereira, Arthur Lonergan.

1967   **El Dorado** (Paramount/Laurel Productions)
dir: Hawks; *prod:* Hawks; *sc:* Leigh Brackett, after the novel by Harry Brown, *The Stars in their Courses; ph:* Harold Rosson; *mus:* Nelson Riddle; *ed:* John Woodcock; *des:* Hal Pereira, Carl Anderson. BYU: Box 5, Folder 10.

1970   **Rio Lobo** (Cinema Center/Malabar Productions)
dir: Hawks; *prod:* Hawks; *sc:* Leigh Brackett, Burton Wohl, after a story by Wohl; *ph:* William H. Clothier; *mus:* Jerry Goldsmith; *ed:* John Woodcock; *des:* William R. Kiernan, Robert Smith.

Unfinished Projects and Uncredited Contributions to Other Films

Documentation for these projects and contributions can be found either in the collection of Hawks papers at the Harold B. Lee Library of Brigham Young University (indicated by **BYU** with Box and Folder numbers), in Hawks's personal interviews, or in Joseph McBride's *Hawks on Hawks*.

Angel Face
    story by Charles Schnee, n.d., **BYU**: Box 2, Folder 8.
The Banshee Shadow Flies
    story by Gordon Grant, n.d., **BYU**: Box 2, Folder 10.
The Battle Cry
    story by William Faulkner, April 21, 1943. **BYU**: Box 2, Folders 12–13.
The Black Door
    original story by Cleve F. Adams, screenplay by Leigh Brackett, January 18, 1945; revised and retitled Stiletto, April 13, 1951. **BYU**: Box 4, Folders 7–9.
Captain's Courageous
    film directed by Victor Fleming (1937). Hawks co-scenarist [uncredited].
Casino Royale
    film produced by Charles K. Feldman (1967). Hawks co-scenarist [uncredited].
The Chariot of the Gods
    scenario by Howard Hawks and L. G. Rigby, n.d. **BYU**: Box 4, Folder 11.
Claudia
    script, n.a., n.d. **BYU**: Box 4, Folder 12.
Dambuster Film
    story, n.a., November 9, 1943. **BYU**: Box 5, Folders 1–2.
Destination Dublin
    screenplay by Stewart Farrar, April 1971. **BYU**: Box 5, Folder 5.
The Detectives
    script by Allan Sloane, n.d. **BYU**: Box 5, Folders 6–7.
Dreadful Hollow
    script by William Faulkner, n.d. **BYU**: Box 5, Folders 8–9.
The Dressmaker from Paris
    film directed by Paul Bern (1925), screenplay by Howard Hawks.
El Paso Red
    stories, n.a., n.d. **BYU**: Box 6, Folder 1.
Father Junipero Serra
    story outline by Jack DeWitt, n.d. **BYU**: Box 6, Folder 2.
The FBI and the Barker-Karpis Gang
    story by Murry Faulkner, n.d. **BYU**: Box 6, Folder 3.
The Food of Love
    script by Zoe Akins, n.d. **BYU**: Box 6, Folder 4.

For Whom the Bell Tolls
film directed by Sam Wood (1943). Hawks co-scenarist [uncredited].
A Ghost Story
script by William Faulkner, n.d. **BYU**: Box 6, Folder 7.
Gone with the Wind
film credited to Victor Fleming (1939). Hawks co-scenarist [uncredited].
Gunga Din
film directed by George Stevens (1939). Screenplay by Ben Hecht, Charles MacArthur, revised by Dudley Nichols and Howard Hawks, June 17, 1937. **BYU**: Box 7, Folder 1.
Honesty—The Best Policy
film directed by Chester Bennett (1926). Hawks co-scenarist [uncredited].
Honor
scripts by William Faulkner, with dialogue from Jules Furthman and Harry Behn, January 24 to March 30, 1933. **BYU**: Box 7, Folder 8; Box 8, Folders 1–2.
Indianapolis Speedway
film directed by Lloyd Bacon (1939) based on a story by Howard Hawks.
The Left Hand of God
film directed by Edward Dmytryk (1955). Screenplay developed by Hawks and William Faulkner, February 7, 1951 to July 18, 1952. **BYU**: Box 8, Folders 4–8; Box 9, Folder 1.
The Little Princess
film directed by Marshall Neilan (1917). Hawks director [uncredited] of several scenes.
Lulu Belle
script, n.a., n.d. **BYU**: Box 9, Folder 2.
Moll
story by Ben Hecht and Gene Fowler, November 4, 1952. **BYU**: Box 9, Folder 5.
Morning Star
story by Robert Carr, n.d., of magazine version in *Saturday Evening Post* of December 6, 1947. **BYU**: Box 9, Folders 8–10.
Morocco
film directed by Josef von Sternberg (1930). Hawks co-scenarist [uncredited]. **BYU**: Box 9, Folder 11.
Moss Rose
film directed by Gregory Ratoff (1947). Hawks co-scenarist [uncredited]. **BYU**: Box 10, Folders 1–2.
Murder in the Air
film directed by Lewis Seiler (1940). Script developed by Hawks [uncredited] from a synopsis by Francis Agnew, n.d. **BYU**: Box 10, Folder 3.
101 Ranch
notes by Joel DeWitt, n.d. **BYU**: Box 10, Folder 4.
Queer People
script, n.a., June 30, 1931. **BYU**: Box 10, Folder 10.

Quicksands
> film directed by Jack Conway (1923). Hawks co-scenarist [uncredited].

Red Dust
> film directed by Victor Fleming (1932). Hawks co-scenarist [uncredited].

The Roughneck and the Lady
> story by Howard Hawks, September 4, 1925. BYU: Box 12, Folder 2.

Rurales
> preliminary script by Robert Carr, June 21, 1952. BYU: Box 12, Folder 3.

Scandal Sheet
> film directed by Phil Karlson (1946). Hawks co-scenarist [uncredited].

Seventh Cavalry
> script by Dudley Nichols, September 5, 1939. BYU: Box 12, Folder 9.

Shanghai Express
> film directed by Josef von Sternberg (1932). Hawks co-scenarist [uncredited].

The Sun Also Rises
> film directed by Henry King (1957). Hawks co-scenarist [uncredited] on the screenplay by Horace Jackson. BYU: Box 13, Folder 4.

Sutter's Gold
> film directed by James Cruze (1936). Hawks co-scenarist [uncredited] on the screenplay by William Faulkner. BYU: Box 13, Folder 5.

Test Pilot
> film directed by Victor Fleming (1938). Hawks co-scenarist [uncredited].

Tiger Love
> film directed by George Melford (1924). Hawks co-scenarist [uncredited].

Two Arabian Knights
> synopsis by Dorothy Robinson, April 5, 1948. BYU: Box 14, Folder 11.

Underworld
> film directed by Josef von Sternberg (1927). Hawks co-scenarist [uncredited].

When It's Hot Play It Cool
> script, Howard Hawks Productions, n.a., July 15, 1976. BYU: Box 14, Folder 12.

Index